Atlas of
OPERATIVE
LAPAROSCOPY AND
HYSTEROSCOPY

Atlas of
OPERATIVE LAPAROSCOPY AND HYSTEROSCOPY

Third Edition

Editor

Jacques Donnez MD PhD
Department of Gynecology
Catholic University of Louvain
Brussels, Belgium

informa
healthcare

© 2007 Informa UK Ltd

First published in the United Kingdom in 1994 by Parthenon Publishing Ltd
Second Edition published in the United Kingdom in 2001 by Parthenon Publishing Ltd
Third Edition published in 2007 by Informa Healthcare, Telephone House, 69-77 Paul Street, London EC2A 4LQ.
Informa Healthcare is a trading division of Informa UK Ltd. Registered Office: 37/41 Mortimer Street, London
W1T 3JH. Registered in England and Wales number 1072954.

Tel: +44 (0)20 7017 5000
Fax: +44 (0)20 7017 6699
Website: www.informahealthcare.com

Reprinted 2008

Although every effort has been made to ensure that all owners of copyright material have been acknowledged in this
publication, we would be glad to acknowledge in subsequent reprints or editions any omissions brought to our
attention.

Although every effort has been made to ensure that drug doses and other information are presented accurately in
this publication, the ultimate responsibility rests with the prescribing physician. Neither the publishers nor the
authors can be held responsible for errors or for any consequences arising from the use of information contained
herein. For detailed prescribing information or instructions on the use of any product or procedure discussed herein,
please consult the prescribing information or instructional material issued by the manufacturer.

A CIP record for this book is available from the British Library.

Library of Congress Cataloging-in-Publication Data

Data available on application

ISBN-10: 0 415 38415 X
ISBN-13: 978 0 415 38415 5

Distributed in North and South America by

Taylor & Francis
6000 Broken Sound Parkway, NW, (Suite 300)
Boca Raton, FL 33487, USA

Within Continental USA
Tel: 1 (800) 272 7737; Fax: 1 (800) 374 3401

Outside Continental USA
Tel: (561) 994 0555; Fax: (561) 361 6018
Email: orders@crcpress.com

Book orders in the rest of the world
Paul Abrahams
Tel: +44 (0)20 7017 4036
Email: bookorders@informa.com

Composition by Parthenon Publishing

Printed and bound in India by Replika Press Pvt Ltd

Contents

List of contributors   ix

Foreword   xiii

1.   Anatomy in relation to gynecological endoscopy   1
     S Ploteau, J Donnez

2.   Instrumentation and operational instructions   17
     J Donnez, P Jadoul

Section I: Operative laparoscopy
Part 1: Endometriosis

3.   Laparoscopic management of peritoneal endometriosis   31
     P Jadoul, J Donnez

4.   Laparoscopic management of ovarian endometriosis   43
     P Jadoul, C Wyns, J Donnez

5.   Douglasectomy, torus excision, uterine suspension   55
     J Donnez, J Squifflet, P Jadoul

6.   Laparoscopic excision of rectovaginal and retrocervical endometriotic lesions   63
     J Donnez, P Jadoul, O Donnez, J Squifflet

7.   Ureteral endometriosis: a frequent complication of rectovaginal and retrocervical endometriosis   77
     J Donnez, P Jadoul, J Squifflet

8.   Bladder endometriosis   85
     J Donnez, J Squifflet, O Donnez, P Jadoul

9.   Laparoscopic hysterectomy including for advanced endometriosis with rectosigmoid disease   93
     H Reich, T Seckin, JM Reich

Part 2: Tubal pathology and ovarian pathology

10.   Fertiloscopy   115
     A Watrelot

11.   Transvaginal laparoscopy   133
     S Gordts

12. CO_2 laser laparoscopic surgery: fimbrioplasty, salpingoneostomy and adhesiolysis   141
     J Donnez, P Jadoul, M Smets, J Squifflet

13.   Ectopic pregnancy following assisted conception treatment and specific sites of ectopic pregnancy   157
     C Pirard, J Donnez

14.   Medical treatment: the place of methotrexate   171
     J Donnez, C Pirard

15.   The laparoscopic management of ectopic pregancy   181
     JL Pouly, G Mage, M Canis, B Rabischong, R Botchorishvili, K Jardon

16. Laparoscopic microsurgical tubal anastomosis 187
CH Koh

17. Laparoscopic management of ovarian cysts 195
J Donnez, J Squifflet, P Jadoul

18. Laparoscopic management of adnexal torsion 211
M Canis, H Manhes, B Rabischong, R Botchorishvili, K Jardon, JL Pouly, G Mage

Part 3: Uterine and pelvic floor pathology

19. Laparoscopic repair of wide and deep uterine scar dehiscence following cesarean section 219
O Donnez, P Jadoul, J Squifflet, J Donnez

20. Laparoscopic myomectomy 227
JB Dubuisson, A Fauconnier

21. Laparoscopic myomectomy and myolysis: to whom should it be proposed? 239
P Jadoul, J Donnez

22. LASH: laparoscopic subtotal hysterectomy – a series of 1400 cases 251
J Donnez, J Squifflet, O Donnez, M Smets, P Jadoul

23. Laparoscopic hysterectomy in benign diseases: a series of 1233 cases 263
J Donnez, M Smets, J Squifflet, P Jadoul

24. Laparoscopic approach for prolapse 277
A Wattiez

25. Laparoscopic sacrocolpexy for severe uterine prolapse and severe vaginal vault prolapse 289
J Donnez, M Smets, J Squifflet, O Donnez, P Jadoul

Part 4: Oncology

26. Borderline tumors of the ovary or epithelial ovarian tumors of borderline malignancy 307
A Münschke, P Jadoul, J Squifflet, J Donnez

27. Laparoscopic reimplantation of cryopreserved ovarian tissue 323
J Donnez, MM Dolmans, D Demylle, P Jadoul, C Pirard, J Squifflet, B Martinez-Madrid, A Van Langendonckt

28. Ovarian tissue cryopreservation and existing alternatives 333
MM Dolmans, B Martinez-Madrid, A Van Langendonckt, A Camboni, D Demylle, J Donnez

29. Technical aspects of ovarian tissue cryopreservation 343
MM Dolmans, B Martinez-Madrid, A Van Langendonckt, A Camboni, D Demylle, J Donnez

30. Laparoscopic ovarian transposition before radiotherapy 349
P Jadoul, J Squifflet, J Donnez

31. Laparoscopic preservation of female fertility 355
H Baakdah, T Tulandi

32. The place of endoscopy in malignancy 359
J Donnez, M Berlière, J Squifflet, P Jadoul

33. Indications for lymphadenectomy in stage I/IIa endometrial cancer 369
J Squifflet, J Donnez

34. Place of laparoscopic surgery in the management of cervical cancer: the Dargent techniques 375
D Dargent, P Mathevet

Part 5: Endoscopy during pregnancy

35. Fetal endoscopy   391
     C Hubinont

36. Laparoscopic abdominal cerclage   403
     R Al-Fadhli, T Tulandi

Part 6: Robotics: the future

37. Improving ergonomics in laparoscopic gynecological surgery   407
     R Polet, J Donnez

38. Robotically assisted gynecological surgery   417
     T Falcone, JM Goldberg

Part 7: Complications

39. Complications of laparoscopic surgery in gynecology   425
     P Jadoul, J Donnez

Section II: Operative hysteroscopy

40. Instrumentation for hysteroscopy   453
     J Donnez

41. Hysterosonography and hysteroscopy in the diagnosis of specific disorders   457
     J Squifflet, J Donnez, P Jadoul

42. Office hysteroscopy   471
     S Bettocchi, O Ceci, L Nappi, G Pontrelli, L Pinto, A Costantino, L Selvaggi

43. Müllerian duct anomalies   483
     P Jadoul, C Pirard, J Donnez

44. Hysteroscopic lysis of intrauterine adhesions   507
     J Donnez, P Jadoul, J Squifflet

45. Hysteroscopic myomectomy   515
     J Donnez, P Jadoul, M Smets, J Squifflet

46. Endometrial resection   527
     BJ van Herendael

47. Global endometrial ablation   533
     GA Vilos

48. Tubal sterilization   549
     BJ van Herendael

49. Complications of hysteroscopic surgery in gynecology   553
     P Jadoul, J Donnez

Index   561

Members of the Department of Gynecology

St. Luc's University Hospital (Catholic University of Louvain)
Brussels, Belgium

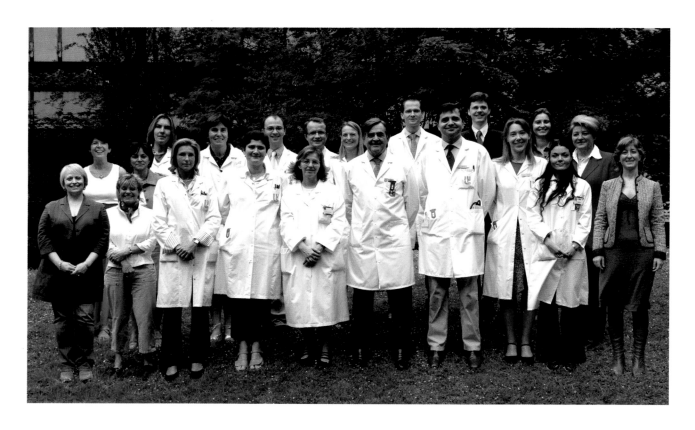

'There is no life without pressure....'

Brussels, July 2006

Contributors

R Al-Fadhli
Department of Obstetrics and Gynecology
McGill University
Montreal
Quebec
Canada

H Baakdah
Department of Obstetrics and Gynecology
McGill University
Montreal
Quebec
Canada

M Berlière
Department of Gynecology
Université Catholique de Louvain
Cliniques Universitaires Saint-Luc
Brussels
Belgium

S Bettocchi
Department of General and Surgical Sciences
Institute of Obstetrics and Gynecology II
University of Bari
Bari
Italy

R Botchorishvili
Department of Obstetrics, Gynaecology and
Reproductive Medicine
Polyclinique de l'Hotel Dieu
Clermont-Ferrand
France

A Camboni
Department of Gynecology
Université Catholique de Louvain
Cliniques Universitaires Saint-Luc
Brussels
Belgium

M Canis
Department of Obstetrics, Gynaecology and
Reproductive Medicine
Polyclinique de l'Hotel Dieu
Clermont-Ferrand
France

O Ceci
Department of General and Surgical Sciences
Institute of Obstetrics and Gynecology II
University of Bari
Bari
Italy

A Costantino
Department of General and Surgical Sciences
Institute of Obstetrics and Gynecology II
University of Bari
Bari
Italy

D Dargent
Deceased

D Demylle
Department of Gynecology
Université Catholique de Louvain
Cliniques Universitaires Saint-Luc
Brussels
Belgium

MM Dolmans
Department of Gynecology
Université Catholique de Louvain
Cliniques Universitaires Saint-Luc
Brussels
Belgium

J Donnez
Department of Gynecology
Université Catholique de Louvain
Cliniques Universitaires Saint-Luc
Brussels
Belgium

O Donnez
Department of Gynecology
Université Catholique de Louvain
Cliniques Universitaires Saint-Luc
Brussels
Belgium

JB Dubuisson
Département de Gynécologie et Obstétrique
Hôpitaux Universitaires de Genève
Genève
Switzerland

T Falcone
Department of Obstetrics and Gynecology-A81
Cleveland Clinic Foundation
Cleveland, OH
USA

A Fauconnier
Département de Gynécologie et Obstétrique
Hôpitaux Universitaires de Genève
Genève
Switzerland

JM Goldberg
Reproductive Endocrinology
Department of Obstetrics and Gynecology-A81
Cleveland Clinic Foundation
Cleveland, OH
USA

S Gordts
Leuven Institute for Fertility and Embryology
Leuven
Belgium

C Hubinont
Department of Obstetrics
Université Catholique de Louvain
Cliniques Universitaires Saint-Luc
Brussels
Belgium

CH Koh
Reproductive Speciality Center
Milwaukee, WI
USA

P Jadoul
Department of Gynecology
Université Catholique de Louvain
Cliniques Universitaires Saint-Luc
Brussels
Belgium

K Jardon
Department of Obstetrics, Gynaecology and
Reproductive Medicine
Polyclinique de l'Hôtel Dieu
Clermont-Ferrand
France

G Mage
Department of Obstetrics, Gynaecology and
Reproductive Medicine
Polyclinique de l'Hôtel Dieu
Clermont-Ferrand
France

H Manhes
Department of Obstetrics, Gynaecology and
Reproductive Medicine
Polyclinique de l'Hôtel Dieu
Clermont-Ferrand
France

B Martinez-Madrid
Department of Gynecology
Université Catholique de Louvain
Cliniques Universitaires Saint-Luc
Brussels
Belgium

P Mathevet
Department of Obstetrics and Gynaecology
Hôpital Edouard Herriot
Lyon
France

A Münschke
Department of Gynecology
Université Catholique de Louvain
Cliniques Universitaires Saint-Luc
Brussels
Belgium

L Nappi
Department of General and Surgical Sciences
Institute of Obstetrics and Gynecology II
University of Bari
Bari
Italy

L Pinto
Department of General and Surgical Sciences
Institute of Obstetrics and Gynecology II
University of Bari
Bari
Italy

C Pirard
Department of Gynecology
Université Catholique de Louvain
Cliniques Universitaires Saint-Luc
Brussels
Belgium

G Pontrelli
Department of General and Surgical Sciences
Institute of Obstetrics and Gynecology II
University of Bari
Bari
Italy

S Ploteau
Department of Gynecology
Université Catholique de Louvain
Cliniques Universitaires Saint-Luc
Brussels
Belgium

R Polet
Department of Gynecology
Université Catholique de Louvain
Cliniques Universitaires Saint-Luc
Brussels
Belgium

JL Pouly
Department of Obstetrics, Gynaecology and
Reproductive Medicine
Polyclinique de l'Hôtel Dieu
Clermont-Ferrand
France

B Rabischong
Department of Obstetrics, Gynaecology and
Reproductive Medicine
Polyclinique de l'Hôtel Dieu
Clermont-Ferrand
France

H Reich
Shavertown, PA
and
Columbia Presbyterian Medical Center
New York, NY
USA

JM Reich
Morristown Memorial Hospital
Morristown, NJ
USA

T Seckin
Lenox Hill Hospital
New York, NY
and
Kingsbrook Jewish Medical Center
Brooklyn, NY
USA

L Selvaggi
Department of General and Surgical Sciences
Institute of Obstetrics and Gynecology II
University of Bari
Bari
Italy

M Smets
Department of Gynecology
Université Catholique de Louvain
Cliniques Universitaires Saint-Luc
Brussels
Belgium

J Squifflet
Department of Gynecology
Université Catholique de Louvain
Cliniques Universitaires Saint-Luc
Brussels
Belgium

T Tulandi
Department of Obstetrics and Gynecology
McGill University
Montreal
Quebec
Canada

BJ van Herendael
ACZA Campus Stuivenberg
Endoscopic Training Center Antwerp
2060 Antwerp
Belgium

A Van Langendonckt
Department of Gynecology
Université Catholique de Louvain
Cliniques Universitaires Saint-Luc
Brussels
Belgium

GA Vilos
Department of Obstetrics and Gynecology
Division of Reproductive Endocrinology and Infertility
The University of Western Ontario
London, Ontario
Canada

A Wattiez
Gynécologie Obstétrique Reproduction Humaine
Polyclinique de l'Hôtel Dieu
Clermont-Ferrand
France

A Watrelot
Centre de Recherche et d'Etude de la Stérilité (CRES)
Lyon
France

C Wyns
Department of Gynecology
Université Catholique de Louvain
Cliniques Universitaires Saint-Luc
Brussels
Belgium

Foreword

The use of laparoscopic and hysteroscopic access for gynecologic surgery is now state of the art. However, acceptance of these surgical access routes and their incorporation into daily gynecologic practice has been slow and took well over two decades. Yet the advantages of laparoscopic access as opposed to conventional laparotomy were already evident more than 30 years ago. These advantages include shortened post-operative hospital stay and recovery period; reduced post-operative discomfort which results in less analgesia requirements; frequently lesser costs; and the ensuing medical and cosmetic gains associated with the avoidance of a laparotomy. Many more complex gynecological procedures can now be successfully performed by laparoscopy. The most telling of these developments has been the use of laparoscopic access for pelvic and para-aortic lymphadenectomy and radical hysterectomy for gynecologic malignancy.

In the 1970s hysteroscopy was described as 'a technique looking for an indication.' The application of the tecnique, which at the time was purely diagnostic, remained limited. This was largely due to significant improvements in non-invasive imaging techniques, especially ultrasonography, and the use of a vaginal transducer for the assessment of the pelvic organs. Yet the impact of hysteroscopy in our specialty has been radical. This came about with the use of hysteroscopy as a surgical access into the uterus. It greatly simplified many procedures that previously required a laparotomy and a hysterectomy to access the uterine cavity: lysis of severe uterine synechiae, metroplasty for septate uterus, excision of symptomatic intrauterine fibroids. These, after all, are common conditions; hysteroscopy has radically simplified these procedures and reduced their morbidity. It has also permitted the introduction of a simple technique of permanent tubal sterilization.

Direct access to the uterus led to the introduction of interventions such as endometrial excision and endometrial ablation that offer a less invasive, yet effective alternative to hysterectomy in the treatment of abnormal (dysfunctional) uterine bleeding refractory to medical treatment. Hysteroscopic endometrial ablation is already being replaced by simpler ablation techniques called "global ablation' or 'non-hysteroscopic ablation' that yields similar outcomes. Schopenhauer said it so well: 'change alone is eternal, perpetual, immortal.'

Progress in medicine frequently follows innovations and improvements in technology. Evolution and acceptance of operative laparoscopy and hysteroscopy and their use in more complex procedures was made possible by such technical progress. Improvement in lens systems resulted in the production of endoscopes of smaller caliber and better optics and the introduction of lightweight mini video cameras and high-resolution television monitors permitted the surgeon and others assisting at the procedure to view the operative field in one or more television monitors and work in concert as a team.

The production of hysteroscopes of smaller caliber permitted hysteroscopy to be performed without anesthesia; this eventually led to the introduction of the so-called 'office hysteroscopy.' Improved optics, together with the production of new and better equipment and instruments, allowed hysteroscopic intrauterine procedures to be performed more easily, more quickly and with greater safety.

The advantages associated with minimal access must not reduce the surgeon's threshold in recommending a surgical procedure. Both laparoscopic and hysteroscopic surgery is minimal access surgery, but what is minimal is only the access; not the level of skill required, nor the rate or the degree of complications. One must be reminded that more than one half of the major vascular complications and nearly one half of the gastrointestinal complications occur during the establishment of the laparoscopic access route. Proper technique and vigilance are of foremost importance.

Neither the use of minimal access, nor technical feasibility is an indication for surgical intervention. A surgical procedure is undertaken to benefit the patient. Patient safety and successful outcome are dependent upon the presence of good surgical indication; proper selection of patient and procedure, ubcluding selection of surgical access; knowledge of the prerequisites, respect of the principles and application of careful techniques by an experienced operator.

The *Atlas of Operative Laparoscopy and Hysteroscopy* is comprehensive; it is well written and superbly illustrated. The book is divided into two sections that are preceded by two pertinent introductory chapters: 'Anatomy in relation to gynecological endoscopy' and 'Instrumentation and operational instructions.' The first section, 'Operative laparoscopy' is composed of seven parts: Endometriosis, Tubal and ovarian pathology, Uterine and pelvic floor pathology, Oncology, Endoscopy during pregnancy, Robotics, and Complications. The second section is on 'Operative hysteroscopy.' The book has been edited by Jacques Donnez. It contains a total of 49 chapters. Twenty-six of these have been contributed by European and North American authors, each one internationally recognized for their expertise in the specific field. The vast majority, 32 chapters, have been authored by Professor Donnez and his associates at the Université Catholique de Louvain, Cliniques Universitaires Saint Luc. Thus, the book largely carries the imprint of the Donnez school.

I am please and honored to have been asked to contribute a foreword for this superb book. I have followed with interest Jacques Donnez career. He has embraced with enthusiasm successive developments in gynecologi c surgery, from microsurgery to the more recent cryopreservation of ovary, with operative laparoscopy, operative hysteroscopy, endometriosis, lasers, etc. in between; experimenting with each and incorporating them into the practice of his own department. I had the privilege of being invited to the academic and social program presented in Brussels last year, in celebration of Professor Donnez 20 years as a chair of department, and the opportunity and pleasure to observe to what extent his visionary leadership is appreciated and respected by members of his institution. The meticulous attention he gives to the tasks he undertakes is very much evident in this book, which I strongly recommend to anyone interested in gynecologic surgery.

Victor Gomel

Professor Department of Obstetrics and Gynecology
Faculty of Medicine, University of British Columbia
Vancouver BC, Canada

Anatomy in relation to gynecological endoscopy

S Ploteau, J Donnez

In gynecology, as in other surgical fields, an excellent knowledge of human anatomy is necessary. Surgical progress makes this even more pertinent; laparoscopy requires, more than ever, a thorough knowledge of all the relationships between anatomic structures. If one injures the ureter, uterine artery or large vessels, or if intra-peritoneal bleeding occurs, it is necessary to be able to react quickly and to convert to open surgery. Experienced surgeons possess the required skills, but younger practitioners with less extensive anatomic knowledge could experience serious difficulties. Laparoscopy reveals the undeniable aspect of anatomy as a tool of work. Without perfect knowledge of the different structures encountered during dissection, and particularly those which one would prefer not to encounter because of the dangers they evoke, laparoscopy can become hazardous due to the surgeon's lack of awareness. We are not about to cover all the anatomic data concerning the pelvis; this information can be found in any anatomic textbook and, in any case, it is well known. What is required is the ability to identify, without hesitation, all the structures grasped or isolated during dissection. We will simply call back to mind some anatomic notions to ensure a safe pelvic approach during laparoscopy, and present some anatomic points which highlight potential dangers and require particular attention during surgery. In this chapter, we describe the different steps of gynecological laparoscopy and some recent surgical techniques such as TOT (transobturator tape) for treatment of stress urinary incontinence and the anatomic basis of pelvic or perineal pain. For each stage of surgery, we explain the dangerous elements which should inspire only one instinct in the surgeon: vigilance. In practice, we describe certain strategic notions which should be perfectly understood before beginning laparoscopy, whatever the pathology: pelvic wall anatomy, pelvic cellular tissue and ureteral and broad ligament relationships.

INSUFFLATION AND PRIMARY TROCAR INSERTION

Pneumoperitoneal needle placement should be performed with rigor because it is responsible for 90% of vascular and visceral injuries. It is advisable to use a blunt needle with a perforated mandrel, mounted on a spring, to avoid any unwelcome surprises. After making the cutaneous incision, the abdominal wall is raised, particularly in thin patients, to distance the large vessels (except in cases of previous surgery in this area). For the same reason, needle placement should be perpendicular to the stretched abdominal wall, which corresponds to an angle of 45° from the horizontal.

The pneumoperitoneal needle penetrates the abdominal cavity, crossing several successive layers (Figure 1.1). At the umbilicus, the aponeurosis is stuck to the peritoneum and is therefore pierced in one go. Further down, on the subumbilical linea alba, the peritoneum is not stuck to the aponeurosis and one can feel the two successive jolts as the needle pierces the aponeurosis and the peritoneum. Tactile identification of these jolts is essential in order not to place the needle between the peritoneum and the aponeurosis and so induce an awkward extra pneumoperitoneum, and also so as not to advance the needle through the viscera or a vessel, when the peritoneum has already been crossed.

At this stage, there are many potential hazards, and the surgeon must remain extremely vigilant at all times. During their abdominal passage, trocars can injure numerous structures. Concerning the insufflation needle, it is very important to be aware of the position of the umbilicus because of the risk of major visceral and vascular injury. The umbilicus most often projects towards the L4 (in 67% of cases), that is to say, at the level of the most anterior point of the lumbar lordosis. In fact, the umbilicus is situated opposite the aortic bifurcation in 80% of cases, to within 2 cm. The most dangerous situation is observed in thin patients when the umbilicus is perpendicular to the aortic bifurcation or, in 50% of cases, perpendicular to the left common iliac vein which crosses the promontory near the midline.

In dorsal decubitus, with flexed legs, the stretched aorta tends to move away from the abdominal wall because of sagging of the lumbar lordosis. With age, as well as in obese patients, the umbilicus tends to descend and its relation to the aorta is altered.

The insufflation needle may injure the following organs: large vessels that are even more vulnerable as they are against bone structures, the omentum, the small intestine, the transverse colon, the sigmoid and, more rarely, the left side of the liver and the stomach. For this reason, insufflation and needle insertion should be performed only after assurance that the patient's stomach and bladder are empty. In case of doubt concerning the presence of adhesions, especially if there is a median subumbilical scar, it is recommended that insufflation be performed in the left hypochondrium area, two fingers'

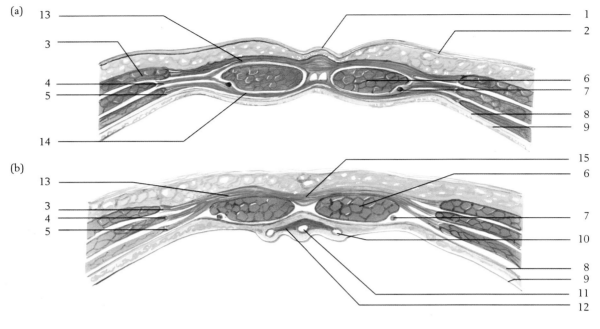

1 Umbilicus
2 Skin
3 Aponeurosis of external abdominal oblique muscle
4 Aponeurosis of internal abdominal oblique muscle
5 Aponeurosis of transversus abdominis muscle

6 Rectus abdominis muscle
7 Epigastric artery
8 Transversalis fascia
9 Peritoneum
10 Medial umbilical ligament

11 Urachus (median umbilical ligament)
12 Umbilical prevesical fascia
13 Anterior layer of rectus sheath
14 Posterior layer of rectus sheath
15 Linea alba

Figure 1.1 Transverse sections of the abdominal wall: (a) at the level of the umbilicus, (b) below the umbilicus

breadth from the costal border, to avoid a large spleen on the lateral side of the rectus abdominis muscle. This is an area of little depression where adhesions are uncommon.

When insufflation has started, one must be vigilant at all times so as to be immediately alerted if a needle is not in the right position. With the pneumoperitoneum established, the subumbilical trocar can be carefully introduced.

ANCILLARY TROCAR PLACEMENT

Ancillary trocar placement requires the Trendelenburg position. This position forces back the bowel, increases pelvic venous circulation, thereby reducing the consequent risk of venous thrombosis, and improves blood flow. We cannot place the patient in this position before insufflation because it may lead to some modifications in the position of the needle, with the consequent risk of vascular injury. During abdominal passage, these trocars may injure two principal structures: the bladder, if it is not empty or if it is attracted to the umbilicus by an anterior scar, and the inferior epigastric vessels. These vessels are situated in the preperitoneal space (between the peritoneum and the transversalis fascia). They originate from the external iliac artery near the deep inguinal ring and go up medially

towards the lateral side of the rectus abdominis muscle; they then rejoin this muscle 5 cm above the pubis. When one of these arteries is injured, it can induce significant bleeding, but the multiplicity of anastomoses in the abdominal wall and the wealth of blood supply mean that it can be sacrificed and ligated, if necessary. On the inside of these epigastric vessels is the median umbilical ligament, a vestige of the urachus, stretched between the umbilicus and the vesical apex, and the medial umbilical ligaments, obliterated umbilical arteries, which extend to the umbilicus. Before ancillary trocar placement, it is important to identify the inferior epigastric vessels along the abdominal wall behind the rectus abdominis muscle. In thin patients, they are usually transparently visible under the peritoneum. However, locating them can be more difficult if there is thick adipose tissue. The distance between the epigastric vessels and the midline is 5–6 cm, located 5 cm above the symphysis pubis; the mean distance between the medial umbilical ligaments and the inferior epigastric vessels is 2 cm. However, humans are not made symmetrically and these distances are significantly greater on the right side than on the left. There is no significant correlation between weight and any measured distance. However, a high body mass index affects the visibility of the inferior epigastric vessels, medial umbilical ligament and ureter on the left. Once the abdominal wall is pierced, the surgeon must take care not to injure the pelvic structures, particularly vascular and visceral structures.

During laparoscopic surgery, two golden rules that must be applied in order to avoid injury to the intra-peritoneal and retroperitoneal structures are knowledge of their normal anatomic localization and their visibility and appearance on the video-monitor. Compared with the laparotomic view, certain anatomic structures in the abdominal and pelvic cavity may look different during laparoscopic procedures because of the effect of pneumo-peritoneal pressure, Trendelenburg positioning and the use of an intrauterine manipulator. However, magnification should enhance visualization of these structures, allowing finer dissection.

PELVIC ANATOMY IN LAPAROSCOPY

Broad ligament or operative peritoneum

When one penetrates the peritoneal cavity, one encounters the digestive viscera which are moved upwards. One is then opposite the pelvic viscera, covered with peritoneum, which define, from front to back, the retropubic space (of Retzius) behind the pubis symphysis, in front of the vesical wall, known for the venous plexus which is situated there; the transverse vesical fold on the vesical corpus; and the vesicouterine pouch situated between the bladder and the uterine isthmus, with its opening leading to the vesicouterine septum. This septum is bordered below by an intimate connection between the ureters and the vagina. The rectouterine pouch described by Douglas is bordered by the rectum and its fascia behind, the vagina and the uterus in front and laterally by rectouterine folds which extend backwards towards the pararectal fossae. Its opening leads to the rectovaginal septum, which is limited by the joining of the two uterosacral ligaments behind the cervix. The retrorectal space is situated between the rectal and the retrorectal fascia.

The broad ligament is situated laterally, a double-layer formation extending from the uterus to the lateral walls of the pelvis. Perfect knowledge of its anatomy is essential to performing adnexal and fertility surgery. It extends like a sheet across clothes-lines, which represent the different subperitoneal elements. Each broad ligament consists of three peritoneal mesos, the funicular meso, the meso-salpinx and the meso-ovarium, which extends with the mesometrium, below and medially.

The funicular meso, raised by the round ligament of the uterus, extends from the uterine horn to the deep inguinal ring. Its removal allows one to approach the paravesical fossae the superior opening of which is situated between the umbilical artery on the inside and the iliac vascular pedicle on the outside. It is a wide and deep space;

its floor consists of the elevator ani muscle and its caudal part of the iliopubic branch and Cooper's ligament. It is crossed by the obturator pedicle which emerges from the interiliac space. The obturator nerve is the most superficial element of the pedicle and converges towards the obturator foramen. It can be recognized by its pearly white color at the level of the lateral pelvic concavity. One sometimes observes, against the superior branch of the pubis, accessory obturator vessels, branches of the inferior epigastric vessels. This paravesical space contains the obturator lymph nodes and the external iliac nodes and is therefore affected by lymphadenectomy. The potential danger at this level is from the inferior hypogastric vessels and the sometimes present accessory obturator vein, which emerges from the obturator pedicle near the foramen and ends on the inferior side of the external iliac vein, 1 or 2 cm from the femoral foramen.

The mesosalpinx, triangular when spread out, is bordered by the Fallopian tube above and the infundibulo-pelvic ligament on the outside. It contains vascular archways (infratubal, infraovarian and tubal branches of ovarian vessels) and the infratubal nervous plexus.

The lateral limit of the mesosalpinx is the tubo-ovarian ligament, partially followed by Richard's fimbrial fringe, whose role it is to connect the fimbria loosely with the ovary. It is essential that the mesosalpinx and tubo-ovarian ligament are free for good ovular capture and subsequent fertilization.

The meso-ovarium contains the ovarian vessels and nerves.

The preovarian fossa is bordered in front by the funicular fold and the mesosalpinx behind. It forms a triangle the relief of which is marked by the external iliac vessels laterally and the uterine horns inside. It covers the obturator fossa and faces the appendix on the right side, and the sigmoid on the left.

The tubo-ovarian recessus is between the mesosalpinx and the meso-ovarium. The ovarian fossa is between the meso-ovarium in front, the iliac vessels on the outside and the discrete fold of the ureter behind. Under its peritoneum is the obturator pedicle. Just behind, the uterine vessels are covered by the dorsal side of the broad ligament, advancing into the parametrium with the ureter.

Lateral to the ovary is the infundibulopelvic ligament, which contains the ovarian vessels. It crosses the external iliac vessels 2 cm in front of the ureter. It ends on the tubal extremity of the ovary. On the inside of the ovary is the proper ovarian ligament which emerges from the uterine horn behind and below the uterine tube, and goes to the uterine side of the ovary. The mesometrium extends behind, as far as the uterosacral ligaments.

The two pararectal fossae, the superior opening of which is narrow in the sacroiliac sinus, are not generally affected by gynecological laparoscopy. They are bordered in front by the paracervix, and inside by the rectum and the uterosacral folds, with the piriformis muscle outside, the levator ani muscle below and the lateral rectal ligament behind. They are covered with peritoneum under which is the ureter. They extend forwards by the paravesical space, passing under the paracervix. Access is difficult because of the presence of internal iliac and rectal vessels.

Laterally, still under the peritoneum, are the iliac vessels. The most accessible structure is the external iliac artery which continues the bifurcation of the common iliac artery (Figure 1.2). If the internal iliac artery is dissected at this level, one inevitably arrives at the anterior branches and some of its visceral branches. Situated more deeply on the inside of the artery is the external iliac vein. More laterally, the pelvic wall consists of the internal obturator muscle and its fascia.

Pelvic cellular tissue

A knowledge of pelvic cellular tissue is essential for the surgeon who operates on the pelvis. This tissue has two forms: slack zones, which can be easily dissected, and dense zones (fascia and visceral ligaments), which must be cut for dissection.

The slack zones are full of areolar tissue, relatively easy to dissect (retropubic space, paravesical fossae, pararectal fossae, retrorectal space, vesicovaginal septum, rectovaginal septum). The pelvic fascia is a dense conjunctive lamina covering the pelvic wall (parietal pelvic fascia), and forms

the adventitia of the viscera (visceral fascia). The pelvic parietal fascia (or urogenital diaphragm) is not greatly affected by laparoscopy. It is, first of all, a conjunctive lamina which constitutes an effective support for the pelvic viscera because of the continuity between the parietal and visceral pelvic fascia.

The visceral pelvic fascia covers the visceral non-peritonealized surface. The thickness of this fascia is variable and it is impaired particularly on the midline in case of prolapse. Only the vaginal fascia is a thick conjunctive layer reinforced by a strong elastic network. All this fascia exchanges fibers which makes anatomic relationships much tighter and dissection more precarious. This generates risks of visceral injury, especially at the level where the connections between the viscera and the urogenital diaphragm are dynamic (at the point where each viscus passes through the pelvic fascia, between the vagina and the vesical cervix, between the vagina and the rectum).

The visceral ligaments are made up of densifications of pelvic cellular tissue whose visceral insertion intermingles with the perivisceral fascia. They are very resistant structures that require ligature and section for visceral mobilization. Pelvic cellular tissue looks like the stitches of a mesh, with traction on a point of this mesh provoking a reduction of the stitches and mesh densification. The

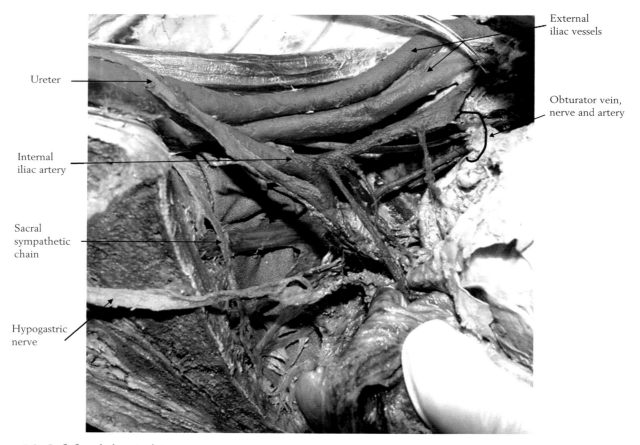

Ureter

External iliac vessels

Internal iliac artery

Obturator vein, nerve and artery

Sacral sympathetic chain

Hypogastric nerve

Figure 1.2 Left female hemipelvis

greater the traction, the more pronounced the densification near the point of traction, in other words, near the viscera. These visceral ligaments are divided into two groups: the lateral ligaments go with the internal iliac artery branches and the sagittal ligaments convey the inferior hypogastric plexus branches.

There are three lateral ligaments: rectal, genital and vesical. The genital ligament is the strongest and constitutes the strongest means of suspension of the uterus. It comprises three continuous parts: the parametrium, the paracervix and the paravagina. They present, near their visceral attachments, a densification of conjunctive tissue, very rich in elastic fibers and smooth muscle fibers. The parametrium situated just above the ureter contains the uterine artery, veins and lymphatics. The sometimes present lateroureteral cervicovaginal arteries can give the parametrium an anterior extension which is near the vesicouteral ligament and even merged with it. The paracervix, situated under the ureter, contains the vaginal arteries, the voluminous venous plexus and the uterovaginal lymph nodes. Contrary to the parametrium, the paracervix is frequently affected by cervical cancers. The genital ligament is also called the cardinal ligament.

The vesical ligament is located around the anterior vesical arteries, branches of the umbilical artery, and is attached to the anterior side of the paracervix. The rectal ligament is located around the middle rectal vessels. It is thick and disposed almost transversally on each side of the rectum. It separates the retrorectal area from the pararectal area.

The sagittal ligaments consist of the uterosacral, vesicouterine and tubovesical ligaments. The uterosacral ligaments are attached to the posterolateral side of the cervix and the vaginal fornix, and run alongside the lateral sides of the rectum to be finally lost, like a broad fan, on the inside of the sacral foramen from S2 to S4. They contain few vessels, but notably the inferior hypogastric plexus nerves described by Lee and Frankenhauser. A little transverse relief joins the points of uterine origin: the torus uterinus. On the whole, the content of these ligaments is principally made up of nerves; vessels are few and often their surgical section does not cause bleeding or necessitate hemostasis. Moreover, the wealth of nervous elements in these ligaments is expressed by their sensitivity. Their section can soothe pain provoked by static uterine defects. They are always extremely resistant and are even very elastic. Their resistance is due to both the nervous elements and the framework of pelvic fascia.

The vesicouterine ligaments extend from the isthmus and the cervix to the meatus uretrae area. They are situated around the arterial and venous cervicovaginal branches and extend in front of the parametrium. In front of them, the pubovesical ligaments extend from the posterior side of the pubis symphysis to the vesical cervix. All these structures form the tendinous arch of the pelvic fascia (the genitopelvic–rectosacral arch).

The parametrium and the paracervix have an extremely important functional role in the support of the uterus and vaginal fornix. These ligaments and fascias share numerous fibers which make their individualization very difficult and their borders imprecise. A typical example is the pericervical and perivaginal fascia which turn into the uterosacral ligaments and the two paracervices, and which share fibers with the parietal pelvic fascia. This explains why removal of the cervix does not provoke prolapse, because the vaginal vault is supported by the fascia.

Vascular relationships

Pelvic visceral vascularization derives from the iliac vessels, but also from the abdominal vessels for the adnexa and the rectum. We only briefly recall these elements and describe in more detail the strategic points which can be risk factors during laparoscopy. It is vital to know the dangerous anatomic areas, and carefully identify the important structures before proceeding with dissection.

Arterial relationships

The principal vascular relationship that is encountered when introducing the optic is represented by the external iliac vessels, which continue outside the viscera against the lateral pelvic wall. Pelvic visceral vascularization is essentially assured by the internal iliac arteries, the ovarian arteries and the superior rectal arteries.

The internal iliac artery divides into the principal visceral pelvic arteries. To see it during laparoscopy, it is necessary to push the infundibulopelvic ligament upwards. It is not necessary to cut it, as it serves as a screen against bowel inrush. It is classically divided into two branches at the level of the greater sciatic foramen. The anterior branch separates into essentially visceral branches. The umbilical artery continues in front along the superior part of the vesical inferolateral side. It constitutes a surgical landmark which leads to the origin of the uterine artery. It then leads to the superior vesical arteries. The uterine artery has three segments (Figure 1.3):

(1) The parietal segment descends forwards from its origin against the pelvic wall as far as the ischiatic spine. It is accompanied by the umbilical and obturator arteries in front and the ureter inside.

(2) The parametrial segment: the artery branches transversally inside, under the parametrium, and crosses the ureter in front. Around this point of crossing, there are some important venous plexus and lymph vessels.

(3) The mesometrial segment is very sinuous, running alongside the lateral side of the uterus in the mesometrium. It is accompanied by the uterine venous plexus, lymphatic vessels and the sometimes present parauterine lymph nodes.

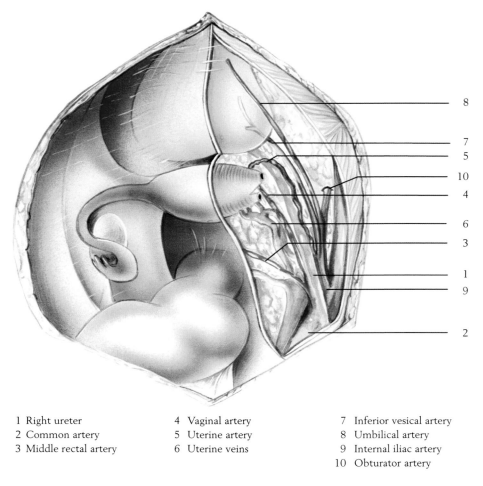

1	Right ureter	4	Vaginal artery	7	Inferior vesical artery
2	Common artery	5	Uterine artery	8	Umbilical artery
3	Middle rectal artery	6	Uterine veins	9	Internal iliac artery
				10	Obturator artery

Figure 1.3 Relationships of the ureter to the blood vessels

The uterine artery leads to several collateral branches, including vesicovaginal branches, the cervicovaginal artery after the ureteral crossing, the sinuous cervical artery, the corporeal artery and the round ligament artery. The vaginal arteries run behind the uterine artery. The obturator artery proceeds forwards, towards the obturator foramen. It is situated against the internal obturator muscle fascia and is bordered by the obturator nerve above and the obturator vein below. Its distal part is opposite the obturator lymph nodes. The middle rectal artery goes down medially towards the lateral side of the rectum, into the lateral rectal ligament. The internal pudendal artery accompanies the pudendal nerve in the perineum. After leaving the pelvis through the greater sciatic foramen, passing around the sciatic spine, penetrating the ischiorectal fossa and traveling along the pudendal canal, it ends in two branches, the deep artery and the dorsal artery of the clitoris. The posterior branch of the internal iliac artery has parietal branches, the iliolumbar artery, the lateral sacral artery and the superior gluteal artery.

The ovarian artery emerges from the abdominal aorta at the L2 level and joins the ovary by means of the infundibulopelvic ligament.

The superior rectal artery emerges from the inferior mesenteric artery and joins the superior rectal ligament.

At the pelvic level, there is an efficient anastomotic arterial system which compensates for all obstruction, even internal iliac.

An important arterial relationship to be aware of is the median sacral artery. It emerges from the posterior side of the aorta just above its bifurcation and descends against the anterior side of L4, L5 and the sacrum. It vascularizes the posterior side of the rectum. During surgical intervention for genital prolapse, we perform vaginal vault sacrofixation. During strip fixation using tackers at the L4–L5 level or promontory, there is always a risk of arterial injury and that is why efficient coagulation of the fixation zone is necessary. One must also take great care not to injure the anterior sacral roots which emerge on each side.

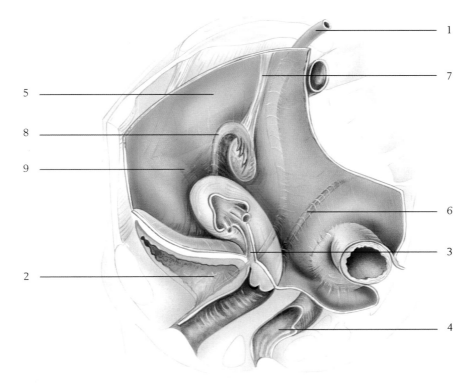

1 Right ureter: crossing at the pelvic brim	3 Broad ligament	5 Peritoneum	7 Infundibulopelvic ligament
2 Bladder	4 Rectum	6 Uterosacral ligament	8 Fallopian tube
			9 Round ligament

Figure 1.4 Relationships of the ureter to other pelvic organs

Venous relationships

The pelvic veins are essentially drained by the internal iliac veins and secondarily by the external iliac, common iliac, superior rectal and ovarian veins. The internal iliac vein does not contain valves, and emerges from the superior side of the greater sciatic foramen and connects to the external iliac vein at the promontory level, to form the common iliac vein. The tributary veins are satellites of the arteries and drain the pelvic venous plexus.

The ureter and its relationships

The lumbar ureter lies on the psoas muscle on each side of the rachis, and is only seen in gynecology by specialists who perform para-aortic lymphadenectomy. It then passes through the superior pelvic strait and becomes pelvic. The right ureter crosses the right external iliac artery in front, near its origin. The left ureter is situated in front of the end of the common iliac artery. On each side, it maintains a close relationship with the infundibulopelvic ligament which crosses it (Figure 1.4). It is therefore vulnerable when hemostasis of this ligament is carried out and during reperitonealization, which are pointless anyway. Laterally,

it is situated opposite the internal iliac vein and next to the obturator nerve and obturator, umbilical, uterine and vaginal vessels. In a thin patient, it is easy to identify under the peritoneum by its characteristic peristaltic motion. In an obese patient, it is necessary to search for it and dissect it in order not to injure it.

The retroligamentary ureter runs forwards and medially, along the posteromedian side of the uterine artery, approaching the uterosacral ligament origin. This course may be modified in the case of attraction to endometriosis, sequelae of infection or previous surgery. It can then come into contact with the ovary or the uterosacral ligament, and its identification is indispensable before continuing the dissection further. The distance between the ureter and the uterosacral homolateral ligament and the infundibulopelvic ligament is small, but significantly greater on the left side. The ureter is located about 1–3 cm from the uterosacral ligament and the infundibulopelvic ligament.

The intraligamentary ureter is of even more concern to the surgeon as it is invisible. It crosses the vessels and the lateral ligaments of the uterus from back to front to join the bladder (Figures 1.3 and 1.5). In fact, in crossing under

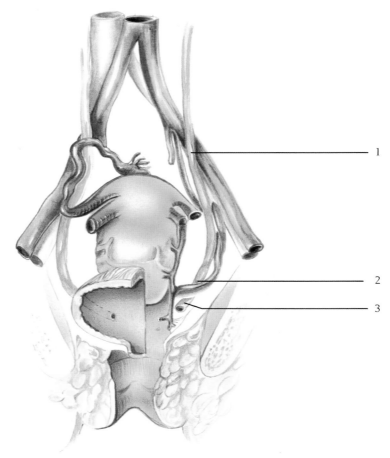

1 At the crossing with the iliac vessels   3 At the angle of the vaginal fornix
2 At the crossing with the uterine artery

Figure 1.5   Localization of ureteric injuries

the uterine artery loop, it passes between the parametrium and the paracervix.

The ureter, however, remains clearly independent of the uterine artery, since the crossing occurs behind the artery, 15 mm from the isthmus and 10 mm from the lateral vaginal fornix. It then joins the vesical extremity of the vesicouterine ligament which attaches above the ureteral meatus (retrovesical ureter).

Knowing that the ureter is at some distance from the isthmus and the vaginal fornix is not enough to guarantee safe surgery. It is necessary to know exactly how to dissect and shelter it. Mobilizing the uterus, it is possible to display the ascending segment of the uterine artery without modifying the position of the ureter, which remains at some distance from the vascular section. One can also use the uterine artery as a guide, cutting it at the isthmus level, and, by moving aside its parietal stump laterally, the ureter is effectively protected. Another way is to open the vesicouterine space and remove the vesicouterine ligament laterally and with it the retrovesical ureter which runs alongside.

Ureteral vascularization (Figure 1.6) merits a brief reminder. It derives from the renal, ovarian, common iliac and uterine arteries. These ureteral branches divide into a T-shape on ureteral contact to form a rich adventitial network the anastomotic system of which compensates for vascular interruption, thus allowing dissection over a long distance.

Digestive system

After moving the bowels upwards, out of the way, the only other awkward digestive elements in laparoscopy are the sigmoid and the rectum. The rectal peritoneum extends forwards to the vagina to form the rectouterine pouch. The lateral sides of the rectal peritoneum extend, with the pelvic wall peritoneum, to form the pararectal fossae which proceed obliquely towards the rectouterine pouch. Injury is rare in gynecology, but possible in some operations which require a prior intestinal wash-out, such as cases of rectovaginal adenomyosis resection by laparoscopy. It is difficult and perilous surgery, reserved for

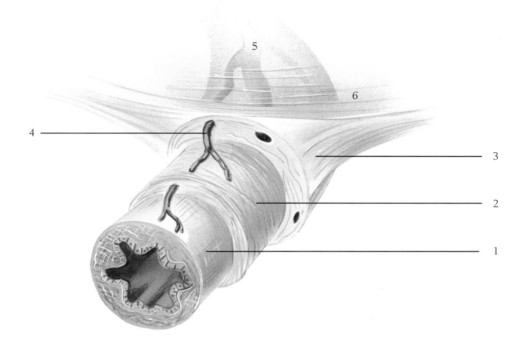

1 Mucosa with urothelium	4 Arteriole between musculosa and adventitial sheath
2 Medial muscular layer	5 Ureteral artery
3 Adventitial sheath	6 Peritoneum

Figure 1.6 Anatomy of the ureter

experienced surgeons, because it requires not only gynecological knowledge but also knowledge of the particular behavior of endometriosis and of digestive surgery. Rectal effraction is a constant risk, and, if any doubt exists, a diagnostic test by air or dye injection in the rectum may be necessary. On the other hand, the spread of these lesions can be considerable, not only on the rectal mucous membrane but also more laterally towards the pelvic wall, sometimes leading to ureteral stenosis and even invasion of the muscle elevator ani.

The rectum can also pose a danger in cancer surgery. Its invasion can make its approach dangerous during dissection. There is another gynecological procedure that is risky for the rectum, namely vaginal vault sacrospinofixation, described by Richter and Dargent in prolapse surgery. It consists of fixing the vagina to the sacrospinal ligament through a vaginal approach. Without a wide opening of the pararectal fossa, the ligatures are placed blindly and a rectal or pudendal nerve injury is possible.

Nervous elements

Pelviperineal innervation is both somatic and vegetative. The peripheral nervous system of the pelvis includes the sacral and pudental plexi. The first, which consists of roots L4, L5, S1, S2 and S3, goes to the inferior limbs and the pelvis. The second, coming from roots S2, S3 and S4, is responsible for the innervation of the perineum and the viscera. These two plexi are closely linked with the vegetative nervous system from the superior and inferior hypogastric plexus. This association between the somatic and vegetative nervous systems exists in all the great visceral functions of the organism, but is more intense at the level of the pelvic viscera.

The laparoscopic surgeon safely avoids, in contrast to the abdominal surgeon, section of the anterior branch of the iliohypogastric and ilioinguinal nerves, which may lead, although reversible, to cutaneous anesthesia of the pubic region, the inside of the thigh and the labium majus, as well as injury to the femoral nerve, which extends along the lateral side of the psoas and may be in danger of compression by the autostatic valves during laparotomy.

The nervous elements that are important to know in laparoscopy include primarily the genitofemoral nerve which emerges from spinal nerves L1 and L2 and crosses the psoas to extend in its sheath behind the ureter and the peritoneum. It then continues along the lateral side of the external iliac artery. Its genital branch provides sensitive innervation to the labia majora and the neighboring areas. Its injury is very rare in laparoscopy.

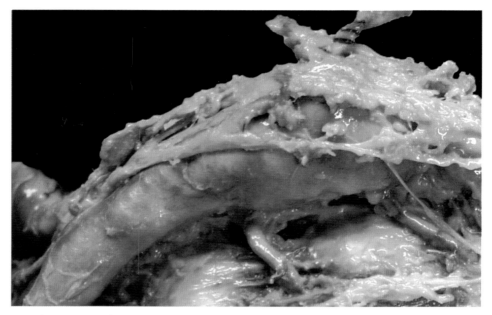

Figure 1.7 Superior hypogastric plexus

The obturator nerve (L2, L3, L4) emerges in the pelvis between the external and internal iliac vessels. It extends against the lateral wall opposite the ovarian fossa, before entering the obturator foramen. It can be affected at this level by endometriosis or adnexal infection, leading to obturator neuralgia on the superomedial side of the thigh and the knee.

Surgical injury to these nerves can be observed during lymphadenectomy, but the functional consequences are minor.

ANATOMIC BASIS OF PELVIC AND PERINEAL PAIN AND THERAPEUTIC APPLICATIONS

Anatomic description

The perineum receives its innervation from the pudental plexus. This plexus also supplies visceral nerves, which are of variable number. They extend forwards towards the lateral walls of the pelvic viscera to the bladder, the rectum and the internal genital organs, either directly, or by the intermediary of the hypogastric plexus. Through these branches, the nervous impulses controlling micturition, defecation and sensory innervation of the pelvic viscera proceed. Vegetative innervation of the pelvic viscera derives essentially from the inferior hypogastric plexi, but also from the superior hypogastric plexus and the ovarian plexus.

The superior hypogastric plexus is situated facing L5 and the promontory, and is the origin of the left and right hypogastric nerves which connect to the corresponding inferior hypogastric plexus (Figure 1.7). This plexus used to be resected according to Cotte's procedure, but the mediocre results obtained have now made this method obsolete.

The inferior hypogastric plexus, or Lee and Frankenhauser's ganglion, is a collection of afferent and efferent fibers going towards the pelviperineal viscera. It is symmetrically paired in the form of a nervous quadrilateral lamina of 4 cm in length and 3 cm in height. It is located in the lateral part of the uterosacral ligament, surrounded by the lateral side of the rectum on the inside and the visceral venous plexus on the outside. Its superior edge is in contact with the ureter, its inferior edge with the pelvic floor, its posterior edge with the sacrum and its anterior edge with the posterior bladder wall. This inferior hypogastric plexus is the central point of a considerable number of nervous branches aimed at all the organs inside the pelvis.

Each inferior hypogastric plexus receives afferent branches: the hypogastric nerve originating from the superior hypogastric plexus, the sacral sympathetic chain (sacral splanchnic nerves), the pelvic splanchnic nerves (nervi erigentes) and the inferior mesenteric plexus (some spindle nerves). Efferent branches make up the pelvic visceral plexus: the uterovaginal plexus, the rectal plexus and the vesical plexus (vesical nerves, when cut during extended hysterectomies, can account for bladder hypotonia).

The ovarian plexus supplies innervation to the ovaries and the distal half of the Fallopian tubes. It originates from the aortic plexus. The parasympathetic fibers come from the pneumogastric nerve, which could explain vagal digestive reactions during adnexal torsion. These plexi contain orthosympathetic and parasympathetic fibers. The pelvic orthosympathetic centers are located inside the intermediolateralis columnae of the medulla, from the tenth thoracic verbebra to the third lumbar vertebra. The efferent branches, the positioning of which is segmental, provide nerve supply to the pelvic viscera. The fibers follow the vessels, leading them to the viscera.

The sacral parasympathetic nucleus is located at the level of the S2–S4 segments, on the basal part of the ventral horn, and takes charge of all pelvic elements except the ovaries. Concerning the orthosympathetic system, the sensitive fibers are individualized and carry influx such as nociception. Thereafter, they join the closest somatic nerve and account for abdominal wall pain originating from visceral discomfort. Concerning the parasympathetic fibers, their sensitive role is still in question, even if their existence itself cannot be disputed. The motor response to nociceptive perceptions correlates with the anatomy: the parietal pain experienced during acute salpingitis is, in fact, pain from a viscus transmitting painful information through the closest somatic nerve into the corresponding iliac fossa. Motor cells under orthosympathetic influence may account for abdominal wall contracture on clinical examination.

Another example of these sensitive functions is the pain experienced by patients who suffer from adeno-myotic nodules of the rectovaginal septum. These are caused by stimulation of the orthosympathetic fibers inside the rectovaginal septum; through the inferior hypogastric plexus, they carry their nociceptive informa-tion to the superior centers. The sympathetic motor cells then induce a reflex contraction of the pelvic diaphragm, closing the vagina and making intercourse even more painful.

Although such pain is no indication for laparoscopic treatment, it is important to evoke the anatomic basis of chronic perineal neuralgia and the role of the pudendal nerve which leads to pain, the etiologic diagnosis of which is sometimes difficult, and often considered as having a psychiatric origin. These patients suffer pain in the area of the pudendal nerve, either uni- or bilaterally, and this pain is exacerbated, if not provoked, by the sitting position. The positional character of this pain in a given area leads us to investigate a compression syndrome of the nerve stem.

These pains can be urogenital, anal or mixed. They involve women in two-thirds of cases and manifest themselves as burning sensations, torsions, heaviness or even intravaginal or intrarectal foreign bodies. They are not satisfactorily treated by different local therapeutic approaches and can be exacerbated by a proctological, urological or gynecological surgical procedure.

The pudendal nerve generally issues from S3, and can intercept contingents from adjoining roots S2 and S4. Emerging in the ventral sacral area, it rapidly penetrates, together with its vessels, the gluteal area under the piriformis muscle, in ligamentary claws formed from the sacrotuberous and sacrospinous ligaments (Figure 1.8). It passes around the sciatic spine between the superior rectal

nerves on the inside and the pudendal vessels on the outside. In the perineal area, the nerve lies on the medial side of the internal obturator muscle in the pudendal canal (described by Alcock), formed by a split in the apo-neurosis. In the posterior part of this canal, it crosses over the falciform process of the sacrotuberous ligament, which is a fibrous lamina with a sharp superior edge, concave above, and parallel to, the medial side of the ischium.

Medially, the abundant fat of the ischioanal fossa occupies all the posterior perineum. Observation of the course of this nerve, as described above, highlights several possible areas of conflict:

- In the ligamentary claws near the sciatic spine, the nerve is pressed between the sacrotuberous and sacrospinous ligaments

- The falciform process of the sacrotuberous ligament can emerge very high and come into contact with the nerve which overlaps it

- The fascia of the internal obturator muscle, when it splits, can be thickened and thus become a potential site of conflict

Several studies have shown that a sitting position provokes an ascent of the ischioanal fat, which presses the sacro-tuberous ligament falciform process laterally and brings it closer to the nerve stem.

Therapeutic applications

LUNA (laser uterine nerve ablation)

This is the practical application of the anatomy of the inferior hypogastric plexus. Uterosacral ligament ablation by laser interrupts the vegetative fibers and thus leads to a diminution in dysmenorrhea and dyspareunia. Some authors believe that the beneficial effect of LUNA is due more to the treatment of endometriosis of the uterosacral ligament than to the fiber ablation itself.

Torus uterinus ablation

According to the same principle, surgery consists of ablation of the area which joins the isthmic origin of the two uterosacral ligaments.

Rectovaginal septum adenomyosis

Apart from ablation of the adenomyotic lesion, surgery also effects suppression of vegetative fibers which provoke pain at the level of the rectovaginal septum.

Chronic perineal pain

Surgical liberation of the pudendal nerve, described by Robert et al., gives excellent results when anesthetic infiltrations fail. Of course, this type of surgery requires

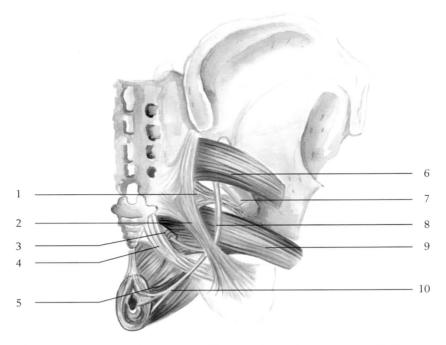

1 Sacrospinous ligament   4 Falciform process of the sacrotuberous ligament   7 Sciatic nerve
2 Sacrotuberous ligament   5 Levator ani muscle   8 Pudendal nerve
3 Pudendal canal   6 Piriformis muscle   9 Internal obturator muscle
                                                                                             10 Inferior rectal nerve

Figure 1.8 Posterior view of the deep gluteal area

perfect knowledge of the regional anatomy. The principle is very simple: by a transgluteal approach, the gluteus maximus muscle is incised in the direction of its fibers, on both sides of a transverse line passing at the level of the coccyx and thus the sciatic spine. The muscular attachments of the posterior side of the sacrotuberous ligament are removed over 2–3 cm. The pudendal pedicle then appears to cross the sacrospinous ligament behind. The latter is sectioned and the nerve can then be transposed forwards to the sciatic spine, gaining precious centimeters. Dissection of the nerve in the pudendal canal is easy, and the internal obturator muscle fascia is incised and the nerve stem and its branches are freed over 3–4 cm. Section of a threatened falciform process is performed if necessary. It is then easy to release the nerve stem in this simple way.

DANGEROUS RELATIONSHIPS DURING ILIAC AND AORTIC LYMPHADENECTOMY BY LAPAROSCOPY

Because of the anatomic complexity and technical difficulty of lymphadenectomy, we devote an entire chapter to this subject. In fact, rare are those gynecologists who perform lymphadenectomy by laparoscopy, because vascular and nervous relationships of pelvic lymph nodes make dissection extremely delicate. The advantages of the laparoscopic approach are the absence of trauma and a decreased risk of adhesions, for the price of specialized training, but without any diminution in the quality of samples taken.

Cancer work-ups and pelvic or lumbar lymph-adenectomy require thorough knowledge of these lymph nodes (Figure 1.9). The indications are essentially diagnostic and prognostic. Lymphadenectomy is the surgical removal of an entire cellulo-lymph node area.

Occasionally present pelvic lymph nodes are situated near the viscera and are drained by the external iliac, obturator, interiliac, internal iliac, common iliac and lumbar nodes. The paravesical nodes are situated in the lateral ligaments of the bladder. The parauterine nodes are found in the parametrium near the uterine artery loop. The paravaginal nodes are located in the paracervix. The pararectal nodes are situated in the lateral ligaments of the rectum. External iliac nodes are eight to ten in number; they are found along the external iliac vessels, and they include three groups:

(1) The lateral group are outside the external iliac vessels.

(2) The intermediate group lie on the external iliac vein or between the artery and the vein. They drain the

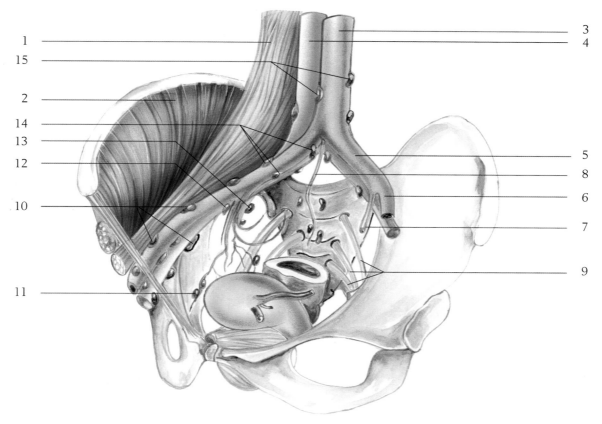

1 Psoas muscle	5 Common iliac artery	9 Sacral plexus	13 Internal iliac nodes
2 Iliacus muscle	6 External iliac artery	10 External iliac nodes	14 Common iliac nodes
3 Abdominal aorta	7 Internal iliac artery	11 Obturator nodes	15 Lumbar nodes
4 Inferior vena cava	8 Median sacral artery	12 Interiliac nodes	

Figure 1.9 Anterior view of the lymph nodes of the pelvis

inguinal nodes and the medial external iliac nodes towards the common iliac nodes.

(3) The medial group are situated under the vein and against the pelvic wall, so it is necessary to lift the vein to reach them. This group receives the lymph vessels of the bladder, the pelvic ureter, the uterus and the vagina.

The obturator nodes are situated against the obturator pedicle and the internal obturator muscle. They receive the lymph vessels of the bladder, the ureter, the uterus and the vagina. The interiliac nodes are situated at the bifurcation of the internal and external iliac vessels. They drain the obturator and external iliac nodes. The also receive the lymph vessels of the bladder, the uterus and the vagina.

The internal iliac nodes are found between the internal iliac artery branches. One can distinguish the sacral nodes, situated along the lateral sacral artery, which receive the lymph vessels of the rectum and the cervix, and the gluteal nodes, which lie on the piriformis muscle, and drain the lymph vessels of the rectum, the deep area of the

perineum and the gluteal area. The common iliac nodes are situated against the common iliac vessels, and drain the external, internal and intermediate iliac nodes. They include five groups:

(1) The lateral group: on the lateral sides of the common iliac artery at the level of the iliolumbar fossa;

(2) The intermediate group: under the common iliac vessels, against the obturator nerve, the ascending lumbar vein and the lumbosacral trunk;

(3) The medial group: situated against the medial side of the right common iliac artery and the right and left common iliac veins;

(4) Promontory nodes;

(5) Subaortic nodes; the lumbar nodes are found around the aorta, the inferior vena cava and between these two vessels.

Lymphadenectomy is performed according to several techniques in laparoscopy: by either a transperitoneal approach to the paravesical fossa, or an extraperitoneal approach, by careful detachment of the peritoneum, beginning with the retropubic space and then the prevascular and preperitoneal areas. Insufflation through the trocar detaches the preperitoneal area. Lymphadenectomy can be extended to several levels, described below.

Level I describes the angle defined by the common iliac artery bifurcation. It removes the medial and intermediate external iliac nodes, obturator and interiliac. These are the sentinel lymph nodes of the front line of the uterine cervix, which can first be identified by the sentinel lymph node technique during surgery for cervical cancer. This level is sufficient for small cervical tumors and endometrial cancers. The risk during dissection of this area is to the inferior obturator vein, the internal iliac vein branches and the obturator vessels.

Level II is astride the pelvis and the abdomen, limited above by the angle of the aortic bifurcation. It includes the common iliac nodes, the lateral external iliac nodes not affected by the first level, the promontory and the subaortic nodes. The risk during lateral external iliac node removal is injury to the genitofemoral nerve which runs alongside the psoas and, particularly, the sometimes present psoic artery, which emerges from the external iliac artery. The epigastric vessels must also be respected near the deep inguinal ring. On the other hand, the retrocrural nodes described by Cloquet are removed. During promontory node dissection, care must be taken with regard to the middle sacral pedicle, the presacral veins and, particularly, the left common iliac vein.

Level III is lower aortic, defined above by the emergence of the inferior mesenteric artery. It is bordered laterally by the lumbar ureters, and behind by the iliac vessels, the sympathetic ganglions and psoas attachment. These elements are generally well visible, and complications are rare if the dissection is carefully performed.

Level IV, infrarenal, does not generally involve laparoscopy and is rarely carried out.

Increasingly, removal of the cellular lymph node tissue of the distal part of the paracervix, known as paracervical lymphadenectomy, is performed. Its purpose is to supplant the removal of the distal part of the paracervix. The affected tissue is removed, preserving the nerves and vessels of the paracervix. It is necessary, at this level, to identify the middle rectal artery at the back and the vegetative nerves in order to protect them.

ANATOMIC BASIS OF URINARY STRESS INCONTINENCE AND THERAPEUTIC APPLICATIONS

Stress incontinence is a frequent and complex symptom in women. It is caused by obstetric trauma to the urogenital perineum, but also dystrophic modifications of the menopause. Finally, it can be the consequence of surgery or radiotherapy to the bladder or urethra. The principal anatomic structures implicated in stress continence are the retropubic space, the base and cervix of the bladder, the urethra and its sphincter. The retropubic space described by Retzius is situated in the preperitoneal space. It is bordered in front by the pubis symphysis, the pubovesical ligaments, the tendinous arch of the pelvic fascia and the retropubic branches of the obturator and pudendal vessels. Laterally is the superior branch of the pubis and a thickening of the periosteum, the pectineal or Cooper's ligament, implicated in pectineal colposuspension described by Burch. Behind is the inferolateral side of the bladder as well as the urethra and the pelvic vagina. This area is closed below by the pelvic diaphragm. It is full of loose tissue, infiltrated by fat and easily cleavable during laparoscopy. The vesical base includes the trigone of the bladder and the retrotrigonal fossa, the depth of which increases with age, which is a factor in post-micturition dribble.

The vesical cervix is essential for urinary continence. It is situated 25 mm from the pubic symphysis and 10 mm above the horizontal, passing along its inferior side. Its anterior fixity is assured by the pubovesical ligaments. The normal urethrovesical angle is 90–100°.

The urethra includes three segments: supradiaphragmatic, diaphragmatic and infradiaphragmatic. It is situated obliquely below and in front, and at an angle of 30° from the vertical. The supradiaphragmatic urethra is supported by the pubovesical ligament; the infradiaphragmatic urethra is supported by the pubourethral ligament and suspensory ligament of the clitoris.

Micturition requires absolute synergy between the bladder, the urethra and abdominal pressure.

During the repletion phase, abdominopelvic pressure constitutes a passive occlusion force of the urethra. It opposes urogenital diaphragmatic resistance against which the urethra pushes. The resultant force exerted by the abdominopelvic pressure and the resistance of the urogenital diaphragm makes its way forward, perpendicularly, to the perineal membrane, which constitutes the essential static structure of diaphragmatic urethral occlusion. Techniques using a perineal sling in urinary stress incontinence surgery illustrate perfectly the biomechanics of the urogenital diaphragm. The TVT and TOT methods (tension-free vaginal tape and transobturator tape), in particular, are among those which, by their physiological and almost non-invasive approach, currently give very good results. This sling exerts retrourethral resistance the orientation of which adjoins that of the pubis. The resultant abdominopelvic pressure and tape resistance is then perpendicular to the perineal membrane. During any effort, abdominopelvic pressure, oriented towards the posterior perineum, leads to a posterior transfer of the supradiaphragmatic urethra. On the other hand, the diaphragmatic urethra opposes the resistance of the tape and bends.

During the micturition phase, the association of both intravesical pressure and intraparietal tension created by detrusor contraction is directed to an area of weak resistance, the vesical cervix. The tonus of the urethra yields and the urethra opens.

In urinary stress incontinence, there is ptosis of the urethrovesical region, and shortening and horizontalization of the urethra. The surgeon's objective is to replace the vesical cervix so that it will maintain its anatomic position, while preserving cervical and urethral flexibility.

The wide use of retropubic tension-free suburethral slings (TVT) has been associated with various peri- and postoperative complications. To reduce these complications, TOT using transobturator passage of the tape has been developed. This technique uses specific instruments for the passage of synthetic tape from beneath the urethra towards the thigh fold. With this technique, the risk of injury to the bladder, the epigastric vein and the external iliac vein is non-existent. By contrast, such injuries may occur if the tape is introduced through the retropubic space. Anatomic dissection shows that the transobturator tape does not enter the retropubic space. The tape is inserted according to a fixed path which penetrates from the suburethral space into a strictly perineal region, limited medially and cranially by the levator ani muscle, caudally by the perineal membrane and laterally by the obturator internus muscle. This region corresponds to the most anterior recess of the ischiorectal fossa. The tape then perforates the obturator membrane and muscles, and exits through the skin after crossing the adductor muscles and subcutaneous tissue. It passes through the obturator foramen along the upper third of the ramus inferior of the pubic bone. The tape courses away from the dorsal nerve of the clitoris located more superficially below the perineal membrane, the obturator nerve and vessels, and the saphenous and femoral vessels. The tape is not visible in the Retzius space; it remains covered with the fasciae of the internal obturator muscle, so that it cannot access the lower pelvis at any time. This is a highly accurate, reproducible and safe technique, which does not require perioperative cystoscopy, as does TVT.

BIBLIOGRAPHY

Bonnet P, Waltregny D, Reul O, de Leval J. Transobturator tape inside out for the surgical treatment of female stress urinary incontinence: anatomical considerations. J Urol 2005; 173: 1223–8

Bradley WE. Neural control of urethrovesical function. Clin Obstet Gynecol 1978; 21: 653–67

Carter JE. Surgical treatment for chronic pelvic pain. J Soc Laparoendosc Surg 1988; 2: 129–39

Dargent D, Salvat J. L'Envahissement Ganglionnaire Pelvien. Paris: Medsi, 1989

Dargent D. Laparoscopic surgery in gynecologic oncology. J Gynecol Obstet Biol Reprod Paris 2000; 29: 282–4

Enhörning G. Simultaneous recording of intravesical and intraurethral pressure. A study on urethral closure pressure in normal and stress incontinent women. Acta Chir Scand Suppl 1961; Suppl 276: 1–68

Faucheron JL. Surgical anatomy of pelvic nerves. Ann Chir 1999; 53: 985–9

Fauconnier A, Delmas V, Lassau JP, et al. Ventral tethering of the vagina and its role in the kinetics of urethra and bladder-neck straining. Surg Radiol Anat 1996; 18: 81–7

Fétiveau G. The inferior hypogastric plexus, Report for MSBM. Anatomy Laboratory, Faculty of Medicine, University of Nantes, France, 2002

Jacquetin B. Use of TVT in surgery for female urinary incontinence. J Gynecol Obstet Biol Reprod Paris 2000; 29: 242–7

Kamina P. Petit bassin et périnée. Rectum et Organes Urogénitaux. Paris: Maloine, 1995; 1, 2

Lazorthes G. Le système nerveux périphérique. Description, Systématisation, Exploration Clinique Abord Chirurgical. Paris: Masson, 1955: Ch XXII

Nezhat CH, Nezhat F, Brill AI, et al. Normal variations of abdominal and pelvic anatomy evaluated at laparoscopy. Obstet Gynecol 1999; 94: 238–42

Ploteau S, Donnez J. Anatomy in relation with gynecological endoscopy. In Donnez J, Nisolle M, eds. An Atlas of Operative Laparoscopy and Hysteroscopy, 2nd edn. Carnforth, UK: Parthenon Publishing, 2001: 33–45

Querleu D. Techniques Chirurgicales en Gynécologie, 2nd edn. Paris: Masson, 1998

Richter K, Dargent D. La spino-fixation dans le traitement des prolapsus du dôme vaginal après hystérectomie. J Gynecol Obstet Biol Reprod 1986; 15: 1081–8

Robert R, Brunet C, Faure A, et al. Surgery of the pudendal nerve in various types of perineal pain: course and results. Chirurgie 1993–94; 119: 535–9

Robert R, Prat-Pradal D, Labat JJ, et al. Anatomic basis of chronic perineal pain: role of the pudendal nerve. Surg Radiol Anat 1998; 20: 93–8

Roberts WH, Hunt GM, Henken HW. Some anatomic factor having to do with urinary continence. Anat Rec 1968; 162: 341–8

Shafik A. Pudendal canal syndrome as a cause of vulvodynia and its treatment by pudendal nerve decompression. Eur J Obstet Gynecol Reprod Biol 1998; 80: 215–20

Testut L, Latarjet A. Traité d'Anatomie Humaine, 9th edn. Paris: G. Doin & Cie, 1949; 3: Book 7; 5: Books 12, 13

Ulmsten U, Falconer C, Johnson P, et al. A multicenter study of tension-free vaginal tape (TVT) for surgical treatment of stress urinary incontinence. Int Urogynecol J Pelvic Floor Dysfunc 1998; 9: 210–13

2

Instrumentation and operational instructions

J Donnez, P Jadoul

ENDOSCOPIC INSTRUMENTS

Telescopes

Telescopes used in laparoscopy are available with different viewing directions, either with or without an instrument channel. The various telescopes and their application range are briefly described below (Figure 2.1):

- 0° straightforward telescope: this telescope has the greatest application range, because it facilitates orientation and conveys an impression of the area inspected. The direction of view corresponds to the natural approach and the usual perspective. The 0° telescope is generally preferred in gynecological interventions

- 30° forward-oblique telescope: this can be rotated to enlarge the field of vision. Use of the 30° telescope can be advantageous during dissection in the Douglas pouch

- 45° telescope

Telescopes without instrument channels are used in the majority of cases in gynecology, as they give a better overview and offer better image resolution. However, in some cases, it may be more reasonable to use telescopes with an integrated instrument channel (telescope with parallel eyepiece, see Figure 2.1, top). These telescopes are generally 0° straightforward telescopes. The diameter of the instrument channel is 5–7 mm; thus, a correspondingly large instrument can be inserted.

Additional devices can also be connected to this laparoscope, such as a CO_2 laser. The best example of this is for laparoscopic sterilization; tissue fragments or biopsy specimens can also be extracted through the telescope trocar with the aid of a grasping forceps, which is introduced through the telescope's instrument channel.

A disadvantage of using telescopes with instrument channels is the deterioration in image quality. This is due to the lower light intensity that can be picked up by the video camera, when compared with telescopes that do not have an instrument channel.

A Verres optical needle with insufflation can be used in some difficult cases (Figure 2.2), or in order to perform 'mini-laparoscopy'.

Trocars

Small passageways through incisions in the abdominal wall are created with the aid of trocars. The use of disposable trocars is clearly in decline, in the era of cost reduction.

In general, trocars with various diameters are used in surgical endoscopy. The standard sizes (Figure 2.3) are 5.5, 11, 12, 15 and 22 mm.

Spherical and flap valves make it possible to change operating instruments quickly, as the change can be carried out without activating the valve mechanism. Trumpet valves are mostly found in telescope trocars. The telescope is protected from contamination by tissue and blood particles during insertion by pressing the trumpet valve. Sharp, pyramidal trocar tips, on the other hand, can be positioned

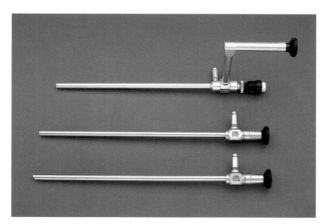

Figure 2.1 Telescopes used in gynecology. From top to bottom: telescope with instrument channel, 30° and 0° telescopes (Karl Storz)

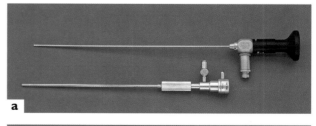

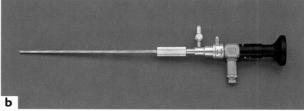

Figure 2.2 (a) and (b) Optical Verres needle

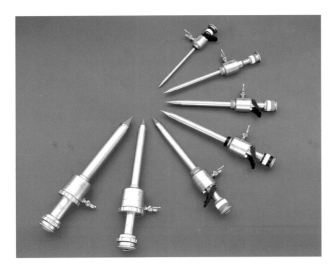

Figure 2.3 Trocars are available in different sizes and with various valve mechanisms (Karl Storz)

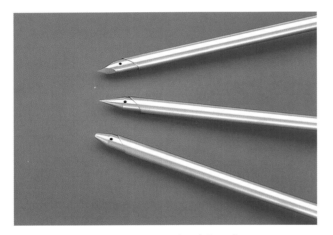

Figure 2.4 Various trocar tips (Karl Storz)

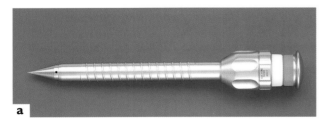

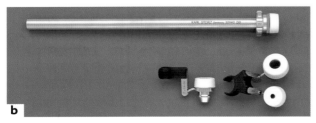

Figure 2.5 (a) Threaded trocars offer a better grip in the abdominal wall (Karl Storz); (b) various trocar reducers (Karl Storz)

relatively easily. The sharp edges can sometimes damage smaller blood vessels and other organs.

There are great differences between trocar tips (Figure 2.4). By using spherical, blunt, trocar tips, the blood vessels are pushed aside and protected to a large degree. Sometimes, however, greater pressure has to be exerted during insertion. Since the skin incision for the auxiliary puncture is carried out under transillumination and the puncture itself is in full view, the choice of trocar tip here can be regarded as being of secondary importance. Better protection to prevent the trocar slipping out of the intraperitoneal space is provided by sheaths with screw threading (Figure 2.5a). However, these cause increased trauma to both the abdominal wall and the peritoneum. Trocar reducers facilitate the surgery (Figure 2.5b).

INDIVIDUAL INSTRUMENTS

Grasping forceps

Atraumatic dissecting and grasping forceps (Figures 2.6 and 2.7) are particularly suitable for grasping and the liberation of hollow organs. The claws are fashioned so that trauma to the tissue should not occur. Atraumatic grasping forceps (multiserrated) are designed for atraumatic and precise tissue grasping, such as of ligaments during diagnosis. Grasping forceps (2 × 4 teeth) are used to grasp and liberate solid organs. Sturdy grasping forceps are indispensable in surgical endoscopy; in the case of endoscopic cyst extirpation, for example, they can help to fix the ovary capsule properly and remove the cystic bag.

Dissecting and grasping forceps (claw forceps) are particularly designed for grasping solid structures (e.g. myomas). These forceps are used where trauma of the tissue does not have to be particularly considered.

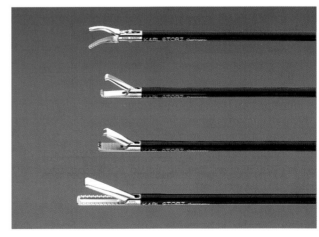

Figure 2.6 Grasping forceps. From top to bottom: Kelly grasping forceps (atraumatic), Manhes grasping forceps (atraumatic), Manhes grasping forceps (traumatic), Schneider lymph node grasping forceps (atraumatic)

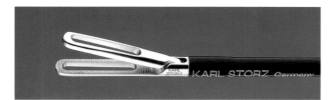

Figure 2.7 Intestinal grasping forceps, diameter 5 mm (Karl Storz)

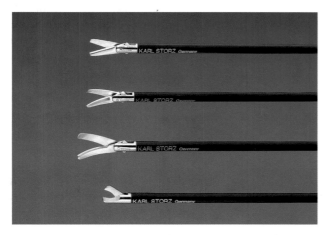

Figure 2.8 Laparoscopic scissors. From top to bottom: straight scissors, curved scissors (different lengths of blades), hook scissors

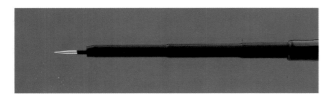

Figure 2.9 Monopolar high-frequency needle (Karl Storz): the tip of the needle can be retracted into the sheath

Scissors

Hook scissors (Figure 2.8) are particularly suitable for transecting ligature fibers and for tissue transection. Delicate dissection can be carried out with straight scissors. Curved scissors, in general, have the same features as for straight scissors. In some cases they are easier to dissect with, because the curvature changes the viewing angle.

Coagulation instruments

The tip of a monopolar high-frequency needle (Figure 2.9) can be retracted into the sheath. Various bipolar forceps (Figures 2.10 and 2.11) can be introduced through a 5-mm trocar.

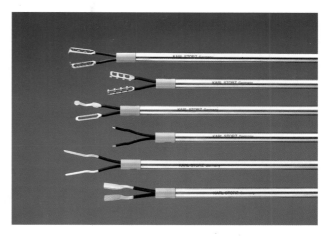

Figure 2.10 Various bipolar forceps (Karl Storz)

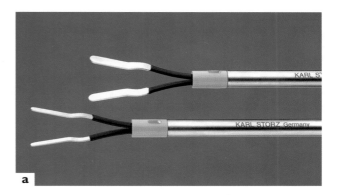

a

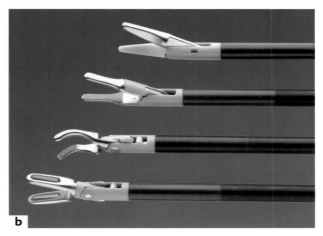

b

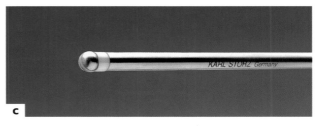

c

Figure 2.11 (a) 1-mm and 3-mm wide bipolar forceps; (b) RoBi™: new generation of rotating bipolar forceps and scissors; (c) bipolar ball electrode

Additional instruments

Other 5-mm instruments are needed for laparoscopic surgery, for example probes (atraumatic), a needle for cyst puncture and an irrigation–suction probe (Figure 2.12).

Biopsy forceps

Biopsy forceps (Figure 2.13) are used during diagnostic laparoscopy in cases of malignant disease (ovarian cancer: before chemotherapy or during second-look laparoscopy) and benign disease such as endometriosis.

Needle holder

Figure 2.14 shows 5-mm and 3-mm needle holders.

Myoma holder

Figure 2.15 shows a myoma fixation instrument.

Atraumatic forceps

Atraumatic forceps (Figure 2.16) are used for prehension of the Fallopian tube or the ureter.

Intestinal probe

The intestinal probe (Figure 2.17) is used to push back the intestines in order to achieve a good view.

MORCELLATORS

In the past, laparoscopic surgeons were faced with the difficult problem of extraction of tissue, and were often

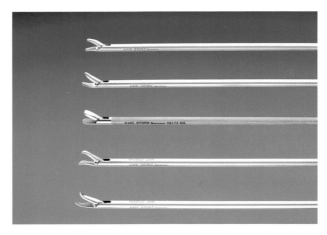

Figure 2.14 Tips of various needle holders

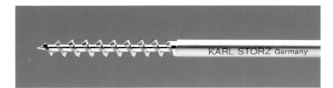

Figure 2.15 Myoma fixation instrument

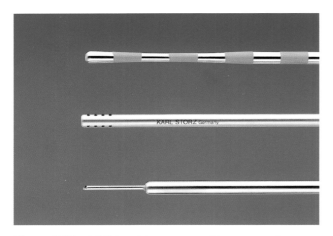

Figure 2.12 Additional instruments. From top to bottom: palpation probe, irrigation and suction tube, puncture needle

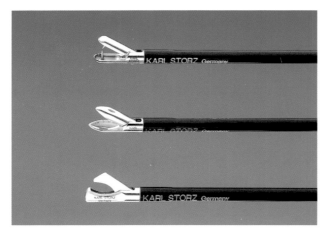

Figure 2.13 Various biopsy forceps

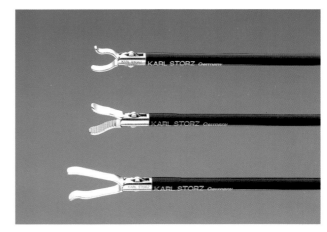

Figure 2.16 Various atraumatic forceps

obliged to perform a suprapubic mini-laparotomy or a transvaginal extraction. The first substantial improvement was the development of the manual morcellator (Semm–Wisap). Much force and time were necessary, depending on the consistency of the tissue.

In collaboration with Storz, Steiner developed the electromechanical morcellator (Figure 2.18), consisting of a motor-driven cutting tube. The speed can be selected in three stages. It is possible, with the aid of this morcellator, to extract even large amounts of tissue from the abdomen, using the size 11 trocar, in a short period of time. With 12-mm and 15-mm trocars (Figure 2.19), large quantities of tissue can be extracted in this way within a few minutes.

Because of the good cutting quality of the rotating morcellator, the tissue structure is minimally damaged. It also enables a reliable histological examination to be carried out.

CO₂ GAS INSUFFLATOR

A pneumoperitoneum must be created so that the organs and tissues are separated from each other and rendered accessible. Conventional gas insufflators are sufficient for a purely diagnostic laparoscopy. However, in surgical laparoscopies performed today, compensation for considerable volume losses must be made in a relatively short period of time, for example due to frequent suction of irrigation solutions using high-performance irrigation–aspiration units. High-flow CO_2 insufflators (Figure 2.20) are a basic prerequisite for surgical laparoscopy, as they offer the only option for reducing operating time to a minimum. Electronically controlled insufflators have become the preferred choice in this respect.

The insufflator's display, which the surgeon should always be able to see, gives continuous information on the following data:

- The patient's intra-abdominal pressure (actual value): the preselected maximum intra-abdominal pressure should never exceed a value of 15 mmHg!

- Flow rate: the required set value for the patient's intra-abdominal pressure must be preselected. The maximum flow rate (set value) must be preset

- Total CO_2 insufflated volume is given

- Gas reserve, is indicated

Some of the state-of-the-art insufflators (Figure 2.20) are equipped with an integrated preheating element which

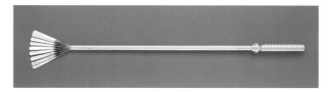

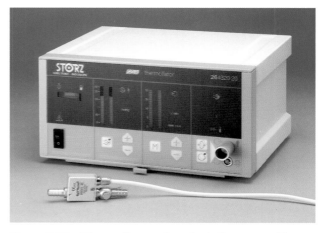

Figure 2.19 Rotocut G1 morcellator in diameters 12 mm and 15 mm

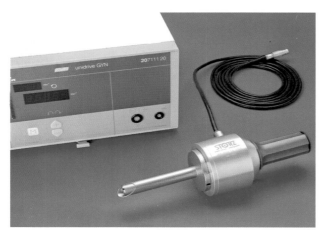

Figure 2.17 Intestinal probe

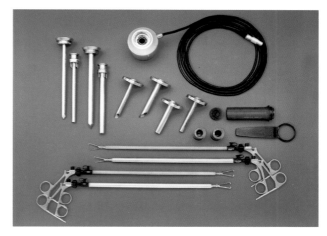

Figure 2.18 Rotocut™ G1 morcellator with Unidrive® Gyn motor system

Figure 2.20 Thermoflator for high-flow insufflation (30 l/min) with Optitherm® heating element

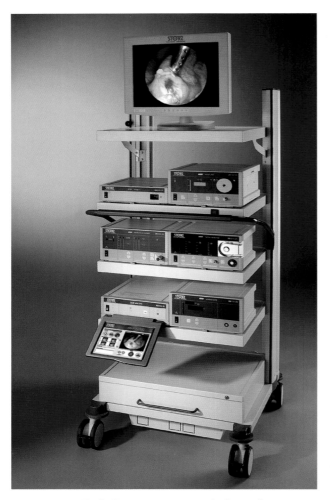

Figure 2.21 EndoCart™ set-up, including: flat screen monitor, digital camera, xenon light source, insufflator, suction–irrigation system, Aida DVD recorder (for digital storage of still images, video sequences and audio files) and motor system for morcellator

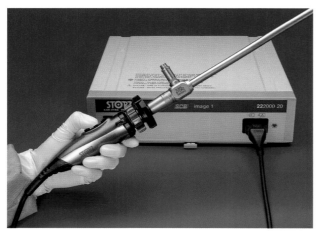

Figure 2.22 Digital three-chip Image1™ camera with camera control unit

keeps the insufflated gas at body temperature, to prevent the patient from cooling down. In order to avoid the disadvantages of CO_2 insufflation, gasless laparoscopy could be an alternative.

IRRIGATION–SUCTION UNIT

Within the framework of diagnostic and surgical laparoscopy, it is often necessary to drain fluids and irrigate wound surfaces until they are clean and can be viewed adequately. Sometimes, effective irrigation can also be used for adhesiolysis (hydrodissection). Suction is performed either with an additional suction pump or by means of a central vacuum supply system. It is important that these solutions are used at body temperature.

In summary, the equipment in an operating theater for endoscopic surgery (laparoscopy) should comprise (Figure 2.21):

- Gas insufflator
- Light source
- Video camera unit (Figure 2.22)
- Suction irrigation device
- Monitor and documentation system (video recorder, printer or photodigitalizer for digital image storage)

LASER INSTRUMENTATION

Utilization of the laser in advanced modern surgery owes its wide dissemination to the fact that lasers commonly used in industrial, military, commercial or scientific applications interact with biological tissue in such a way that localized and precisely controlled alterations of the cellular structure are effected irreversibly. In the hands of the skilled surgeon, the laser becomes an instrument capable of inducing desired therapeutic effects, far beyond the scope of conventional surgical tools such as cold knives or electrocautery probes. The laser enables the surgeon to utilize a variety of operational modalities for the treatment of diseased tissue. Precise incisions can be performed, lesions extending over large areas can be vaporized and voluminous lesions can be debulked and destroyed by ablation or necrotization. Very often, it is possible to target the therapeutic energy selectively at cells characterized by a well-defined property (e.g. color), implementing the selectivity of the interaction process between laser and tissue.

Laser energy can be delivered to tissue in a variety of ways: by contact or from a distance, in conjunction with an operative microscope, through an endoscope or with the aid of freehand tools.

Finally, laser treatments provide significant advantages, unmatched by competitive techniques; in the majority of cases the operation is largely hemostatic. Thus, the surgeon enjoys the convenience of a dry and clear field, even when operating in an environment of high vascularity.

Moreover, the contamination of adjacent areas is considerably reduced because of the sealing of blood and lymph vessels. The extent of injury to surrounding tissue is, to a large degree, controllable. Consequently, the risk of postoperative pain, complications or irreversible damage is diminished considerably. In some cases, the recurrence rate of the disease also appears to be reduced. The laser enables the surgeon to reach anatomic structures the size or location of which renders them inaccessible to any other known surgical instrument.

The reasons for this impressive procedural variety and wealth of benefits lie in the particular properties of the laser as a special source of energy

Physical effects of laser on tissue

The laser effect on a tissue sample is one of transmission, reflection, scattering or absorption (Figure 2.23). The effect on tissue achieved by any laser commonly used in therapeutic medicine is a consequence of its absorption therein. In particular, the energy deposited by most of the commonly used lasers is transformed into heat, thereby obtaining a thermal effect on the tissue. The types of lasers used in therapeutic medicine are confined to the visible, ultraviolet and infrared regions of the spectrum. Figure 2.24 presents a list of these lasers with their respective wavelengths.

The infrared lasers constitute the primary subject of this book. They are widely recognized by the medical community as part of the armamentarium of modern surgery. Therefore, we elaborate further on their interaction with biological tissue.

Figure 2.25 illustrates the relative absorption of light in water as a function of wavelength. Because water is a major component of the cellular structure, its interaction with the laser is predominant. The CO_2 laser features a wave-length of $10.6\,\mu m$ in the far infrared range. It is strongly absorbed by water, as indicated in Figure 2.25. CO_2 laser radiation is readily absorbed by the first few cellular layers of tissue, constituting the first $100\,\mu m$. Consequently, this is a laser used for superficial treatments.

The neodymium : yttrium–aluminum–garnet (Nd : YAG) laser features a wavelength of $1.06\,\mu m$ (near infrared). Water is completely transparent to this type of radiation. Consequently, the Nd : YAG laser is ideal for the treatment of lesions located in liquid-filled cavities, such as the bladder and the uterus (filled with a distension liquid). The Nd : YAG laser is, however, strongly scattered by the tissue. Penetrating beams are scattered and folded at multiple sites, increasing the effective path length of the beam through the tissue. Nd : YAG laser light, which is absorbed to some degree by the proteins within the tissue bed, deposits energy each time absorption takes place. The end result is the creation of a deep and laterally extended ball of affected tissue, 3–5 mm in diameter.

Contact fibers allow a more controlled incisional effect with Nd : YAG lasers, with only about 1 mm of surrounding thermal necrosis.

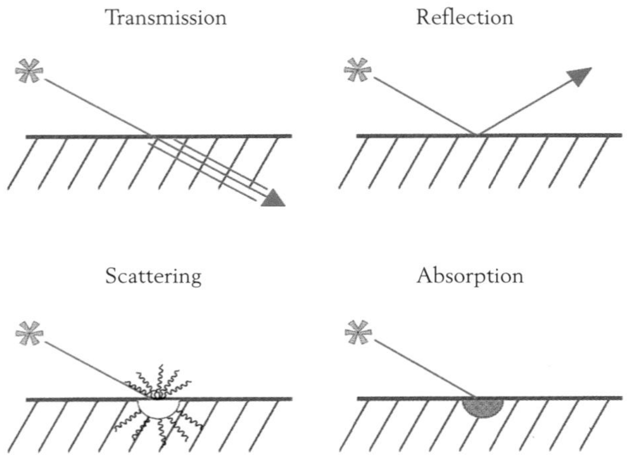

Name	Color	Wavelength
Excimers	Ultraviolet	200–400 nm
Argon	Blue	400 nm
	Green	515 nm
532 Yag	Green	532 nm
Krypton	Green	531 nm
	Yellow	566 nm
Dye laser	Yellow-green	577 nm
	Red	630 nm
Helium–neon	Red	630 nm
Gold vapor	Red	630 nm
Krypton	Red	647 nm
Ruby	Deep red	694 nm
Diode	Infrared	810–980 nm
Nd : YAG	Infrared	1064 nm
	Infrared	1318 nm
CO_2	Infrared	10 600 nm

(V I S I B L E)

Figure 2.24 Lasers used in therapeutic medicine

Transmission

Reflection

Scattering

Absorption

Figure 2.23 Laser–tissue interaction

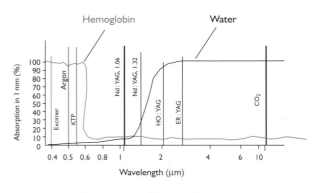

Figure 2.25 Absorption of laser radiation

More recently, high-power diode lasers have become available, emitting wavelengths of either 810 or 980 nm. Tissue interaction at these wavelengths resembles the interaction of the Nd : YAG laser; therefore, these diode lasers are replacing the Nd : YAG lasers in certain medical applications.

Thermal effects on tissue

Heat deposited in tissue elevates its temperature. Figure 2.26 summarizes how the tissue is affected, both visually and biologically, by the increase in its temperature. As long as the temperature does not reach 60°C, there is no visual change in the appearance of the tissue. Up to 45°C, the changes that occur are all reversible. Beyond that temperature, some of the cellular enzymes are destroyed and the functional operation of the cell is impaired. Between 60 and 65°C, capillary blood vessels shrink and the tissue undergoes extensive coagulation, showing distinct blanching.

It is noteworthy that the coagulation process induced by the CO_2 laser is rather different from that effected by the Nd : YAG laser. Shrinkage of the capillary vessel caused by the CO_2 laser is a result of vaporization of the water contained in the walls of the blood vessel. If, however, the CO_2 laser beam hits a vessel, it is readily absorbed by the liquid blood at its exit from the initially desiccated wall. Thus, it will never have the chance to hit the opposite wall, leaving the vessel open and, thereby, causing extensive bleeding. Hence, it is important to remember that the sharply focused beams of CO_2 lasers are inadequate for the treatment of highly vascular tissue.

Conversely, Nd : YAG lasers are unhindered by the presence of the liquid medium; consequently, they can very effectively accomplish complete coagulation of the bulk of the tissue. Nd : YAG lasers are excellent coagulators.

Temperatures between 65 and 90°C completely denature the proteins. The tissue turns a whitish color, indicative of dead cells, which subsequently slough off.

At 100°C, vaporization of the cellular water occurs. The high vapor pressure (generated by rapid expansion of the cellular content that undergoes transformation from liquid to vapor) pushes against the cell membrane, which eventually ruptures, vigorously expelling the resulting fragments in an outgoing plume. The end effect of the entire process is the local removal of tissue matter.

If temperatures are raised much above boiling point, carbonization ultimately occurs.

Energy, power and power density

The rise in temperature of the tissue matter depends primarily on the amount of energy deposited on the target site, as well as on the capability of the tissue to rid itself of heat by dissipating it to surrounding areas. If a large quantity of energy is deposited in the tissue before it can dissipate the heat, a rise in temperature will occur.

Energy, power and power density are the physical parameters that determine the eventual rise in temperature. Energy is measured in joules. Power is the amount of energy delivered per second and is measured in watts (joules/s). The thermal effect of the laser is local. Thus, the physical quantity which governs the thermal response of the tissue is the amount of power delivered to a unit of area; this quantity is called power density, and is measured in W/cm^2.

The higher is the power density, the more rapid is the temperature rise on and around the area where the laser beam impinges upon the tissue. In order to obtain the desired surgical effect, both power and power density can be adjusted easily. All commercial laser systems enable the user to vary the power to the tissue in a continuous manner. At constant output powers, the power density can be varied with the aid of optical devices, which either bring the laser beam into focus on the target site, or defocus it intentionally (Figure 2.27).

The shape of the cross-section of the beam in most commercial systems is approximately circular. The diameter of the beam can be decreased or increased by the respective focusing/defocusing method. Reducing the diameter of the beam spot by a factor of two represents a reduction of the spot area by a factor of four and,

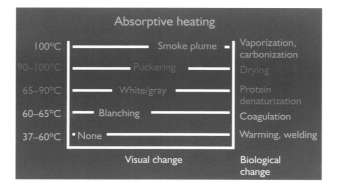

Figure 2.26 Thermal effects on tissue

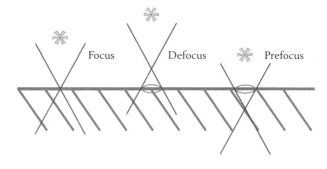

Figure 2.27 Focusing/defocusing the laser beam on tissue

consequently, a four-fold increase in the power density (Figure 2.28).

The optical system through which the CO_2 laser beam is delivered incorporates specially designed lenses. This system is responsible for bringing the beam into focus on the tissue at the operative site. For a given optical system at a given power, the maximum power density is obtained when the beam is completely focused.

If the surgical circumstances require lower power densities, the surgeon can achieve this by defocusing the beam, i.e. by increasing the diameter of the spot size and, consequently, increasing its area. Defocusing is normally effected by manually retracting the optical system from its focused position, or by employing a focusing/defocusing device.

High-power densities are required when fine incisions must be performed. Traction is applied to the tissue on both sides of the desired incision and a focused beam is aimed at the required location. The depth of the incision is a function of the power delivered and of the dwell time of the laser on each and every point of the incision. The longer is the dwell time, the larger is the volume of tissue removed by the laser and, therefore, the deeper is the cut. However, the dwell time is inversely proportional to the speed of movement of the cutting tool. In short, the depth of the incision increases with the power of the beam and decreases with the speed of movement. Vaporization may be performed with a defocused beam and high power. However, in this mode, tissue ablation is not well controlled, and is accompanied by excessive carbonization and deeper thermal necrosis. A significantly more effective CO_2 laser vaporization technique is based on rapid scanning of a focused beam over the area to be vaporized. This Flashscan™ technology allows extremely uniform, char-free, layer-by-layer vaporization with minimal residual thermal necrosis.

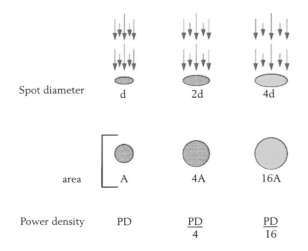

Figure 2.28 Diameter (d) and area (A) of the spot versus power density (PD)

CO_2 laser systems and accessories

The CO_2 laser beam is generated by a sealed gas-filled tube. The lasing gas is CO_2, and it is mixed with other types of gases which are required for different technological reasons. The excitation of the CO_2 molecules is effected by an electrical discharge.

One of the limitations of the CO_2 laser beam is that it cannot propagate very effectively through flexible fibers. Consequently, the delivery system ordinarily used in commercial products consists of a lightweight articulated arm, composed of straight, hollow, segmental tubes with reflective mirrors mounted at the joints. Hence, the CO_2 laser beam propagates in straight lines and bounces off each consecutive joint, eventually reaching the target tissue through an optical device attached to the end joint. As the CO_2 laser is invisible to the human eye, each laser system is equipped with a red helium–neon (He–Ne) laser tube, the direction of propagation of which is coincident with the infrared beam. The red He–Ne beam enables the surgeon to aim at the target area and simulate visually, on the tissue, the position and the extent of the therapeutic beam.

Manufacturers offer CO_2 laser units featuring various maximum powers from 15 to 150 W. CO_2 laser systems are composed of:

- A laser tube
- A power supply which provides the necessary electrical energy to excite the lasing gas
- A closed-circuit water-cooling system which removes excess heat from the tube and its surroundings
- A control system based on a microcomputer
- An articulated-arm delivery system
- A He–Ne laser tube

Figures 2.29 and 2.30 show, respectively, a schematic diagram and a photograph of a state-of-the-art CO_2 laser system.

The latest generation of CO_2 lasers employs SurgiTouch™ Flashscan technology, which significantly improves the laser's tissue vaporization capabilities. This technology, introduced by Lumenis, allows uniform, char-free, layer-by-layer tissue vaporization control with minimal residual thermal necrosis. Tissue layers as thin as 100 μm may be removed with extreme precision and excellent visual control.

The 'Flashscanner' is a miniature optomechanical scanner compatible with any Lumenis microprocessor-controlled laser (Figure 2.31). It consists of two almost, but not exactly, parallel folding mirrors. Optical reflections of the CO_2 laser beam from the mirrors cause the beam to deviate from its original direction by an angle θ (Figure 2.32). The mirrors constantly rotate at slightly different angular velocities, thereby rapidly varying with time

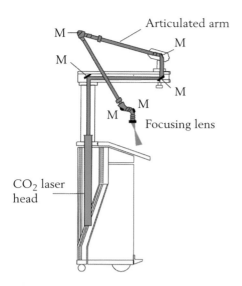

Figure 2.29 Schematic structure of a CO_2 laser. M, mirror

Since therapeutic CO_2 medical lasers typically generate a focused beam smaller than 0.9 mm in diameter at the laparoscope working distance, use of the SurgiTouch with a laser power level of 30 W will generate an optical power density of greater than 50 W/mm² on tissue. This is considerably higher than the threshold for the vaporization of tissue without residual carbon charring (the threshold for char-free tissue ablation is about 30 W/mm²). The time required for the SurgiTouch to cover homogeneously a 2.5-mm round area is about 100 ms. During this time, the 30-W operating laser will deliver 3000 mJ to the tissue. Since the typical energy required to ablate tissue completely is about 3000 mJ/mm³, keeping the laparoscope precisely on a single site for 0.1 s will generate a clean, char-free crater of 0.2 mm in depth.

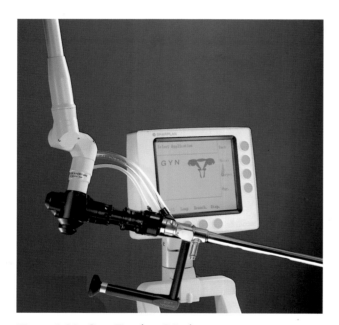

Figure 2.30 SurgiTouch™ CO_2 laser system

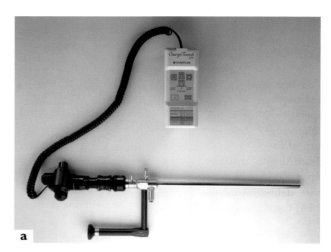

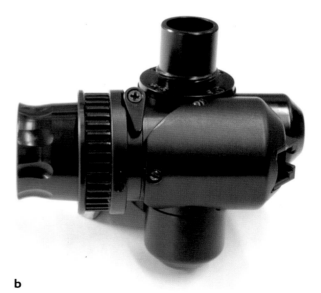

between zero and a maximal value, θ_{max}. By attaching the laparoscope-focusing coupler of focal length F to the Flashscan, the CO_2 laser generates a focal spot which rapidly and homogeneously scans and covers a round area of diameter $2F\tan\theta_{max}$ at the distal end of the laparoscope.

For a single-puncture laparoscope ($F = 300$ mm), θ_{max} is selected to provide a round treatment area of 2.5 mm diameter. The rapid movement of the beam over the tissue ensures a short duration of exposure on individual sites within the area, and very shallow ablation.

Figure 2.31 (a) SurgiTouch optomechanical scanner consisting of two almost, but not exactly, parallel microprocessor-controlled mirrors; (b) 'Flashscanner', connected to the direct coupler (ESC Lumenis)

Nd : YAG laser and accessories

Manufacturers offer Nd : YAG laser units featuring different maximum powers, from 40 to 100 W. Nd : YAG laser systems are composed of:

- A laser head or resonator

- A power supply, which furnishes the flashlight lamp with the necessary electrical energy

- A closed-circuit water-cooling system, further chilled by a radiator which removes excess heat from the resonator

- A control system, based on a microcomputer

- A He–Ne laser tube

- An output port optical assembly to which the external glass fiber is attached

Several types of fibers are offered with the Nd : YAG laser.

THE OPERATING LAPAROSCOPE

The operating laparoscope for laser laparoscopy is an instrument which is 11 mm in diameter with a 7.3-mm operative channel. To use the CO_2 laser through the laparoscope, the operator simply swings the articulated arm of the laser over the operative field and attaches the BeamAlign™ coupler to the operative channel of the laparoscope (Figure 2.33) or to a special second-puncture laser delivery tube. The laser coupler assembly (Figure 2.34) consists of the following:

- Direct coupler housing: this contains a mechanical alignment mechanism which must be preadjusted for the specific operating laparoscope used. Once adjusted, alignment remains for multiple uses with the same laparoscope

- Interchangeable lens housing:

  – 200-mm working distance lens housing to match beam focal length to nominal length of standard second-puncture tube, giving spot size diameter of 0.64 mm; laser beam may also be defocused

  – 300-mm working distance lens housing to match beam length to nominal length of single-puncture tube (and optional 300-mm second-puncture tube), giving spot size diameter of 0.70 mm; laser beam may also be defocused

  – Each lens housing has a groove around it for convenient attachment of the sterile drape

- Laser arm attachment

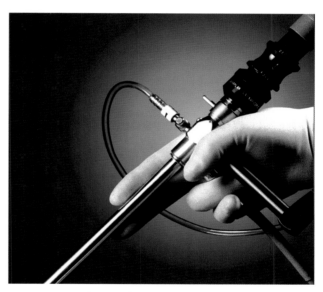

Figure 2.33 The single-puncture operating laparoscope for laser laparoscopy. The direct coupler containing the focusing lens is attached to the operative channel of the laparoscope

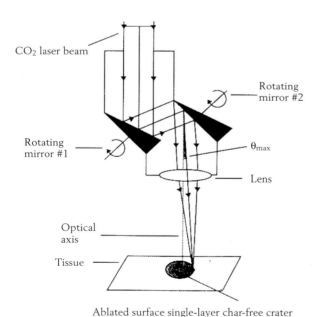

Figure 2.32 Optical reflections of the beam from the two mirrors cause it to be deflected from its original direction by $\theta°$

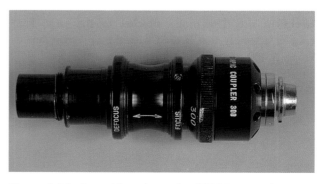

Figure 2.34 Laser 'direct' coupler (ESC Lumenis)

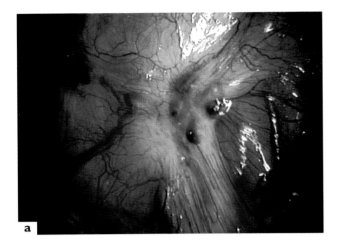

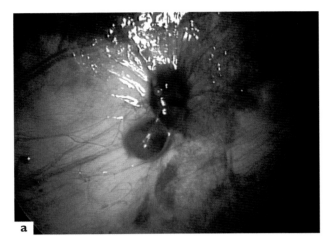

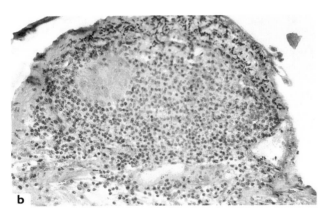

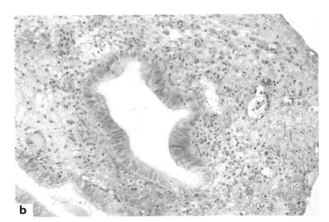

Figure 3.1 Puckered black lesion. (a) Laparoscopic aspect; (b) histology: presence of endometrial glands and typical stroma; note the presence of intraluminal debris (Gomori's trichrome ×110)

Figure 3.2 Red flame-like lesion of the peritoneum. (a) Laparoscopic aspect; (b) histology: active endometriotic glands surrounded by stroma (Gomori's trichrome ×110)

(3) Subovarian adhesions, or adherence between the ovary and the peritoneum of the ovarian fossa, as distinct from adhesions characteristic of previous salpingitis or peritonitis: they are the consequence of an inflammatory reaction induced by active lesions (Figure 3.4a and b).

(4) Areas of petechial peritoneum or areas with hypervascularization, diagnosed as endometriosis in one of our previous studies[1,8,12]: these lesions resemble petechial lesions resulting from manipulation of the peritoneum or from hypervascularization of the peritoneum (Figure 3.5a). They generally affect the bladder and the broad ligament; histologically, red blood cells are numerous and endometrial glands are scarce (Figure 3.5b).

White lesions

Sometimes, subtle endometriotic lesions are the only lesions seen at laparoscopy and appear as:

(1) White opacification of the peritoneum (Figure 3.6a), which looks like peritoneal scarring or circumscribed patches, often thickened and sometimes raised: histologically, white opacified peritoneum is due to the presence of an occasional retroperitoneal glandular structure and scanty stroma surrounded by fibrotic tissue or connective tissue (Figure 3.6b).

(2) Yellow-brown peritoneal patches resembling 'café au lait' patches (Figure 3.7a): the histological characteristics are similar to those observed in white opacification but, in yellow-brown patches, the presence of the blood pigment hemosiderin among the stromal cells produces the 'café au lait' color (Figure 3.7b).

(3) Circular peritoneal defects, as described by Chatman[4] (Figure 3.8a): serial section demonstrates the presence of endometrial glands in more than 50% of cases (Figure 3.8b).

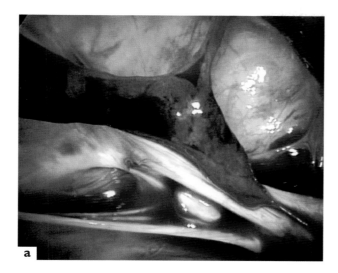

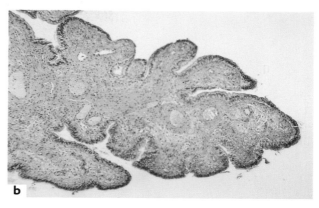

Figure 3.3 Glandular excrescences on the peritoneal surface. (a) Laparoscopic view; (b) histology: presence of numerous endometrial glands (Gomori's trichrome ×56)

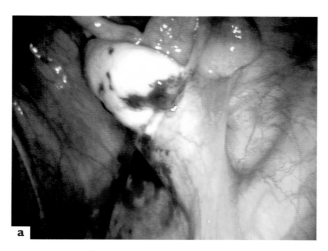

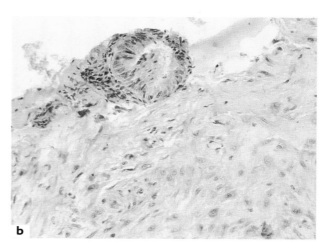

Figure 3.4 Subovarian adhesion. (a) Laparoscopic aspect: adherence between the ovary and peritoneum of the ovarian fossa; (b) connective tissue with sparse endometrial glands (Gomori's trichrome ×110)

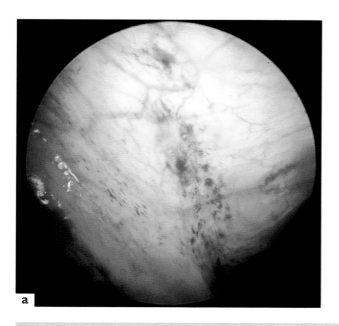

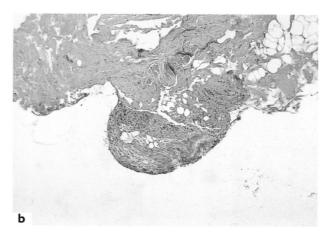

Figure 3.5 Areas of petechial peritoneum. (a) Laparoscopic aspect; (b) histology: note the typical endometrial glands and stroma (Gomori's trichrome ×56)

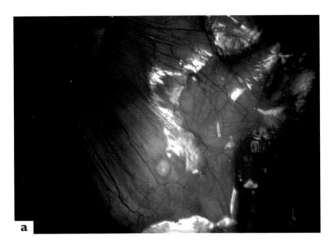

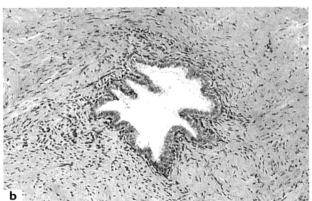

Figure 3.6 White opacification of the peritoneum. (a) Laparoscopic aspect; (b) histology: rare retroperitoneal glandular structure and scanty stroma surrounded by fibrotic tissue (Gomori's trichrome × 110)

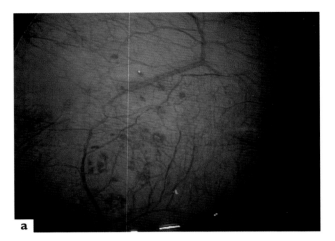

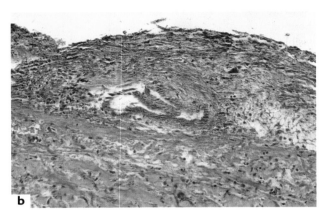

Figure 3.7 Yellow-brown peritoneal patches of the peritoneum. (a) Laparoscopic aspect; (b) histology: the presence of blood pigment (hemosiderin) among the stromal cells produces the 'café au lait' color (Gomori's trichrome × 110)

Non-visible endometriosis

In one of our studies[8] (Table 3.2), biopsies were taken from visually normal peritoneum of the uterosacral ligaments. Histological study revealed the presence of endometriotic tissue in two out of 32 infertile women without endometriosis. This rate (6%) was less than half the rate (13%) observed in normal peritoneum taken from 52 women with visible endometriosis, but shows that unsuspected peritoneal endometriosis can be found in the visually normal peritoneum of infertile women, with or without known associated endometriosis. The size of endometriotic lesions in visually normal peritoneum, ranging from 88 to 720 μm (mean 313 μm, SEM 185 μm), probably explains why the peritoneum had a normal aspect and why the lesions were not visible, even though a meticulous inspection was carried out to identify small and non-hemorrhagic lesions.

Since our first publication in 1990, the findings of others, such as Nezhat *et al.*[13], and more recently Walter *et al.*[14], have reinforced the concept of invisible lesions.

The concept of 'non-visible' endometriosis was recently reviewed by Redwine[15]. His conclusion was that 'invisible microscopic endometriosis' or IME is a rare and clinically unimportant entity and that allegations of its existence are almost always due to inexperience and lack of magnification at surgery.

According to Redwine, human visual acuity is remarkable, and a human hair (100 μm in diameter) can be seen at arm's length at a distance of 70 cm; he therefore suggests that the non-visible lesions described in our study (ranging from 88 to 720 μm) were actually large enough to be seen.

Redwine forgets to mention, however, that all the non-visible lesions identified in our study were in the retroperitoneal space, beneath the mesothelium, at a distance varying from about 100 to 900 μm. Furthermore, we can safely assume that every gynecologist, every medical doctor and indeed every human-being would agree that it is very difficult to see a human hair under a thin sheet of paper!

In spite of the scant evidence put forward by Redwine, the presence of microscopic endometriosis in visually normal pelvic peritoneum has become a generally accepted concept[16]. Evers *et al.*[17] go one step further, suggesting that invisible endometriosis is much more frequent than generally suspected: 'If in every patient in the studies on invisible endometriosis, the researchers had taken 8–16 biopsies instead of a single one, all the women with normal peritoneum would have shown evidence of endometriosis.'

The take-home message is that laparoscopy is fallible. Inspecting the peritoneum through the looking glass of a laparoscope has high false-positive and false-negative rates: not all we see is endometriosis; and if we do not see it, it may still be there. But the presence of non-visible lesions is surely not an argument for prescribing postoperative hormonal treatment, nor does it explain recurrence. Non-visible endometriotic lesions are quiescent lesions. They are non-active and, at this stage, clinically irrelevant. Nevertheless, nobody knows the exact evolution of these lesions.

Vascularization of endometriotic implants is probably one of the most important factors in the growth and invasion of other tissue by endometrial glands. We evaluated histologically the vascularization of typical peritoneal endometriosis and its modifications, according to the macroscopic appearance of peritoneal endometriosis[18,19].

Our study demonstrated significant differences between the typical (black or bluish) lesion and the 'subtle' lesion. Subtle lesions were classified as red lesions (vesicular, red flame-like and glandular excrescences) and white lesions (white opacification, yellow-brown patches and circular peritoneal defects). When compared with typical lesion data, vascularization was found to be significantly higher in red lesions and significantly lower in white lesions. This was due to an increase (red) or decrease (white) in the volume occupied by the vessels, as proved by both the mean capillary surface area and the ratio of capillaries/stroma surface area.

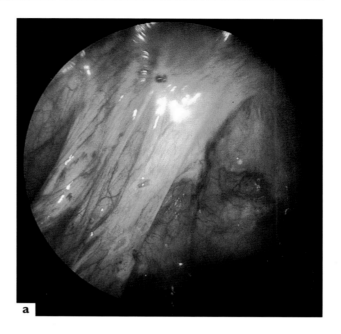

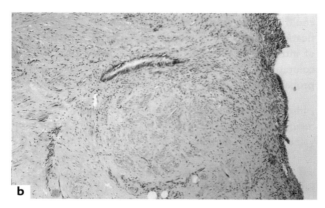

Figure 3.8 Circular peritoneal defects. (a) Laparoscopic aspect; (b) histology: typical endometrial glands are found in more than 50% of cases (Gomori's trichrome ×25)

Table 3.2 Morphological characteristics of peritoneal endometriosis

	Group I (n = 52)	Group II (n = 32)
Number of biopsies		
from visible endometriotic lesions*	86	—
from normal-looking peritoneum*	52	32
Histological proof of endometriosis		
in visible lesions*	80/86 (93%)	—
in normal-looking peritoneum*	7/52 (13%)	2/32 (6%)

*Macroscopic appearance

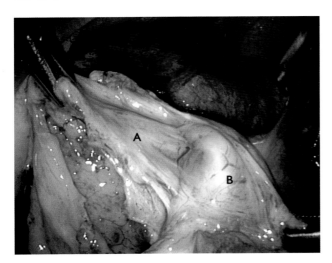

Figure 4.15 Ovarian cystectomy. A, endometrioma capsule. B, ovarian cortex

Although these were randomized controlled studies, we believe it is not possible to draw accurate conclusions from them. First of all, the number of cases was small (164 patients). Second, ablation was performed by bipolar coagulation, not by laser. Third, no preoperative drugs were used to decrease cyst size or reduce the thickness and hypervascularization of the cyst wall. Finally, neither study addressed ovarian function after surgery.

When we attempt to address the question of ovarian function after surgery, data in the literature are contradictory.

Indeed, Canis et al.[39], Marconi et al.[40], Donnez et al.[41] and Wyns and Donnez[42] found no effect on ovarian response in IVF after cystectomy or vaporization of endometriomas. Canis et al.[39] showed that the number of oocytes retrieved and the number of embryos obtained did not significantly decrease after ovarian cystectomy. Ovarian response was not affected after cystectomy in Marconi's study either[40].

In one of our studies[41], endometrioma wall vaporization did not negatively affect IVF outcome. A later study actually suggested that both cystectomy and cyst wall vaporization allow preservation of a good ovarian response to stimulation by gonadotropins[42].

Our studies led us to conclude that (1) vaporization of the internal cyst wall does not impair ovarian function in terms of IVF parameters and outcome; (2) theoretical risks of loss of viable ovarian tissue during cystectomy exist but may be avoided by a 'microsurgical' laparoscopic technique, taking care to preserve the normal residual ovarian cortex; and (3) after removal or destruction of endometriomas, IVF outcomes are similar in endometriosis patients compared with women with tubal factor or idiopathic infertility.

Other studies in the literature, however, point to the risk of ovarian damage due to ovarian cystectomy for

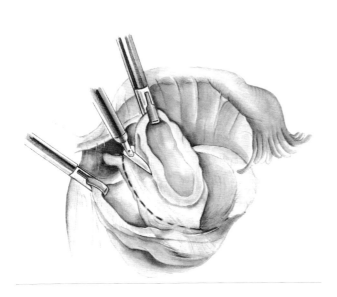

a

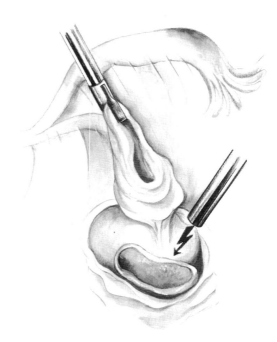

b

Figure 4.16 Combined technique. (a) A partial cystectomy is carried out. (b) To avoid excessive bleeding close to the hilus, vaporization of the residual cyst is carried out

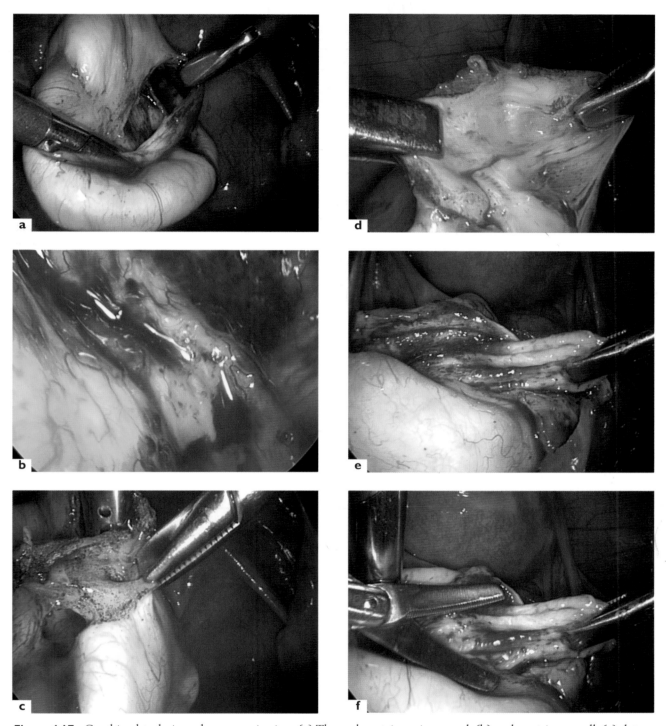

Figure 4.17 Combined technique: laparoscopic view. (a) The endometrioma is opened; (b) endometrioma wall; (c) detection of plane of cleavage between the endometrioma wall and ovarian cortex; (d) cystectomy of the endometrioma; (e)–(g) partial cystectomy: section of the endometrioma wall;

endometriomas. Several studies have shown reduced follicular response after cystectomy. Nargund *et al.*[28] showed that in cycles with ovulation induction after cystectomy, the normal ovary yielded a significantly higher number of follicles and oocytes compared with the contralateral ovary which had undergone cystectomy.

Loh *et al.*[29] demonstrated that post-cystectomy ovaries showed reduced follicular response in natural and clomiphene citrate-stimulated cycles in women <35 years of age. Ho *et al.*[30] concluded that surgery for ovarian endometriomas induces poor ovarian response to controlled ovarian hyperstimulation, compared with the

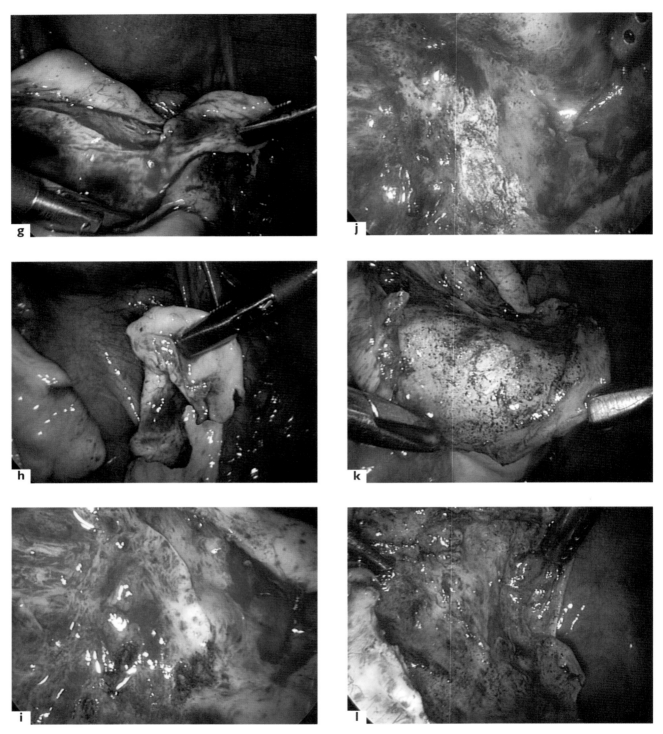

Figure 4.17 *continued* (h) resected part of the endometrioma; (i) remaining endometrioma wall on the left side, ovarian cortex after cystectomy on the right side; (j) and (k) vaporization of the remaining endometrioma wall; (l) final view: vaporized endometrioma wall on the left, ovarian cortex after cystectomy on the right

response of the contralateral normal ovary in the same individual. In Geber's group, patients <35 years of age with previous ovarian surgery had fewer retrieved oocytes than patients in the control group[31]. Others showed reduced ovarian volume after cystectomy. Exacoustos *et* *al.*[34] showed that ovarian stripping of endometriomas, but not of ovarian dermoids, is associated with a significant decrease in residual ovarian volume, which may result in diminished ovarian reserve and function. Histological studies demonstrated the presence of follicles in the excised tissue. One or several primordial follicles were found in 68.9% of endometrioma capsules removed by cystectomy in a study by Hachisuga and Kawarabayashi[32]. Compared with cystectomy for dermoid cysts, cystectomy for endometriomas was associated much more frequently with the ablation of follicles[32]. Close to the ovarian hilus, the ovarian tissue removed along the endometrioma wall consisted mostly of tissue which contained primordial, primary and secondary follicles in 69% of cases[35].

In the light of all this evidence, we can conclude that excisional surgery and ablative surgery are valuable techniques, but that they should be performed by experienced surgeons.

In the hands of inexperienced surgeons, cystectomy can be destructive for the ovary, whereas ablation may be incomplete, with a greater risk of recurrence. The combined technique appears to take the best of both techniques, while avoiding the risks, but requires further evaluation.

REFERENCES

1. Brosens I, Gordon A. Endometriosis: ovarian endometriosis. In Brosens I, Gordon A, eds. Tubal Infertility. London: Gower Medical Publishing, 1989: 313–17

2. Nisolle M, Casanas-Roux F, Donnez J. Histologic study of ovarian endometriosis after hormonal therapy. Fertil Steril 1988; 49: 423–6

3. Sampson JA. Heterotopic or misplaced endometrial tissue. Am J Obstet Gynecol 1925; 10: 649–64

4. Hughesdon PE. The structure of endometrial cysts of the ovary. J Obstet Gynecol Br Emp 1957; 44: 69–84

5. Brosens IA. Is mild endometriosis a disease? Is mild endometriosis a progressive disease? Hum Reprod 1994; 9: 2209–11

6. Brosens IA. Classification of endometriosis. Endoscopic exploration and classification of the chocolate cysts. Hum Reprod 1994; 9: 2213–14

7. Brosens IA. Ovarian endometriosis. In Shaw RW, ed. Endometriosis – Current Understanding and Management. London: Blackwell Science, 1995: 97–111

8. Nezhat F, Nezhat C, Allan CJ, et al. A clinical and histological classification of endometriomas: implications for a mechanism of pathogenesis. J Reprod Med 1992; 37: 771–6

9. Donnez J, Nisolle M. L'endométriose péritonéale, le kyste endométriotique ovarien et le nodule de la lame rectovaginale sont trois pathologies différentes [Editorial]. Réf Gynécol Obstét 1995; 3: 121–3

10. Donnez J, Nisolle M, Gillet N, et al. Large ovarian endometriomas. Hum Reprod 1996; 11: 641–6

11. Serov SF, Scully RE, Sobin LH. Histological Typing of Ovarian Tumors. International Histological Classification of Tumors, No 9. Geneva: World Health Organization, 1973: 17–21

12. Motta PM, Van Blerkom J, Mekabe S. Changes in the surface morphology of ovarian germinal epithelium during the reproductive life and in some pathological conditions. Submicrosc Cytol 1992; 99: 664–7

13. Nisolle M. Peritoneal, ovarian and rectovaginal endometriosis are three distinct entities. Thèse d'Agrégation de l'Enseignement Supérieur. Louvain, Belgium: Université Catholique de Louvain, 1996

14. Nisolle M, Donnez J. Peritoneal, Ovarian and Rectovaginal Endometriosis: the Identification of Three Separate Diseases. Carnforth, UK: Parthenon Publishing, 1996

15. Rosenfeld DL, Lecher BD. Endometriosis in a patient with Rokitansky–Kuster–Hauser syndrome. Am J Obstet Gynecol 1981; 139: 105–7

16. Donnez J, Nisolle M, Casanas-Roux F, et al. Endometriosis: rationale for surgery. In Brosens I, Donnez J, eds. Current Status of Endometriosis. Research and Management. Carnforth, UK: Parthenon Publishing, 1993: 385–95

17. Donnez J, Lemaire-Rubbers M, Karaman Y, et al. Combined (hormonal and microsurgical) therapy in infertile women with endometriosis. Fertil Steril 1987; 48: 239–42

18. Sutton CJ, Ewen SP, Jacobs SA, et al. Laser laparosopic surgery in the treatment of ovarian endometriomas. J Am Gynecol Laparosc 1997; 4: 319–23

19. Jones KD, Sutton CJ. Pregnancy rates following ablative laparoscopic surgery for endometriomas. Hum Reprod 2002; 17: 782–5

20. Milingos S, Kallipolitis G, Loutradis D, et al. Affecting postoperative pregnancy rate after endoscopic management of large endometriomata. Int J Gynaecol Obstet 1998; 63: 129–37

21. Pouly JL. Endometriomas and in vitro fertilization outcomes. J Gynecol Obstet Biol Reprod (Paris) 2003; 32: S37–41

22. Calhaz-Jorge C, Chaveiro E, Nunes J, et al. Implications of the diagnosis of endometriosis on the success of infertility treatment. Clin Exp Obstet Gynecol 2004; 31: 25–30

23. Garcia-Velasco JA, Mahutte NG, Corona J, et al. Removal of endometriomas before in vitro fertilization does not improve fertility outcomes: a matched, case-control study. Fertil Steril 2004; 81: 1194–7

24. Kuivasaari P, Hippelainen M, Anttila M, et al. Effect of endometriosis on IVF/ICSI outcome: stage III/IV endometriosis worsens cumulative pregnancy and live-born rates. Hum Reprod 2005; 20: 3130–5

25. Kennedy S, Bergqvist A, Chapron C, et al. ESHRE guideline for the diagnosis and treatment of endometriosis. Hum Reprod 2005; 20: 2698–704

26. Younis JS, Ezra Y, Laufer N, et al. Late manifestation of pelvic abscess following oocyte retrieval, for in vitro fertilization, in patients with severe endometriosis and ovarian endometriomata. J Assist Reprod Genet 1997; 14: 343–6

27. Wei CF, Chen SC. Pelvic abscess after ultrasound-guided aspiration of endometrioma: a case report. Zhonghua Yi Xue Za Zhi 1998; 61: 603–7

28. Nargund G, Cheng WC, Parsons J. The impact of ovarian cystectomy on ovarian response to

PELVIC CONGESTION SYNDROME

Pelvic congestion syndrome has often been associated with uterine retroversion. In Taylor's original description of the syndrome in 1949, only 35% of patients were found to have uterine retroversion[9,10]. Taylor believed that vascular congestion of the pelvic organs explained the fact that pelvic veins can easily become dilated because they lack valves, since the surrounding adventitial tissue in the broad ligaments is weak. Taylor did not recommend hysterectomy or uterine suspension for these patients. He recognized the frequency with which his patients also suffered from psychosomatic and psychiatric complaints. It is not known how many patients with vascular congestion of pelvic organs are asymptomatic. Some authors have recommended embolization of the pelvic veins as treatment for pelvic congestion syndrome. Others, such as Manhes (personal communication), have suggested photocoagulating the veins in order to shrink them.

INDICATIONS FOR UTERINE SUSPENSION

Since the 19th century, uterine suspension has been practiced to relieve pelvic pain, dyspareunia and infertility.

Numerous methods and variations have been described in the medical literature, wherein the round ligament is folded, plaited, ligated, transplanted, banded or shirred[11]. Uterine suspension has been suggested to be very effective in the relief of deep dyspareunia or pelvic pain due to uterine retroversion. Primary suspension of the retroverted uterus is not necessary for adequate gynecological practice. Uterine suspension is most often indicated in connection with conservative operations such as those carried out for endometriosis or tubal pregnancy, or with microsurgical tubal reconstruction procedures for relief of infertility. The goal is to avoid leaving the uterus of an infertile patient in the cul-de-sac, where tubal adhesions may recur, while performing other conservative procedures. The presence of uterine retrodisplacement alone in an asymptomatic patient is not an indication for prophylactic uterine suspension. Symptomatic anatomic vaginal wall relaxation and uterine descensus are rarely associated with uterine retroversion. In such cases, we prefer to perform laparoscopic uterine sacrofixation (see Chapter 25).

Mild pelvic pain with dyspareunia is described as mild abdominal discomfort and fullness on intercourse, while moderate pelvic pain with dyspareunia is described as mild tolerable pain, whereupon the patient still enjoys the sexual act.

Pelvic examinations are systematically performed to evaluate the uterine position, degree of misalignment of the uterus and the severity of adhesions. We also try to reproduce the described pelvic pain and dyspareunia by palpation of the retroverted uterus. Ultrasound is performed to confirm the initial findings and to rule out myomas, adenomyosis or any uterine or ovarian abnormalities.

CHOICE OF OPERATION

To a great extent, choice of operative technique depends on the patient's desire for future pregnancy. The modified Gillian suspension is a good technique for suspending the uterus while preserving the potential for pregnancy.

The modified Gillian suspension procedure[12] draws each round ligament through an aperture in the peritoneum near the internal inguinal ring, and brings each ligament beneath the anterior rectus sheath. Although some patients experience transient round ligament pain with vigorous physical activity or uterine enlargement, there is no evidence that the suspension is detrimental to subsequent pregnancy.

In the Olshausen operation[13], on the other hand, the uterus is fixed to the anterior abdominal wall. This procedure precludes the possibility of a future intrauterine pregnancy because the anchored uterus will produce severe abdominal pain as the uterus enlarges with advancing pregnancy. This operation should never be performed.

In the Webster–Baldy procedure[14], the round ligaments are passed through the anterior and posterior leaves of the broad ligament and sutured to the posterior surface of the uterus. The extraperitoneal technique of shortening each round ligament in the inguinal canal described by Alexander[15] and Adams[16] is no longer used in the United States, although it is still in use in some European countries. The operation is blind because the uterus is not visualized unless a laparotomy is performed. The extraperitoneal approach is its only advantage.

Some authors suggest another procedure to provide additional support, whereby the uterosacral ligaments are shortened. This procedure is especially valuable when some descensus is present or when the cervix has been displaced anteriorly. We have never performed this procedure.

Operative technique (Figure 5.1)

After general anesthesia with endotracheal intubation has been established, the patient is placed in the lithotomy position or the Trendelenburg position. The bladder is emptied with a Foley catheter. A laparoscopic trocar is introduced into the peritoneal cavity. The pelvis is then visualized. The right and then left lower quadrants are transilluminated, and an avascular region is selected about 5–6 cm from the midline incision and 2 cm above the inguinal ligament.

Laparoscopic grasping forceps may be inserted through the trocar, or a Kelly clamp may be pushed through the incisions into the peritoneal cavity. The round ligaments are grasped (Figure 5.2) at about the midpoint and gently

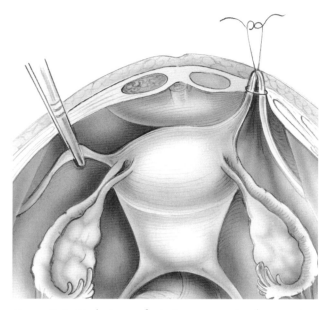

Figure 5.1 Technique of uterine suspension by grasping and fixation of the round ligament

pulled through the fascia as the pneumoperitoneum is allowed to deflate partially (Figure 5.3). The round ligaments are sutured to the aponevrosis with Vicryl® 1-0 suture material (Figure 5.4).

Complications of uterine suspension

Occasionally, evulsion of the round ligament may result when pulling the ligament up to the anterior rectus sheath. The ensuing bleeding must be controlled. If there is undue tension placed on the round ligaments, incisional pain may occur. It is usually mild and temporary and controlled with analgesics, muscle relaxants and heat.

Results (Table 5.1)

The operating time of both procedures is less than an hour.

Mild incisional pain and mild abdominal discomfort are frequently encountered and readily relieved with mild analgesics.

While in the study by Yoon[17], 51.5% and 18.6–45.5% of patients felt better at 6 weeks and 6 months,

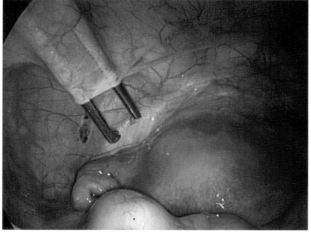

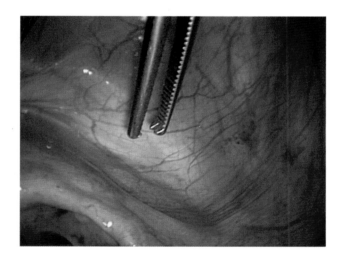

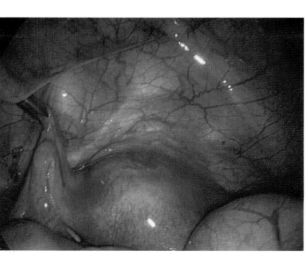

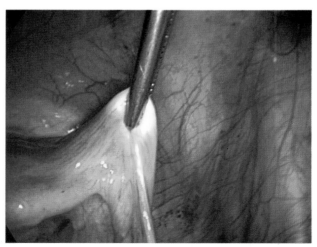

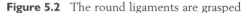

Figure 5.2 The round ligaments are grasped

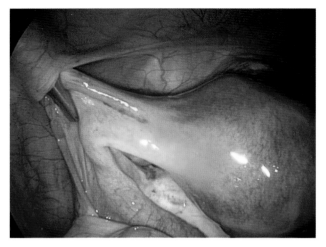

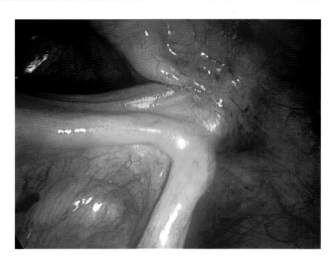

Figure 5.3 The round ligaments are pulled through the fascia

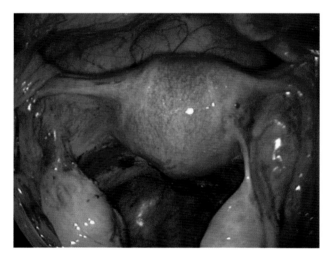

Figure 5.4 The round ligaments have been sutured to the aponevrosis

Table 5.1 Age and parity of 35 patients; indications for pelviscopic uterine suspension, combined with torus excision

Mean age (years)	29.5
Mean parity	1.8
Number of women with deep dyspareunia and chronic pelvic pain	31 (88%)
Improved	32 (91%)
Same	3 (9%)

respectively, following surgery, with no obvious cause for their deep dyspareunia or pelvic pain, all of our patients (100%) experienced a marked improvement at 6 weeks after the operation. Their sex-life improved immensely. After 6 months to 2 years of follow-up in the study by Koh

et al.[18], 17 patients with the Webster–Baldy technique and five patients with Franke's technique (88%) enjoyed an improved sex-life, while three patients were lost to follow-up.

Discussion

Among the many procedures published in the medical literature are Halben's vesical suspension, the Schmid–Matthiesen suspension, Werth's interfascial plication, uterine suspension using Fallopian rings, the modified Gillian method, the Mann–Stenger suspension and the Webster–Baldy and Franke techniques.

Laparoscopy is a valuable tool to determine the cause of pelvic pain, and, when dyspareunia and pelvic pain are caused by a retroverted uterus, we believe that uterine suspension using various procedures will certainly relieve the problem.

In one study[18], the Webster–Baldy method was found to be more time-consuming with more bleeding, but causing less kinking to the Fallopian tubes; thus, this method is preferred in patients who still wish to bear children.

Although Franke's method is simpler, less time-consuming and with less bleeding, since it causes more kinking to the Fallopian tubes, this procedure is more appropriate for patients who no longer wish to become pregnant.

ASSOCIATED SURGERY

Laser uterine nerve ablation (LUNA)

Uterine neurectomy was initially performed by electro-cautery, but there was always concern about the spread of electric current in this area due to the close proximity of the ureter and the uterine artery. Since 1989, we have, by preference, vaporized with CO_2 laser energy transmitted directly through the operating channel[19,20]. The posterior leaves of the broad ligaments are carefully inspected to identify the course of the ureters, which usually run 1–2 cm laterally. They can usually be 'palpated' via a probe, and often the characteristic peristaltic movements can be recognized beneath the peritoneal surface.

The uterosacral ligaments are pulled under tension by manipulating the uterus with an intrauterine manipulator. The laser is set at a relatively high power density of 60 W, and the uterosacral ligaments are vaporized 1 cm from their point of attachment to the posterior aspect of the cervix over a length of 1.5 cm. The idea of the procedure is to destroy the sensory nerve fibers and their secondary ganglia as they leave the uterus. Because of the divergence of these fibers in the uterosacral ligaments, they should be vaporized as close to the cervix as possible. Care must be taken not to vaporize too laterally, to avoid damage to the vessels running alongside the uterosacral ligaments.

Prospective double-blind randomized controlled studies have demonstrated that laparoscopic transection of the uterosacral ligaments close to their point of insertion on the posterior side of the cervix is an effective treatment for dysmenorrhea that has been unresponsive to drug therapy[21].

Torus excision

Another procedure is to lase deeply the posterior aspects of the cervix between the ligament insertions, to interrupt fibers crossing to the contralateral side. It is relatively easy to vaporize to the correct depth when the uterosacral ligaments are well formed. Sometimes, however, their limits are poorly defined.

Douglasectomy

As previously seen (see Chapter 1), parasympathetic fibers are identified in the anterior two-thirds of the uterosacral

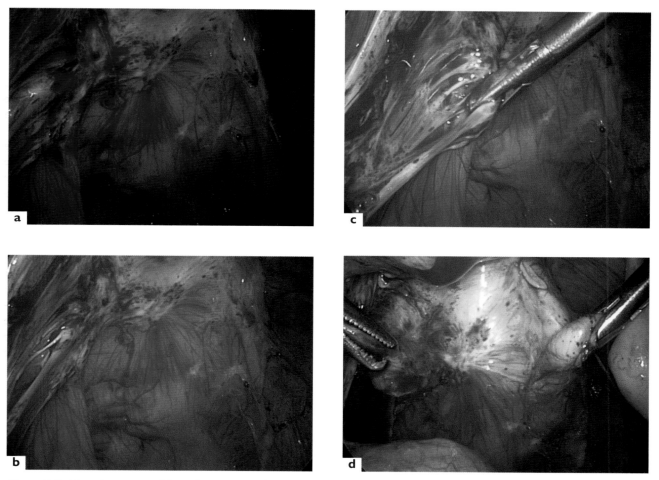

Figure 5.5 Douglasectomy. (a) Endometriosis of uterosacral ligaments and Douglas pouch; (b) vaporization of the right uterosacral ligament; (c) grasping (and vaporization) of the left uterosacral ligament; (d) both uterosacral ligaments have been cut;

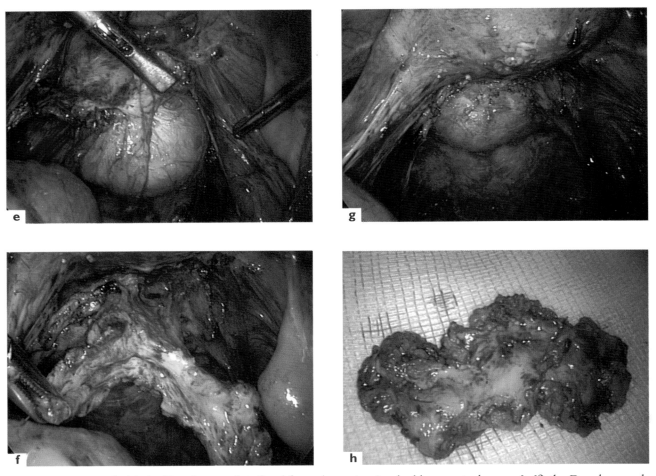

Figure 5.5 *continued*   (e) the Douglas pouch is freed from the vagina (pushed by a vaginal sponge); (f) the Douglas pouch is freed from the cervix; (g) final view after Douglasectomy; (h) the removed uterosacral ligaments and torus uterinum

ligaments. In some patients with deep and severe dyspareunia and secondary dysmenorrhea, or presenting with endometriosis of the uterosacral ligaments at laparoscopy or recurrence of symptoms after LUNA, we propose a Douglasectomy by laparoscopy (Figure 5.5).

The technique starts in the same way as LUNA, vaporizing the uterosacral ligaments as close to the cervix as possible, creating a crater about 2 cm in diameter and 1 cm deep. It is always very important to identify the course of the ureter.

Once this step is completed, the assistant manipulating the uterus places a sponge in the posterior fornix of the vagina in order to individualize the peritoneum of the cul-de-sac of Douglas. In some cases, a 22-mm Hegar dilator is placed in the rectum in order to identify its position. Once the LUNA procedure is completed, we start on one side, pulling the peritoneum of the cul-de-sac of Douglas progressively with the grasping forceps, and separating it from the perirectal fat and the fat below the peritoneum with the CO_2 laser until the peritoneal leaf is completely

removed on the contralateral side. If the cleavage plane between the peritoneum and the fat below has been well defined, there should not be any hemostatic problems. Otherwise, careful bipolar coagulation could be carried out.

Forty-one laparoscopic Douglasectomies with uterosacral ligamentopexy were performed in the Department of Gynecology at the University Hospital of Caen during the period between 1990 and 1995 in patients with painful retroverted uteri[22]. The surgical endoscopic procedure, identical to the operation first promoted by Jamain and Letessier in 1967[23] using laparotomy, is described. Douglasectomy is the only definitive procedure for restoring normal anatomy of the pelvic floor in the case of painful uterine retroversion in a setting of Allen–Masters syndrome. Furthermore, it allows pathological analysis of the excised peritoneum. The results of this procedure are excellent when the indications are correctly met, particularly with regard to positive pessary testing.

Prevesical neurectomy

Resection of the presacral nerve plexus is associated with significant relief from symptoms. The pain impulses from the uterus, which travel through the inferior hypogastric plexus into the intermediate hypogastric plexus and the superior hypogastric plexus, can be interrupted by performing this procedure laparoscopically. The intermediate hypogastric plexus, composed of two or three trunks lying on the vertebral body of L5, is the most appropriate place for resection. Presacral neurectomy is not appropriate treatment for the relief of lateral or back pain. Patients with midline pain, however, will experience significant relief following this procedure[24].

Chen *et al.*[25] compared laparoscopic presacral neurectomy (LPSN) and LUNA for primary dysmenorrhea. One group (33 patients) underwent LPSN and the other group (35 patients), LUNA. There were no complications and all the patients left hospital within 24 h of surgery. The efficacy of both surgical methods was almost the same (87.9% vs. 82.9%) at the 9-month postoperative follow-up visit, but LPSN proved to be significantly more effective than LUNA (81.8% vs. 51.4%) at the 12-month visit.

REFERENCES

1. Nisolle M, Casanas-Roux F, Anaf V, et al. Morphometric study of the stromal vascularization in peritoneal endometriosis. Fertil Steril 1993; 59: 681–4

2. Nisolle M, Paindaveine B, Bourdon A, et al. Histologic study of peritoneal endometriosis in infertile women. Fertil Steril 1990; 53: 984–8

3. Donnez J, Nisolle M, Casanas-Roux F. Three-dimensional architecture of peritoneal endometriosis. Fertil Steril 1992; 57: 980–3

4. Koninckx PD. Deeply infiltrating endometriosis. In Brosens I, Donnez J, eds. Current Status of Endometriosis. Research and Management. Carnforth, UK: Parthenon Publishing, 1993: 437–46

5. Sturgis E, All BJ. Endometriosis peritonei – relationship of pain to functional activity. Am J Obstet Gynecol 1954; 68: 1421–31

6. White JC. Conduction of visceral pain. N Engl J Med 1952; 156: 686–90

7. Allen WM, Masters WH. Traumatic lacerations of uterine supports: the clinical syndrome and operative treatment. Am J Obstet Gynecol 1955; 70: 500

8. Donnez J, Nisolle M, Anaf V, et al. Endoscopic management of peritoneal and ovarian endometriosis. In Donnez J, ed. Atlas of Laser Operative Laparoscopy and Hysteroscopy. Carnforth, UK: Parthenon Publishing, 1994: 63–74

9. Taylor HC Jr. Vascular congestion and hyperemia: their effect on structure and function in the female reproductive system. Am J Obstet Gynecol 1949; 57: 211

10. Taylor HC Jr. Vascular congestion and hyperemia. II. The clinical aspects of the congestion fibrosis syndrome. Am J Obstet Gynecol 1949; 57: 637

11. Fluhman CF. The rise and fall of suspension operations for uterine retrodisplacement. Bull Johns Hopkins Hosp 1955; 96: 59–70

12. Gillian DR. Round-ligament ventrosuspension of the uterus: a new method. Am J Obstet Gynecol 1900; 41: 299

13. Olshausen R. Uber ventrale operation bei prolapsus und retroversio uteri. Sbl Gynakol 1886; 10: 698

14. Baldy JM. Treatment of uterine retrodisplacements. Surg Gynecol Obstet 1909; 8: 421

15. Alexander W. [Cited by] Curtis AH, ed. Obstetrics and Gynecology. Philadelphia: WB Saunders, 1937

16. Adams JA. [Cited by] Graves WP. Gynecology. Philadelphia: WB Saunders, 1916

17. Yoon FE. Laparoscopic ventrosuspension. A review of 72 cases. Am J Obstet Gynecol 1990; 163: 1151–3

18. Koh LM, Tang FC, Huang MH. Preliminary experience in pelviscopic uterine suspension using Webster–Baldy and Franke's method. Acta Obstet Gynecol Scand 1996; 75: 575–6

19. Donnez J, Nisolle M. Carbon-dioxide laser laparoscopy in pelvic pain and infertility. In Sutton C, ed. Laparoscopic Surgery. Baillière's Clinical Obstetrics and Gynaecology. London: Baillière Tindall, 1989: 525–44

20. Sutton CJG. Laser uterine nerve ablation. In Donnez J, ed. Laser Operative Laparoscopy and Hysteroscopy. Leuven: Nauwelaerts, 1989: 43–52

21. Sutton CJ, Pooley AS, Ewen SP, et al. Follow-up report on a randomized controlled trial of laser laparoscopy in the treatment of pelvic pain associated with minimal to moderate endometriosis. Fertil Steril 1997; 68: 1070–4

22. Von Theobald P, Barjot P, Levy G. Laparoscopic Douglasectomy in the treatment of painful uterine retroversion. Surg Endosc 1997; 11: 639–42

23. Jamain B, Letessier A. Douglasectomy in gynecology. Sem Hop 1967; 43: 157–72

24. Carter JE. Laparoscopic presacral neurectomy utilizing contact-tip Nd:YAG laser. Keio J Med 1996; 45: 332–5

25. Chen FP, Chang SD, Chu KK, et al. Comparison of laparoscopic presacral neurectomy and laparoscopic uterine nerve ablation for primary dysmenorrhea. J Reprod Med 1996; 41: 463–6

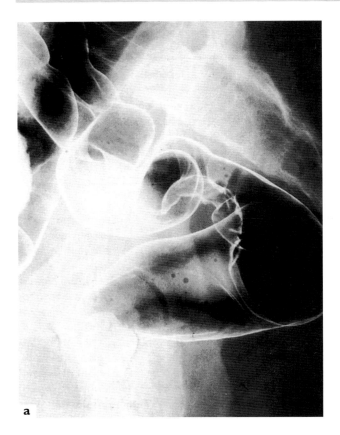

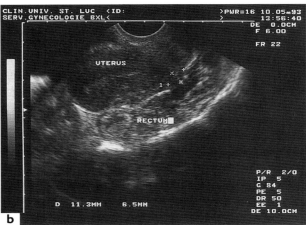

Figure 6.4 Barium enema: profile radiography offers the best evaluation of infiltration of the anterior rectal wall. (a) Typical 'endometriotic' infiltration of the anterior rectal wall without stenosis; intact mucosa. (b) The same patient, showing evaluation of rectal infiltration by vaginal echography

of the lesion could be evaluated. Palpation is very often painful, and the presence of a nodule accounts for symptoms such as deep dyspareunia and dysmenorrhea.

A combination of rectal endoscopic sonography (RES) and MRI has also been advocated to evaluate deep endometriotic lesions[44–47], but most studies to date have

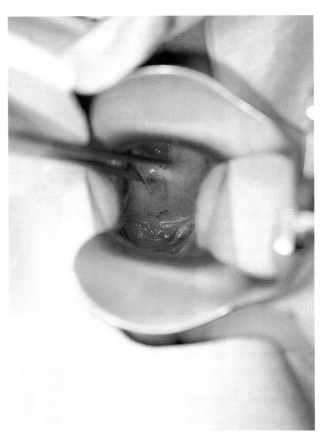

Figure 6.5 Speculum examination: sometimes a bluish lesion is seen protruding into the vaginal fornix

been retrospective and not blind. More recently, Squifflet et al.[28], Darai et al.[48], Bazot and Darai[49] and Delpy et al.[50] demonstrated the important role of both RES and MRI in the detection of deep nodular endometriotic lesions. By injecting jelly for ultrasonography into the vagina and rectum, Takeuchi et al.[51] were able preoperatively to diagnose high rates of not only deep rectovaginal endometriotic lesions, but also complete cul-de-sac obliteration. Squifflet et al. recently proposed a classification of deep lesions into three subtypes, based on transrectal ultrasonography (TRUS) and MRI[28].

Classification of deep lesions (Figure 6.3)

Squifflet et al.[28] distinguished three types of deep retroperitoneal lesions by analyzing their location, as defined precisely by transrectal ultrasonography and MRI[34]. These three types are: (1) type I: rectovaginal septum lesions, (2) type II: posterior vaginal fornix lesions and (3) type III: hourglass-shaped lesions (Table 6.2).

Rectovaginal septum lesions are situated within the rectovaginal septum between the posterior wall of the vaginal mucosa and the anterior wall of the rectal muscularis. Cranially, the rectovaginal septum is limited by

Table 6.2 Prevalence of the three types of deep lesions

Type I*	10%
Type II	58%
Type III	32%

*Only 10% of deep lesions are clearly separated from the cervix and located in the rectovaginal septum (type I)

the joining of the two uterosacral ligaments behind the cervix. According to our classification[34], the lesion is not linked or attached to the cervix. It is situated under the peritoneal fold of the cul-de-sac of Douglas. The caudal portion of the septum is the perineal body. Most cases are located in the cranial part of the septum. This type is observed in only 10% of cases (Table 6.2). Probably only this type is due to metaplasia of Müllerian remnants present in the rectovaginal septum[2,21]. Rectovaginal septum lesions are usually found to be smaller in size. They are distant from the cervix, and their median size estimated by clinical examination is 2 cm. Most of the lesions are exophytic in the vaginal mucosa, and appear bluish on speculum examination. On clinical examination, a free space is found to exist between the lesion and the cervix.

Posterior vaginal fornix lesions are the most frequent type of deep lesions (58%). They develop from the posterior fornix towards the rectovaginal septum. The posterior fornix is retrocervical and corresponds, in its attachment to the vaginal wall, to the posterior wall of the posterior lip of the cervix. It is bordered by the joining of the two uterosacral ligaments behind the cervix; cranially, it is limited by the peritoneal Douglas pouch, and posteriorly, by the anterior wall of the middle third of the rectum. Crossing of the ureter and the uterine artery occurs 10–15 mm from the lateral vaginal fornix. Posterior vaginal fornix lesions are often small, their average size being assessed by clinical examination. There is no extension to the rectovaginal septum or the rectal wall, and so, most of the time, a barium enema reveals a normal rectosigmoid junction, but large posterior fornix lesions can be associated with extension to the rectovaginal septum.

Hourglass-shaped or diabolo-like lesions occur when posterior fornix lesions extend cranially to the anterior rectal wall. Their prevalence is 32%. Clinical evaluation usually reveals a larger lesion, more than 3 cm in size, with a greater risk of extension to the rectal wall (barium enema showed perivisceritis in 78% of cases). This continuum between the rectal muscularis and the cervix was found to obliterate the rectovaginal septum cranially. In this type, the part of the adenomyotic lesion situated in the anterior rectal wall is the same size as the part of the lesion situated near the posterior fornix. A small but well-observed continuum exists between these two parts of the lesion.

This is why we termed these lesions diabolo-like or hourglass-shaped. These lesions always occur under the peritoneal fold of the rectouterine pouch of Douglas. Infiltration of the rectal muscularis is systematically observed in this subtype, as demonstrated by profile radiography or barium enema (Figure 6.4a) and transrectal ultrasonography (TRUS) (Figure 6.4b).

SURGERY

Surgery for deep rectovaginal endometriosis was first described by Reich *et al.*[15] and Donnez[52] in 1991, and the two first large series including 231 and 500 women, respectively, were published in 1995[10] and 1997[11].

Surprisingly, recent studies very often fail to refer to these first papers. Even more surprising, increasingly aggressive surgery, including bowel resection (Figure 6.6a), is systematically proposed in the case of rectovaginal endometriosis and muscularis involvement, even if there is no mucosal involvement[30,48,53–56]. All of these studies, however, were non-randomized and do not evaluate the long-term results of this surgery compared with debulking or shaving surgery (Figure 6.6b).

Our series of 2147 cases of rectovaginal septum adenomyosis treated by laparoscopy is presented in Table 6.3.

Whenever extensive involvement of the cul-de-sac was suspected preoperatively, either because of the clinical presentation or from another physician's operative record, a mechanical bowel preparation (Fleet® Phospho-soda®) was administered orally before surgery to induce brisk, self-limiting diarrhea that rapidly cleansed the bowel without disrupting the electrolyte balance.

In the case of lesions of the anterior rectal wall (diagnosed by radiography or echography), a bowel preparation was proposed as for conventional bowel resection.

SURGICAL TECHNIQUE: 'SHAVING'

All the laparoscopic procedures were performed under general anesthesia. A 12-mm operative laparoscope was inserted through a vertical intraumbilical incision. Three other puncture sites were made: 2–3 cm above the pubis in the midline, and in the areas adjacent to the deep inferior epigastric vessels, which were visualized directly.

Deep fibrotic nodular adenomyosis involving the cul-de-sac required excision of the nodular tissue from the posterior vagina, rectum, posterior cervix and uterosacral ligaments.

To determine the diagnosis of cul-de-sac obliteration during laparoscopy, a sponge on a ring forceps was inserted into the posterior vaginal fornix (Figures 6.7 and 6.8). A dilator (Hegar 25) or a rectal probe was systematically inserted into the rectum (Figure 6.9). Complete obliteration

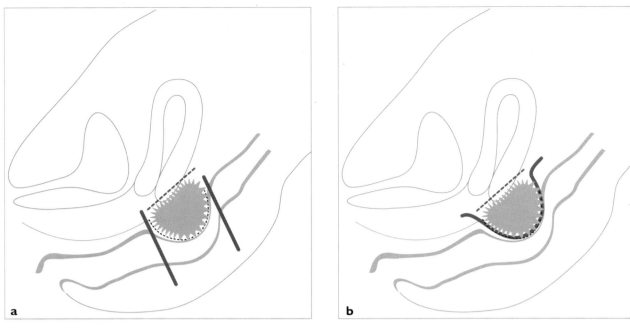

Figure 6.6 (a) Radical surgery: resection of the nodule with a bowel segment. (b) Shaving technique

Table 6.3 A series of 2179 cases: rectovaginal adenomyosis treated by laparoscopic debulking surgery without segmental resection ($n = 2147$) or by segmental bowel resection ($n = 32$). Values are expressed as mean (range) or n (%)

Laparoscopic debulking or 'shaving' surgery* ($n = 2147$)	
Size of lesion (cm)	2.8 (1–6)
Duration of surgery (min)	78 (31–248)
Hospitalization (days)	2.7 (2–7)
Complications	
rectal perforation	12 (0.5%)
fecal peritonitis	1 (0.05%)
delayed hemorrhage (< 24 h postoperative)	3 (0.1%)
ureteral injury	7 (0.3%)
urinary retention	10 (0.5%)
Segmental bowel resection (laparotomy or mini-laparotomy, assisted by laparoscopy ($n = 32$)[†]	
Size of lesion (cm)	3.2 (2–4.5)
Duration of surgery (min)	152 (138–240)
Hospitalization (days)	8.5 (7–10)
Complications	
'incomplete' surgery (vaginal fornix not resected)	32 (100%)
ureteral injury	1 (3%)
urinary retention	6 (18%)
fistula	0

*Not entering the rectal lumen; [†]in 32 cases, bowel resection was carried out by laparotomy because of bowel stenosis with mucosal involvement (these cases are not included in the series of 2147 patients)

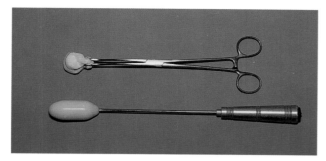

Figure 6.7 Sponge grasped by forceps (top); rectal probe (bottom)

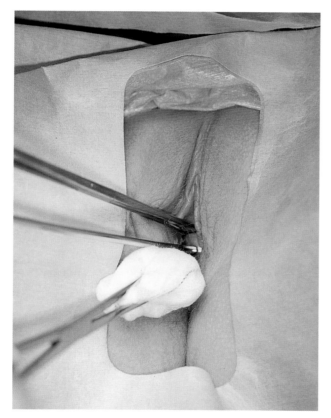

Figure 6.8 Vaginal sponge is inserted into the vagina in order to see the cleavage plane between the rectum, the vagina and the nodule

was diagnosed when the outline of the posterior fornix could not be seen through the laparoscope.

Cul-de-sac obliteration was partial when rectal tenting was visible but a protrusion of the sponge into the posterior vaginal fornix was identified between the rectum and the inverted U of the uterosacral ligaments. Sometimes, however, a deep lesion of the rectovaginal septum is only barely visible by laparoscopy.

Surgical techniques have evolved gradually, but all of them involve separation of the anterior rectum from the posterior vagina and excision or ablation of the

endometriosis in that area. Hydrodissection, scissor dissection and electrosurgery with an unmodulated (cutting) current are used by some authors[15,18], while others[8–12,16,17] prefer the CO_2 laser.

As described by Reich et al.[15] and Donnez et al.[8–12], attention was first directed towards complete dissection of the anterior rectum throughout its area of involvement, until the loose tissue of the rectovaginal space was reached. A sponge on a ring forceps was inserted into the posterior vaginal fornix and a rectal probe was placed in the rectum. In addition, a cannula was inserted into the endometrial cavity to antevert the uterus markedly. The peritoneum covering the cul-de-sac of Douglas was opened between the 'adenomyotic' lesion (Figure 6.10) and the rectum.

We used a technique of first freeing the anterior rectum from the loose areolar tissue of the rectovaginal septum, prior to excising visible and palpable deep fibrotic endometriosis, using the so-called 'shaving technique'. This approach was possible even when anterior rectal muscle infiltration was present. Careful dissection was then carried out using the hydrodissector, and the CO_2 laser for sharp dissection, until the rectum was completely freed (Figure 6.11) and identifiable below the lesion (Figure 6.12).

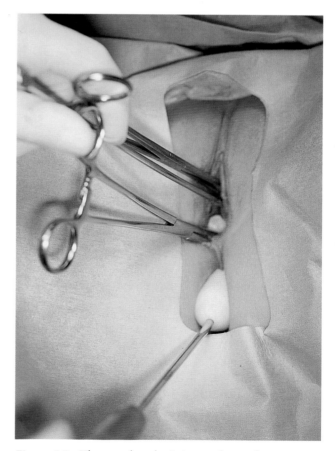

Figure 6.9 The rectal probe is inserted into the rectum

Excision of the fibrotic tissue on the side of the rectum was attempted only after the rectal dissection was complete. In the case of deep lesions, the vaginal wall was more or less penetrated by the adenomyosis and excision of part of the vagina was essential (Figures 6.13 and 6.14).

Dissection was performed accordingly, not only with the removal of all visible adenomyotic lesions (Figure 6.15), but also the vaginal mucosa with at least a 0.5-cm disease-free margin (caudally) (Figure 6.16). Lesions

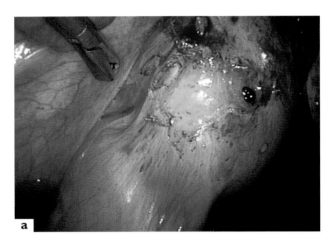

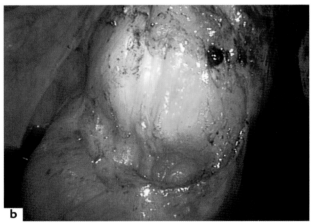

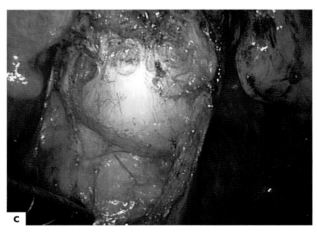

Figure 6.10   (a), (b) and (c) Dissection of the rectum with a CO_2 laser

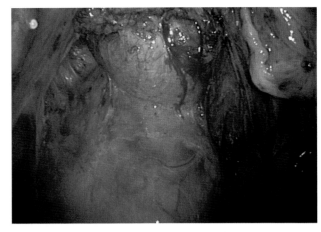

Figure 6.11   The rectum is completely freed

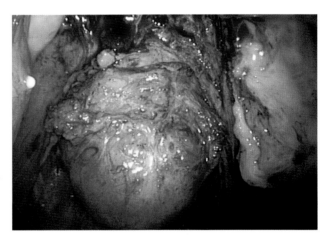

Figure 6.12   Adenomyotic nodule after dissection of the rectum

extending totally through the vagina were treated with *en bloc* laparoscopic resection from the cul-de-sac to the posterior vaginal wall (Figure 6.17); the pneumo-peritoneum was maintained and the posterior vaginal wall was closed vaginally (Figure 6.18).

The anterior rectum was not reperitonealized. Interceed® (Figure 6.19) was used to cover the deperitonealized area[8–11]. Deep rectal muscle defects could be closed with suture (Vicryl® 2-0 or 3-0) (Figure 6.20).

Keckstein and Wiesinger[57] recently reported a series of 202 patients who underwent partial intestinal resection for deep endometriosis. With such surgery, complications are not uncommon and certainly more frequent than with the shaving technique. Much of the recent literature[30,53–56], however, seems to encourage very invasive techniques, including bowel resection in the case of rectal muscularis involvement. In our view, removing part of the rectum is simply not justified, since we know that the technique increases the risk of complications. Furthermore, no

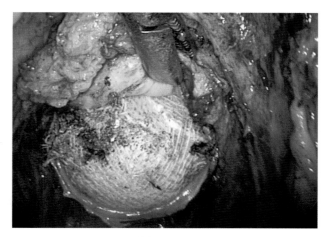

Figure 6.13 Opening of the vagina beneath the nodule on the vaginal sponge

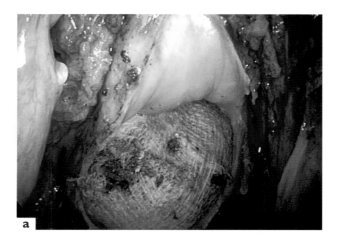

a

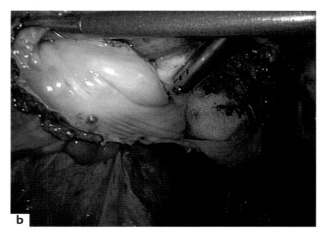

b

Figure 6.14 (a) and (b) Excision of the nodule and a part of the vagina

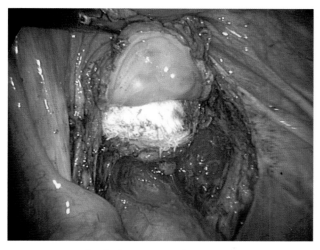

Figure 6.15 Bluish lesion on the vaginal part of the nodule

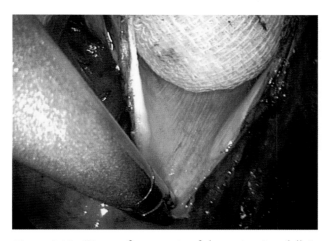

Figure 6.16 Disease-free margin of the vagina (caudally)

randomized studies to date have been able to prove that it is any more effective than the shaving technique.

In our series of 2147 patients (Table 6.3), laparoscopic dissection was performed successfully in all cases, even when radiography of the colon showed bowel involve-ment. Bowel resection is not usually required, and our 'debulking' or 'shaving' surgical approach is often more than adequate. In most cases, perirectal perivisceritis observed in all cases of type III lesions may be left in place. The residual lesion in the muscularis of the rectum does not evolve, and remains constant for a long time. As patients are usually free of symptoms, we consider systematic bowel resection in the case of perirectal visceritis and rectal muscularis involvement unnecessary. Moreover, such surgery increases morbidity, and is responsible for more adhesions due to extensive lateral dissection.

In the case of bowel occlusion and rectal bleeding with rectal mucosa involvement, resection of the rectosigmoid junction must be carried out. It was performed in 32 cases in our series (Table 6.3). These 32 patients, who had rectal endometriosis with stenosis or substenosis with mucosal involvement and rectal menstrual bleeding, were operated on by laparotomy. Bowel resection with anastomosis was then carried out.

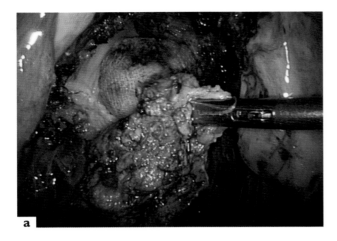

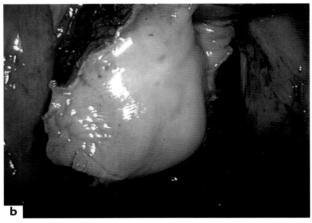

Figure 6.17 Resected nodule: (a) rectal side, (b) vaginal side

COMPLICATIONS

In our series of 2147 cases, laparoscopic rectal perforation occurred in 12 of them. All perforations were diagnosed at the time of laparoscopy. In the first three cases (occurring in the early 1990s), the rectum was repaired by laparotomy, and in the others, by laparoscopy.

One case of fecal peritonitis occurred 7 days after surgery. During surgery, bleeding at the site of lateral dissection of the rectum required extensive bipolar coagulation. At the end of surgery, bowel integrity was checked by CO_2 intrarectal insufflation and the blue test. No rectal defect was diagnosed. Seven days later, a hole of 2.5 cm in size was detected. Extensive coagulation probably provoked thermal rectal injury with subsequent necrosis and a fistula.

Seven cases of ureteral injury were noted in our patients. Two cases of ureteral transection were diagnosed on the first postoperative day by the presence of abundant fluid in the peritoneal cavity. High levels of urea and creatinine in the 'peritoneal' fluid and intravenous pyelog-

raphy (IVP) confirmed the diagnosis. Nephrostomy was carried out. One case resolved spontaneously, with complete healing of the ureter 2 months later. The other case required vesicoureteral reimplantation.

The remaining five cases of ureteral injury were due to thermal damage (bipolar coagulation), and were treated by insertion of a JJ stent.

Urinary retention for a maximum of 2 weeks occurred in ten women. It was probably due to the extensive lateral and prerectal dissection.

RECURRENCE

In one of our previous publications[58], the recurrence rate of deep endometriosis was 3.7% with excision of the nodule and resection of the posterior vaginal fornix, 16% when the vaginal fornix was not resected and 20% when the bowel, but not the vaginal fornix, was resected. Our study led us to suggest strongly that the shaving technique (for the rectum) and the resection technique (for the

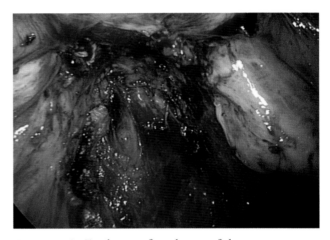

Figure 6.18 Final view after closure of the vagina

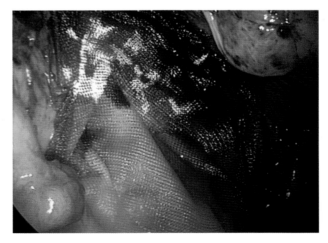

Figure 6.19 Interceed® is used to cover the deperitonealized area

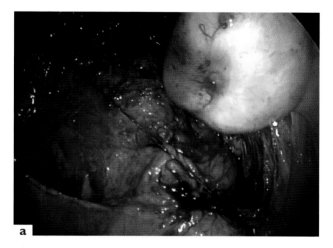

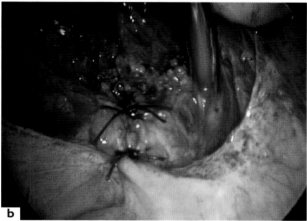

Figure 6.20 (a) and (b) Deep rectal muscle defect should be closed with suture

vagina) must be considered as first-line therapy. Side-wall endometriosis and *ureteral endometriosis* are the consequence of retroperitoneal adenomyotic disease[59]. In the case of rectovaginal adenomyotic nodules or nodules developed more extensively laterally, and in the case of large uterosacral endometriotic nodules (>2.5 cm), patients should systematically undergo preoperative diagnosis of ureteral endometriosis. Lateral extension from the rectovaginal space to the side-wall through the cardinal ligaments also occurs in the retroperitoneal space, sometimes provoking ureteral stenosis, erroneously called ureteral endometriosis. This was observed in nearly 10% of deep lesions of more than 3 cm in size[26]. In such cases, laparoscopic dissection of the ureter is required (see Chapter 7).

CONCLUSION

Deep endometriosis is essentially characterized by the presence of a rectovaginal or retrocervical nodule, which is a circumscribed, nodular aggregate of smooth muscle, endometrial glands and, usually, endometrial stroma.

Histologically, scanty endometrial-type stroma and glandular epithelium are disseminated in muscular tissue. The very similar histological descriptions have led us to suggest that the so-called 'endometriotic nodule of the rectovaginal septum' is, in fact, just like an adenomyoma or adenomyotic nodule, originating from the posterior part of the cervix in the majority of cases and invading the retroperitoneal space.

We therefore suggest that the posterior part of the cervix in the retroperitoneal space should definitely be considered as the origin of this disease. We have, in this chapter, reviewed the classification, the diagnosis and the surgical technique of deep endometriosis, which is an adenomyotic disease of the cervix.

A comprehensive laparoscopic procedure, while not eradicating all the endometriosis, may result in considerable pain relief or a desired pregnancy. Although we recognize that bowel resection may be necessary in rare cases (1.8%), it seems prudent to curtail, rather than encourage, the widespread use of an aggressive, potentially morbid procedure.

REFERENCES

1. Donnez J, Nisolle M, Casanas-Roux F. Three-dimensional architecture of peritoneal endometriosis. Fertil Steril 1992; 57: 980–3
2. Nisolle M, Donnez J. Peritoneal endometriosis, ovarian endometriosis, and adenomyotic nodules of the rectovaginal septum are three different entities. Fertil Steril 1997; 68: 585–96
3. Donnez J, Nisolle M. Appearances of peritoneal endometriosis. Presented at the 3rd International Laser Surgery Symposium, Brussels, 1988
4. Nisolle M, Paindaveine B, Bourdon A, et al. Histologic study of peritoneal endometriosis in infertile women. Fertil Steril 1990; 53: 984–8
5. Nisolle M, Casanas-Roux F, Anaf V, et al. Morphometric study of the stromal vascularization in peritoneal endometriosis. Fertil Steril 1993; 59: 681–4
6. Hughesdon PE. The structure of endometrial cysts of the ovary. J Obstet Gynaecol Br Emp 1957; 64: 481–7
7. Donnez J, Nisolle M, Gillet N, et al. Large ovarian endometriomas. Hum Reprod 1996; 11: 641–6
8. Donnez J, Nisolle M, Casanas-Roux F, et al. Laparoscopic treatment of rectovaginal septum endometriosis. In Donnez J, Nisolle M, eds. An Atlas of Laser Operative Laparoscopy and Hysteroscopy. Carnforth, UK: Parthenon Publishing, 1994: 75–85
9. Donnez J, Nisolle M. Advanced laparoscopic surgery for the removal of rectovaginal septum endometriotic and adenomyotic nodules. Baillieres Clin Obstet Gynecol 1995; 9: 769–74

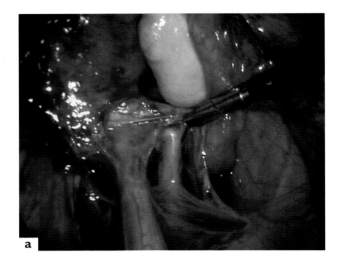

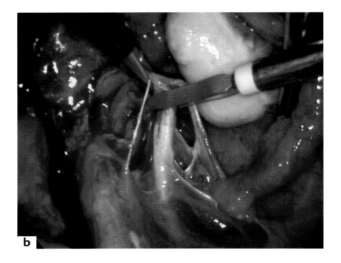

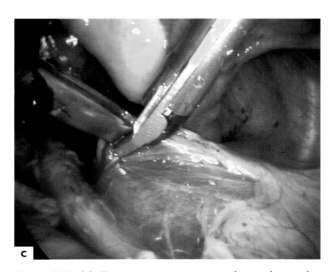

When partial ureteral resection was required (because of the presence of complete stenosis of more than 3 cm in length), laparotomy with ureteroureterostomy and bladder surgery was carried out. Between 1992 and 2004, this occurred in just three cases, and resection and reimplantation were performed using the psoas hitch technique. This means that, in total, 75 cases (96%) of ureteral endometriosis were conservatively treated by laparoscopy.

In patients who underwent preoperative or intra-operative retrograde stent placement, the catheter was left in place for 1–3 months, depending on the severity of the disease. After that period, the JJ stent was removed, and IVP demonstrated the absence of any ureteral stricture.

DISCUSSION

In the past, ureteral endometriosis was uncommon, accounting for less than 0.3% of all endometriotic lesions.

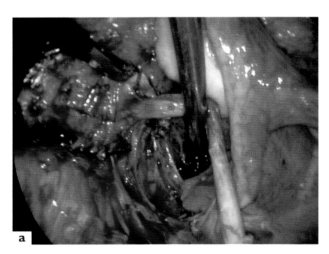

Figure 7.5 (a) Dissection is progressively made in the direction of the uterosacral ligament. Coagulation (b) and ligation (c) of the uterine artery

Figure 7.6 (a) and (b) At the end of dissection, the ureter is free of disease

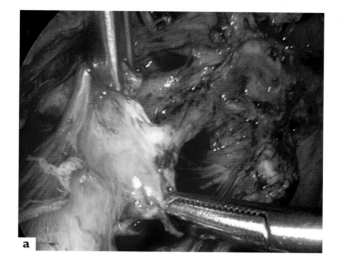

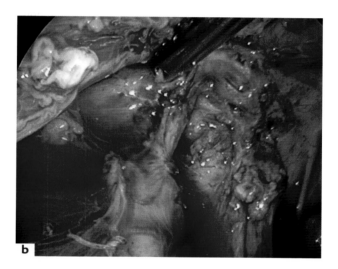

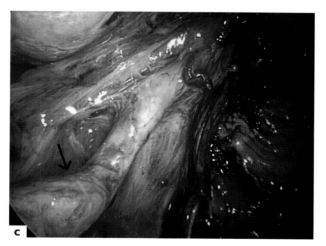

Figure 7.7 (a) The ureteral fibrotic ring, responsible for ureteral stenosis and dilatation, is grasped with forceps; (b) ureteral ring dissection; (c) after dissection, the ureter is free. The ureteral dilatation (arrow) is still visible

Now, its prevalence has reached almost 14% in the case of large (≥3 cm), deep, rectovaginal nodules. Ureteral lesions have thus become much more frequent in recent times, and they are a very serious condition because they may cause silent loss of renal function.

There are two types of ureteral endometriosis, extrinsic and intrinsic[9–11]. Intrinsic ureteral obstruction is characterized by the presence of endometriotic glands and stroma in the ureteral wall, due to primary endometriotic involvement of the ureteral wall. This type of ureteral endometriosis is less common, however, than ureteral obstruction, caused by external compression by surrounding endometriosis, which is known as extrinsic ureteral endometriosis. According to Donnez et al.[12], endometriosis of the ureter usually arises by extension from deep endometriotic (adenomyotic) nodules, or, more rarely, from adhesions with ovarian endometriosis.

Prevalence

Indeed, in a retrospective study from 1988 to 1997, the prevalence of ureteral endometriosis was estimated to be less than 0.1% in cases of endometriosis[9]. In women suffering from rectovaginal adenomyosis, it was found to be 0.9% (6/711). In a prospective study from 1998 to 2000, however, the prevalence was 4.5% in a series of 306 cases of rectovaginal endometriosis or adenomyosis. The latest findings (2005) point to an incidence as high as 14%. The dramatically increasing prevalence of ureteral endometriosis is directly related to the increasing prevalence of severe deep endometriosis, and this must be emphasized.

Surrounding endometriotic lesions responsible for external ureteral compression, without histological evidence of endometriotic glands and stroma in the ureteral wall, are thus mostly the consequence of lateral extension of rectovaginal adenomyotic nodules. These patients also showed other localizations of endometriosis, but ovarian endometriomas were rarely considered solely responsible for ureteral endometriosis, as they were always associated with rectovaginal adenomyosis.

The concept of adenomyosis of the retroperitoneal space should therefore cover not only the rectovaginal space and the vesicovaginal space, but also the area extending laterally in the direction of the cardinal ligaments[11–16]. Deep endometriotic (adenomyotic) nodules should be considered as a benign cancer originating from the posterior part of the cervix, which spreads laterally like cervical cancer.

Left or right?

In a large review of the literature on retrospective series of ureteral endometriosis, the proportion of lesions located on the left was found to be significantly higher than on the right[17]. In one of our previous studies, a higher proportion was also found on the left, but the difference was not significant, the prevalence being 3% and 2%, respectively. In the series of Nezhat et al., a non-significant difference in the prevalence of ureteral endometriosis was also observed between the left and right sides[8]. In our present study, bilateral ureteral anomalies (medialization, lumen irregularities, substenosis or stenosis) were observed in 24 cases. In this large series, a significantly higher proportion of ureteral lesions were found on the left (48.7%) than on the right side (20.5%). The difference was significant ($p < 0.05$) in this series.

In a publication by Vercellini et al.[17], six cases of ureteral endometriosis were described as being associated with ovarian endometriomas. In the opinion of the authors, however, neither the celomic metaplasia theory, nor the embryonic cell rest theory, could explain such a clear-cut difference in the frequency of the distribution of ovarian and ureteral lesions between the two pelvic sites. On the contrary, in our study, adenomyotic disease of the retroperitoneal space, originating from metaplasia of the cervix, was obviously the cause of extrinsic ureteral endometriosis, proved by clinical examination and histological serial sections.

Techniques

In 1996, Nezhat et al. described a series of 17 cases of partial ureteral obstruction[8]. Laparoscopic ureterolysis was performed in ten women, but seven of the 17 women (41%) required partial wall resection. They also reported use of the laparoscopic psoas hitch procedure for infiltrative ureteral endometriosis, to obtain tension-free anastomosis of the bladder[18,19]. A report described one case of recurrent ureteral endometriosis after partial laparoscopic ureteral resection and ureteroneocystostomy. This approach should be considered only in a case of intrinsic ureteral endometriosis involving a long segment of the ureter, to avoid laparotomy.

According to our results, conservative surgery should be proposed in the majority of patients. We do not agree with Yohannes[20], who recommend first hormonal treatment and surgery only in the case of the failure of hormonal treatment or severe stenosis. Indeed, even severe ureteral stenosis usually remains asymptomatic[21], and a delay in efficient therapy may result in the loss of a kidney. Therefore, we recommend performing laparoscopic ureterolysis and removal of the adenomyotic lesions responsible for the ureteral stenosis, even in the case of moderate or severe pyelic dilatation. In the majority of cases, ureteral dissection, with or without uterine artery ligation, is sufficient to free the ureter. In all cases, ureterohydronephrosis was found to be decreased after this procedure. Resection of part of the ureter should only be performed in exceptional cases (4% in our series) or in the case of recurrence. Partial ureteral resection and ureteroneocystostomy can be performed by laparoscopy[19,22].

In conclusion, obstructive uropathy is more frequently provoked by 'extrinsic' rather than 'intrinsic' endometriosis. The approximate ratio of four cases of extrinsic to one case of intrinsic disease, as previously described, has to be re-evaluated according to our study[8]. Obstructive uropathy should be suspected in patients with a rectovaginal adenomyotic nodule of more than 3 cm, because of its high prevalence in such cases. In this group of patients, there is a need to perform non-invasive urinary tract exploration to detect obstructive uropathy and prevent silent loss of renal function, which necessitated nephrectomy in 11% of cases in our series.

Conservative surgery with relief of the ureteral obstruction and the removal of adenomyosis or endometriosis should be the management of choice.

REFERENCES

1. Heilier JF, Ha A-T, Lison D, et al. Increased serum PCB levels in Belgian women with adenomyotic nodules of rectovaginal septum. Fertil Steril 2004; 81: 456–8

2. Heilier JF, Nackers F, Verougstraete V, et al. Increased dioxin-like compounds in the serum of women with peritoneal endometriosis and deep endometriotic (adenomyotic) nodules. Fertil Steril 2005; 84: 305–12

3. Donnez J, Thomas K. Incidence of the luteinized unruptured follicle syndrome in fertile women and in women with endometriosis. Eur J Obstet Gynecol Reprod Biol 1982; 14: 187–90

4. Strathy JH, Molgaard GA, Coulam CB, et al. Endometriosis and infertility: a laparoscopic study of endometriosis among fertile and infertile women. Fertil Steril 1982; 38: 667–72

5. Haney AF. Endometriosis: pathogenesis and pathophysiology. In Wilson EA, ed. Endometriosis. New York: Alan R Liss, 1987: 23–51

6. Nisolle M, Donnez J. Peritoneal endometriosis, ovarian endometriosis and adenomyotic nodules of the rectovaginal septum are three different entities. Fertil Steril 1997; 68: 585–96

7. Stillwell TJ, Kramer SAZ, Lee RA. Endometriosis of the ureter. Urology 1986; 26: 81–5

8. Nezhat C, Nezhat F, Nezhat C, et al. Urinary tract endometriosis treated by laparoscopy. Fertil Steril 1996; 66: 920–4

9. Donnez J, Brosens I. Definition of ureteral endometriosis? Fertil Steril 1997; 68: 178–9

10. Donnez J, Nisolle M, Casanas-Roux F. Endometriosis: rationale for surgery. In Donnez J, Nisolle M, eds. An Atlas of Laser Operative Laparoscopy and Hysteroscopy. Carnforth, UK: Parthenon Publishing, 1994: 53–62

11. Clement PB. Disease of the peritoneum. In Kurman RJ, ed. Blaustein's Pathology of the Female Genital Tract. New York: Springer-Verlag, 1994: 647–703

12. Donnez J, Nisolle M, Squifflet J. Ureteral endometriosis: a complication of rectovaginal endometriotic (adenomyotic) nodules. Fertil Steril 2002; 77: 32–7

13. Donnez J, Nisolle M, Casanas-Roux F, et al. Rectovaginal septum endometriosis or adenomyosis: laparoscopic management in a series of 231 patients. Hum Reprod 1995; 10: 630–5

14. Donnez J, Nisolle M, Gillerot S, et al. Rectovaginal septum adenomyotic nodules: a series of 500 cases. Br J Obstet Gynaecol 1997; 104: 1014–18

15. Donnez J, Spada F, Squifflet J, et al. Bladder endometriosis must be considered as bladder adenomyosis. Fertil Steril 2000; 74: 1175–81

16. Donnez J, Nisolle M, Casanas-Roux F, et al. Endometriosis: rationale for surgery. In Brosens I, Donnez J, eds. Current Status of Endometriosis. Research and Management. Carnforth, UK: Parthenon Publishing, 1993: 385–95

17. Vercellini P, Pisacreta A, Pesole A, et al. Is ureteral endometriosis an asymmetric disease? Br J Obstet Gynaecol 2000; 107: 559–61

18. Nezhat C, Nezhat F, Freiha F, et al. Laparoscopic vesicopsoas hitch for infiltrative ureteral endometriosis. Fertil Steril 1999; 71: 376–9

19. Nezhat CH, Malik S, Nezhat F, et al. Laparoscopic ureteroneocystostomy and vesicopsoas hitch for infiltrative endometriosis. JSLS 2004; 8: 3–7

20. Yohannes P. Ureteral endometriosis. J Urol 2003; 170: 20–5

21. Antonelli A, Simeone C, Frego E, et al. Surgical treatment of ureteral obstruction from endometriosis: our experience with thirteen cases. Int Urogynecol J Pelvic Floor Dysfunct 2004; 15: 407–12

22. Ou CS, Huang IA, Rowbotham R. Laparoscopic ureteroureteral anastomosis for repair of ureteral injury involving stricture. Int Urogynecol J Pelvic Floor Dysfunct 2005; 16: 155–7

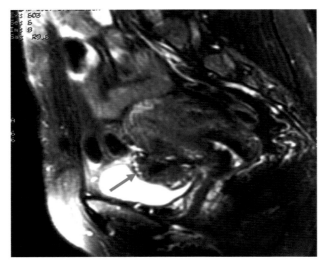

Figure 8.6 Magnetic resonance imaging shows a nodular mass in the anterior fornix adjacent to the uterine wall (arrow), causing extensive compression of the posterior bladder wall (note the absence of concomitant uterine adenomyosis): sagittal image

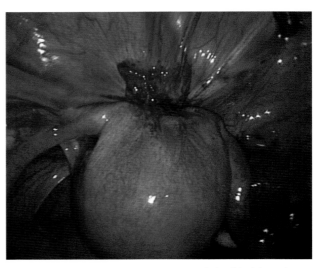

Figure 8.7 First laparoscopic view of the bladder adenomyotic nodule. Both round ligaments are systematically medially attached

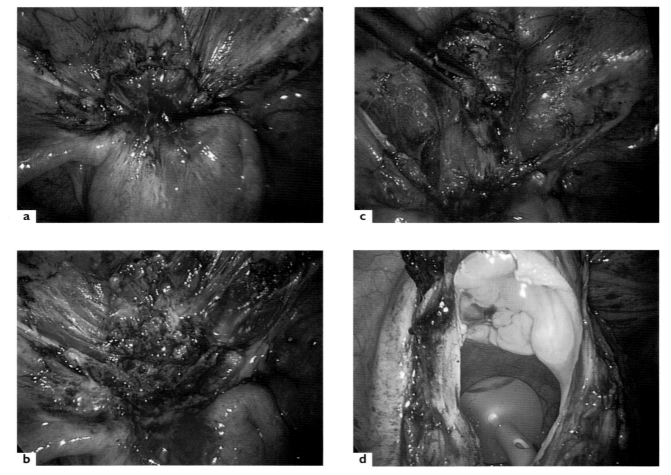

Figure 8.8 Laparoscopic excision of the nodule. (a) Incision of the peritoneum; (b) dissection of the nodule from the anterior wall of the uterus; (c) the nodule is grasped by forceps; (d) the bladder is opened and the submucosal bluish nodule is visualized in the bladder;

diluted methylene blue solution was injected, to ensure watertightness of the sutures.

In some cases, a control cystoscopy was carried out to check the bladder defect closure. In all cases, retrograde cystography was performed 10 days postoperatively to confirm complete recovery of the bladder wall and to exclude any liquid leakage.

The bladder catheter was left in place for 10 days.

In our series, no long-term complications, such as vesical fistulas, were encountered.

HISTOLOGY

Serial sections were obtained and colored with hematoxylin–eosin, or analyzed to evaluate steroid receptor (estrogen and progestogen) content according to a previously described method[9]. On microscopic examination (Figure 8.10), the lesion was characterized by the presence of scarce glands, with active endometrial-type epithelium and scanty stroma. No secretory changes were observed, even when the patient was undergoing progestogen therapy or during the luteal phase. More than 90% of the lesion consisted of smooth-muscle hyperplasia. The bladder nodule was localized throughout the whole thickness of the bladder wall. By serial section, we were able to demonstrate that endometrial glands were not connected to the peritoneal serosa but were almost in the subperitoneal space, again proving that a bladder endometriotic nodule is not the consequence of deep-infiltrating endometriosis.

RESULTS AND DISCUSSION

Several authors have described two types of bladder endometriosis, the first occurring in women who have not previously undergone any uterine surgery (primary) and the second following cesarean section (iatrogenic or secondary)[10,11].

Koninckx and Martin[12] suggested that extraperitoneal endometriosis derives from endoperitoneal disease. In the opinion of Vercellini et al.[10,13,14], peritoneal lesions are able to penetrate under the peritoneum and develop into deep-

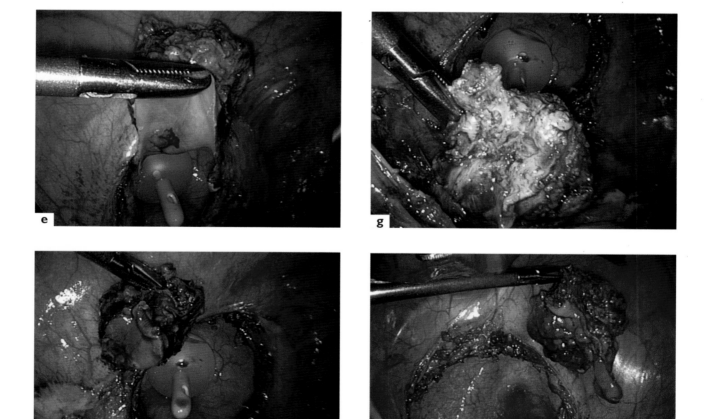

Figure 8.8 *continued* (e) note the thickness of the nodule caused by hyperplasia of the bladder muscularis; (f) resected nodule (bladder mucosa side); (g) resected nodule (uterine side); (h) bladder defect after nodule resection can reach 5–6 cm

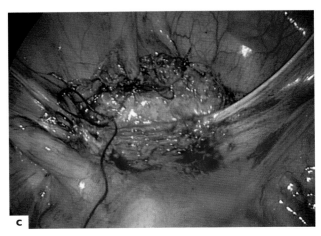

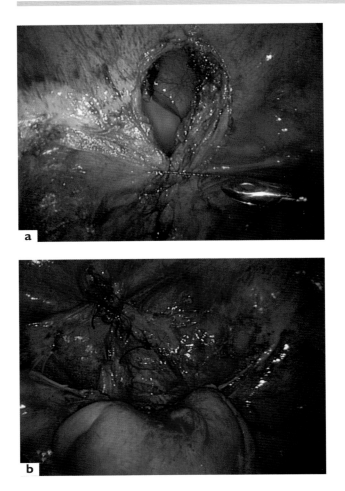

Figure 8.9 (a)–(c) Extramucosal vesical suture by separate or continuous Vicryl® 2-0 stitches

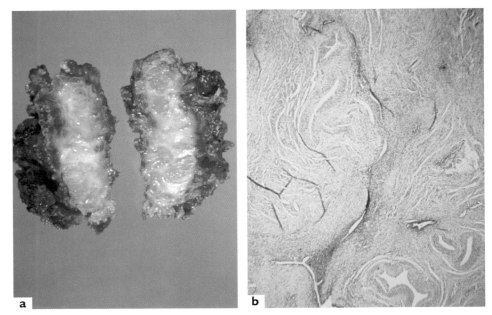

Figure 8.10 Vesical adenomyosis: (a) 90% of the lesion consists of smooth-muscle hyperplasia. (b) Scarce glands with active endometrial-type epithelium and scanty stroma are visible

infiltrating endometriosis. If this were the case, we would have found peritoneal endometriosis in all cases. In our series, 35% of patients had no associated endometriotic lesions, while 65% of women had associated rectovaginal adenomyotic nodules, which we clearly described as a distinct retroperitoneal entity[1,15]. Indeed, the rectovaginal septum nodule was described, like the adenomyoma, as a circumscribed nodular aggregate of smooth muscle and endometrial glands, surrounded by scanty stroma. We have previously suggested that a rectovaginal nodule may be the consequence of metaplasia of Müllerian remnants. Not surprisingly, a bladder nodule appeared exactly the same as a rectovaginal nodule when viewed microscopically.

This frequent association, as well as the similar histological findings observed in our study, lead us to suggest strongly that bladder endometriosis is actually bladder adenomyosis, and also the consequence of metaplasia of Müllerian remnants that can be found in both the rectovaginal septum and vesicovaginal septum, or the result of metaplasia of the retroperitoneal space, again originating from the cervix. Indeed, we systematically found a clear attachment between the cervix and the nodule, and the absence of any real plane of cleavage.

One of the hypotheses advanced by Fedele *et al.*[4], claiming that detrusor endometriosis could result from the extension of adenomyotic lesions from the anterior uterine wall to the bladder, is not supported by our study. Indeed, although the adenomyotic vesical nodule was systematically found to be adherent to the uterine wall or to the cervix, no adenomyotic nodules of the anterior uterine wall were found. These data, observed at surgery, were corroborated by the absence of uterine adenomyosis on echography and MRI, when available.

With regard to treatment, although medical therapy has proven effective in relieving symptoms, the quick recurrence of irritative urinary symptoms after cessation of therapy indicates that surgery is required. In the literature so far, partial cystectomy (or segmental bladder resection) has been considered the treatment of choice[11,16,17]. Successful treatment depends, however, on achieving radical, deep surgical exeresis of the nodule[18,19].

In conclusion, so-called primary bladder endometriosis must be considered as retroperitoneal adenomyotic disease, which is the consequence of metaplasia of the bladder muscularis and can be resected using a laparoscopic approach[5].

REFERENCES

1. Nisolle M, Donnez J. Peritoneal endometriosis, ovarian endometriosis and adenomyotic nodules of the rectovaginal septum are three different entities. Fertil Steril 1997; 68: 585–96
2. Judd ES. Adenomyomata presenting as a tumor of the bladder. Surg Clin North Am 1921; 1: 1271–8
3. Fianu S, Ingelman-Sundberg A, Nasiell K, et al. Surgical treatment of post abortum endometriosis of the bladder and postoperative bladder function. Scand J Urol Nephrol 1980; 14: 151–5
4. Fedele L, Piazzola E, Raffaeli R, et al. Bladder endometriosis: deep infiltrating endometriosis or adenomyosis? Fertil Steril 1998; 69: 972–5
5. Donnez J, Spada F, Squifflet J, et al. Bladder endometriosis must be considered as bladder adenomyosis. Fertil Steril 2000; 74: 1175–81
6. Heilier JF, Ha A-T, Lison D, et al. Increased serum PCB levels in Belgian women with adenomyotic nodules of rectovaginal septum. Fertil Steril 2004; 81: 456–8
7. Balleyguier C, Chapron C, Dubuisson JB, et al. Comparison of magnetic resonance imaging and transvaginal ultrasonography in diagnosing bladder endometriosis. J Am Assoc Gynecol Laparosc 2002; 9: 15–23
8. Donnez J, Nisolle M, Anaf V, et al. Endoscopic management of peritoneal and ovarian endometriosis. In Donnez J, Nisolle M, eds. An Atlas of Laser Operative Laparoscopy and Hysteroscopy. Carnforth, UK: Parthenon Publishing, 1994: 63–74
9. Nisolle M, Casanas-Roux F, Wyns C, et al. Immunohistochemical analysis of estrogen and progesterone receptors in endometrium and peritoneal endometriosis: a new quantitative method. Fertil Steril 1994; 62: 751–9
10. Vercellini P, Meschia M, De Giorgi O, et al. Bladder detrusor endometriosis: clinical and pathogenetic implication. J Urol 1996; 155: 84–6
11. Brosens IA, Puttemans P, Deprest J, et al. The endometriosis cycle and its derailments. Hum Reprod 1994; 9: 770–1
12. Koninckx PR, Martin D. Deep endometriosis: a consequence of infiltration or retraction or possible adenomyosis externa. Fertil Steril 1992; 85: 924–8
13. Vercellini P, Frontino G, Pisacreta A, et al. The pathogenesis of bladder detrusor endometriosis. Am J Obstet Gynecol 2002; 187: 538–42
14. Vercellini P, Frontino G, Pietropaolo G, et al. Deep endometriosis: definition, pathogenesis, and clinical management. J Am Assoc Gynecol Laparosc 2004; 11: 153–61
15. Donnez J, Nisolle M, Smoes P, et al. Peritoneal endometriosis and 'endometriotic' nodules of the rectovaginal septum are two different entities. Fertil Steril 1996; 66: 362–8
16. Zaloudek C, Norris HJ. Mesenchymal tumors of the uterus. In Kurman R, ed. Blaustein's Pathology of the Female Genital Tract. New York: Springer-Verlag, 1987: 373–408
17. Nezhat C, Nehzat F. Laparoscopic segmental bladder resection for endometriosis: a report of two cases. Obstet Gynecol 1993; 81: 882–4
18. Chapron C, Chopin N, Borghese B, et al. Surgical management of deeply infiltrating endometriosis: an update. Ann NY Acad Sci 2004; 1034: 326–37
19. Fedele L, Bianchi S, Zanconato G, et al. Long-term follow-up after conservative surgery for bladder endometriosis. Fertil Steril 2005; 83: 1729–33

small uterus and can be done vaginally. Our profession should discourage abdominal hysterectomy for this indication. If the vaginal approach is not available, laparoscopic total or supracervical hysterectomy can be done.

Of course, there are now many different techniques to reduce bleeding by destroying uterine endometrium. This has resulted in a new indication for hysterectomy: endometrial ablation failure. Many women who have ablations continue to have a bleeding problem, resolved by hysterectomy. Most women seeking an ablation should also be given the alternative of a vaginal or a laparoscopic hysterectomy.

In the UK, national figures show an increase in the total numbers of operations for dysfunctional uterine bleeding (DUB) from 1989 to 1996. Hysterectomy rates have remained steady. Ablation has not been a replacement technique for hysterectomy, but an alternative technique. Endometrial ablation rates have fallen since 1993[16].

Laparoscopic treatment is best carried out in women with endometrial cancer. In most cases of endometrial cancer, the uterus is relatively small, and thus the laparoscopic surgeon can take out the uterus and then examine the inside of it. If the depth of myometrial penetration is less than one-half, the patient is probably cured just by the simple hysterectomy. If there is invasion of the muscle greater than one-half through the myometrium, the surgeon should perform a pelvic lymphadenectomy.

Few relative contraindications to laparoscopic surgery, for which most surgeons would be better served by doing a laparotomy, exist in gynecology. With the assistance of expert laparoscopic training, the majority of these patients can be spared a laparotomy. In most cases in which vaginal access or access to the uterine vessels is limited, and little or no uterine mobility exists, a laparoscopic hysterectomy can be considered.

One should remember that concerning the operative indication, laparoscopic hysterectomy is a substitute for abdominal hysterectomy, including difficult abdominal hysterectomy. Hysterectomy by laparotomy is not preferable in most cases with distorted anatomy or a large uterus.

TOTAL LAPAROSCOPIC HYSTERECTOMY TECHNIQUE

Our technique for a TLH is described, since other types of laparoscopic hysterectomy (e.g. LAVH or LH) are simply modifications of this more extensive procedure. These steps are designed to prevent complications.

Preoperative preparation

The patient is optimized medically for coexistent problems. Preoperative ovarian suppression is sometimes used. Patients are encouraged to hydrate with clear liquids the day before surgery. Fleet® Phospho-soda® 90 ml, divided into two doses, is given at 15.30 and 19.30 to evacuate the lower bowel. If the patient is prone to nausea, Phenergan® 25 mg is taken orally 25 minutes before the bowel prep. Lower-abdominal, pubic and perineal hair is not shaved.

All laparoscopic procedures are done using general endotracheal anesthesia, with orogastric tube suction to minimize bowel distension. The patient's arms are placed at her side (no armboards), and shoulder braces are positioned at the acromioclavicular joint. Nitrous oxide anesthesia gas is avoided because it may cause small-bowel distension. The bladder is emptied when filled. The Trendelenburg position up to 40° is available. We use one dose of a prophylactic antibiotic after induction of anesthesia in all patients.

Incisions

Three laparoscopic puncture sites including the umbilicus are used: 10 mm umbilical, 5 mm right and 5 mm left lower quadrant. Pneumoperitoneum to 25–30 mmHg is obtained before primary umbilical trocar insertion, and reduced to 15 mm afterwards. The lower quadrant trocar sleeves are placed under direct laparoscopic vision above the pubic hairline and lateral to the rectus abdominis muscles (and thus, the deep epigastric vessels). These are placed just beside the anterior superior iliac spines in patients with large fibroids. The left lower quadrant puncture is the major portal for operative manipulation as the surgeon stands on the patient's left side. The right trocar sleeve is used for retraction with atraumatic grasping forceps.

Reduction in wound morbidity and scar integrity as well as cosmesis is enhanced using 5-mm sites. The use of 12-mm incisions when a 5-mm one will suffice is not an advance in minimally invasive surgery.

Vaginal preparation

There will always be room for new innovations in uterine and vaginal manipulation to help the surgeon visualize pelvic anatomy. In the USA, many centers have only old, basic devices available such as the Cohen cannula and HUMI (Harris–Kronner uterine manipulator/injector). The Valtchev uterine manipulator (Conkin Surgical Instruments, Toronto, Canada) has been around for more than 15 years, and is a huge advance. It allows anterior, posterior and lateral manipulation of the uterus, and permits the surgeon to visualize the posterior cervix and vagina. Newer devices are currently available developed by Pelosi, Wattiez, Hourcabie, Koninckx, Koh, McCartney, Donnez and Reich. We still use the Valtchev and the Wolf tube. When using the Valtchev uterine mobilizer in the anteverted position, the cervix sits on a wide pedestal, making the vagina readily visible between the uterosacral ligaments when the cul-de-sac is viewed laparoscopically.

Exploration

The upper abdomen is inspected, and the appendix is identified. Clear vision is maintained throughout the operation using the IC Medical smoke evacuator (Phoenix, AZ). If appendiceal pathology is present, i.e. dilatation, adhesions or endometriosis, appendectomy is done. The appendix is mobilized, its blood supply isolated by making a window in the mesoappendix near the cecum with reusable Metzenbaum-type scissors, and ligated by passing a Vicryl® 2-0 free ligature through this window and securing it extracorporeally with the Clarke–Reich knot pusher. Three endoloops (chromic gut ligature; Ethicon, Somerville, NJ) are then placed at the appendiceal–cecal junction after desiccating the appendix just above this juncture. The appendix is left attached to the cecum. Its stump is divided later in the procedure, after opening the cul-de-sac, so that vaginal removal from the peritoneal cavity can be accomplished.

Retroperitoneal dissection

The peritoneum is opened.

The uterus is pushed cephalad and to one side from below using the uterine manipulator, and the anterior broad ligament is put into tension by pulling the Fallopian tube medially. Scissors are used to make an incision in the peritoneum in front of the round ligament. CO_2 from the pneumoperitoneum rushes into the retroperitoneum and distends it. The tip of the laparoscope is then used to perform 'optical dissection' of the retroperitoneal space by pushing it into the loosely distended areolar tissue parallel to the uterus. This blunt dissection technique is usually successful in identifying the uterine vessels, ureter or both. The uterine artery is often ligated at this time, especially in large-uterus patients.

Ureteral dissection (optional)

Three approaches have been used for laparoscopic ureteric identification, which may be called medial, superior and lateral. Stents are not used, as they cause hematuria and ureteric spasm in some patients. The laparoscopic surgeon should dissect (skeletonize) either the ureter or the uterine vessels during the performance of a laparoscopic hysterectomy.

The medial approach

Immediately after exploration of the upper abdomen and pelvis, each ureter is isolated deep in the pelvis, when possible. Ureteral dissection is performed early on in the operation before the pelvic side-wall peritoneum becomes edematous and opaque from irritation by the CO_2 pneumoperitoneum or hydrodissection, and before ureteral peristalsis is inhibited by surgical stress, pressure or the Trendelenburg position[1].

If the uterus is anteverted using a uterine manipulator, the ureter can usually be easily visualized in its natural position on the pelvic side wall (posterior leaf of the broad ligament), provided that no significant cul-de-sac or adnexal abnormality is present. This maneuver allows the peritoneum immediately above the ureter to be incised to create a peritoneal 'window' in order to make division of the infundibulopelvic ligament or adnexal pedicle safer. The ureter and its overlying peritoneum are grasped deep in the pelvis below and caudad to the ovary, lateral to the uterosacral ligament. An atraumatic grasping forceps is used from the opposite-sided cannula. Scissors are used to divide the peritoneum overlying the ureter, and are inserted into the incision created and spread. Thereafter, one blade of the scissors is placed on top of the ureter, its blade visualized through the peritoneum, and the peritoneum divided. In this manner, the ureter and its surrounding longitudinal endopelvic fascia sheath are dissected together away from the peritoneum without compromising its blood supply. This dissection is continued into the deep pelvis where the uterine vessels cross the ureter, lateral to the cardinal ligament insertion into the cervix. Connective tissue between the ureter and the vessels is separated with scissors. Bleeding is controlled with microbipolar forceps. Often, the uterine artery is ligated at this time to diminish back-bleeding from the upper pedicles.

The superior approach

The superior approach entails dissecting the colon (rectosigmoid on the left, cecum on the right) from the pelvic brim and freeing the infundibulopelvic ligament vessels from the roof of the broad ligament to allow the ureter that lies below it to be identified. The ureter is found as it crosses the iliac vessels (or below them between the hypogastric and superior rectal vessels on the left). The ureter is then reflected off the broad ligament and traced into the pelvis.

The lateral approach

The lateral approach makes use of the pararectal space to identify the ureter, and the ureter does not have to be peeled off the broad ligament for its entire pelvic course to be visible. The tip of the laparoscope is often the best blunt dissector in this area, and may be inserted alongside and just lateral to the pelvic side-wall peritoneum into the loose areolar tissue already distended by retroperitoneal CO_2 (see above) until the ureter and uterine vessels are identified.

After displacing the uterus to the contralateral side, a pelvic side-wall triangle is identified formed by the round ligament, lateral border by the external iliac artery and medial border by the infundibulopelvic ligament. The peritoneum in the middle of the triangle is incised with scissors and the broad ligament opened by bluntly separating the extraperitoneal areolar tissues. The infundibulopelvic ligament is pulled medially with grasping forceps to expose the ureter at the pelvic brim where it crosses the common or external iliac artery. The operator then searches for the ureter distal to the pelvic brim and lateral to the infundibulopelvic ligament. The dissection is carried bluntly underneath and caudad to the round ligament, until the obliterated hypogastric artery is identified extraperitoneally. If difficulty is encountered, the artery is first identified intraperitoneally where it hangs from the anterior abdominal wall, and traced proximally to where it passes behind the round ligament. Then, with both its intraperitoneal portion and the dissected space under the round ligament in view, the intraperitoneal part of the ligament is moved back and forth. After the obliterated hypogastric artery has been identified extraperitoneally, it is an easy matter to develop the paravesical space by bluntly separating the areolar tissue on either side of the artery. The obliterated hypogastric artery is next traced proximally to where it is joined by the uterine artery, and the pararectal space opened by blunt dissection proximal and medial to the uterine vessels, which lie on top of the cardinal ligament. After the pararectal space has been opened, the ureter is identified easily on the medial leaf of the broad ligament (really posterior leaf), which forms the medial border of the pararectal space. The uterine artery and cardinal ligament at the distal (caudal) border of the space, and the internal iliac artery on its lateral border, also become clearly visible.

Bladder mobilization

The round ligaments are divided at their mid-portion using a well-insulated spoon electrode set at 150 W cutting current or with scissors after bipolar desiccation. Persistent bleeding is controlled with bipolar desiccation at 30 W cutting current. Thereafter, scissors or the same electrode are used to divide the vesicouterine peritoneal fold, starting at the left side and continuing across the midline to the right round ligament. The upper junction of the vesicouterine fold is identified as a white line firmly attached to the uterus, with 2–3 cm between it and the bladder dome. The initial incision is made below the white line while lifting the peritoneum covering the bladder. The bladder is mobilized off the uterus and upper vagina using scissors, or bluntly with the same spoon electrode or a suction-irrigator, until the anterior vagina is identified by elevating it from below with ring forceps. The tendinous attachments of the bladder in this area may be desiccated or dissected.

In most cases, incising the peritoneum in front of the round ligaments results in the development of a retroperitoneal pneumoperitoneum. It is very easy to isolate the uterine arteries adjacent to the uterus in this loose, gas-filled areolar tissue.

Upper uterine blood supply (Figures 9.1–9.5)

When ovarian preservation is desired, the utero-ovarian ligament and Fallopian tube are coagulated until desiccated with bipolar forceps, at 25–35 W cutting current, and then divided. Alternatively, the utero-ovarian ligament and Fallopian tube pedicles are suture-ligated adjacent to the uterus with Vicryl 2-0, using a free ligature passed through a window created around the ligament. To create the window, the peritoneum is opened just lateral to the tubal cornua, and the Metzenbaum-type scissors slid down lateral to the utero-ovarian vessels until its tip can be seen through the posterior broad ligament peritoneum.

When oophorectomy is indicated or ovarian preservation not desired, the anterior and posterior leaves of the broad ligament are opened lateral and below the infundibulopelvic ligament with a laparoscopic Metzenbaum-type scissors, and a Vicryl 2-0 free ligature passed through the window thus created and tied

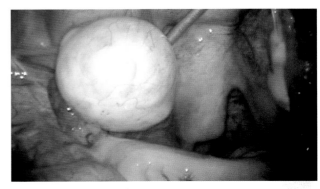

Figure 9.1 A cystic left ovary is seen at the start of total laparoscopic hysterectomy. Left salpingo-oophorectomy will be done. Note the uterus, cervix and upper vagina held anteriorly by the Valtchev uterine manipulator

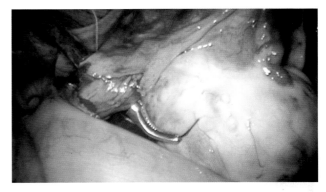

Figure 9.2 A window is made by incising the peritoneum medial and lateral to the infundibulopelvic ligament. A Vicryl® 2-0 suture ligature is placed around the left infundibulopelvic ligament in preparation for its ligation

extracorporeally using the Clarke–Reich knot pusher[17]. This maneuver is repeated twice around the ovarian vessels so that two proximal ties and one distal tie are placed, and the ligament then divided. While applying traction to the cut distal pedicle, the broad ligament is

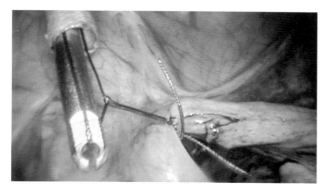

Figure 9.3 An extracorporeal knot is passed down to secure the infundibulopelvic ligament using a Clarke–Reich knot pusher

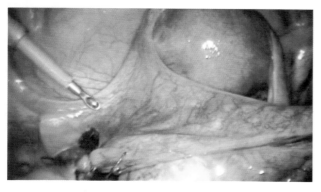

Figure 9.4 After ligation of the infundibulopelvic ligament, a spoon electrode at 100 W cutting current is used to divide it

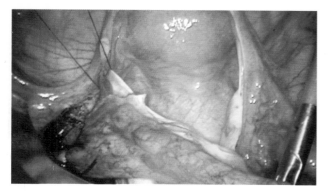

Figure 9.5 Alternatively, the suture ligature can be placed around the utero-ovarian ligament and the ovary preserved

divided to the round ligament just lateral to the utero-ovarian artery anastomosis using scissors or cutting current through a spoon electrode. We rarely desiccate the infundibulopelvic ligament, as it results in too much smoke early on in the operation. If suturing skills are not developed and the tube and ovary are to be removed, the infundibulopelvic ligament is mobilized, and bipolar forceps are used to compress and desiccate its vessels. Stapling devices are rarely used.

If the ovary is to be preserved and the uterus is large, the utero-ovarian ligament/round ligament/Fallopian tube junction may be divided with a 30- or 45-mm GIA™-type stapler. This may be time-saving for this portion of the procedure, thus justifying its increased cost.

Many complications are related to use of the Endo GIA or similar-type staplers. Whereas it decreases operation time, it also increases the risk for hemorrhage and injury to the ureter. At many institutions, complications are associated with the Endo GIA stapler, including postoperative hemorrhage, with resultant re-exploration and transfusion. Ligation or coagulation of the vascular pedicles is safer.

Uterine vessel ligation (Figures 9.6–9.11)

The uterine vessels may be ligated at their origin, at the site where they cross the ureter, where they join the uterus or on the side of the uterus. Most surgeons use bipolar desiccation to ligate these vessels, but these authors prefer suture.

In most cases, the uterine vessels are suture-ligated as they ascend the sides of the uterus. The broad ligament on each side is skeletonized down to the uterine vessels. Each uterine vessel pedicle is suture-ligated with Vicryl 0 on a CTB-1 blunt needle (Ethicon JB260; 27 in, ~68 cm). Use of a blunt needle markedly reduces uterine venous bleeding. The needles are introduced into the peritoneal cavity

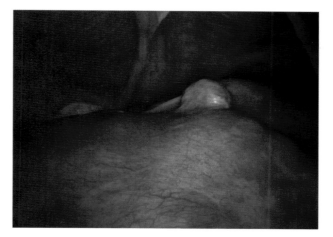

Figure 9.6 A large multiple fibroid uterus fills the peritoneal cavity to well above the umbilicus

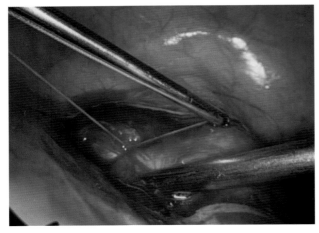

Figure 9.7 The anterior broad ligament is opened as is the vesicouterine peritoneal fold. An extracorporeal knot is passed to secure the left uterine artery with a Clarke–Reich knot pusher

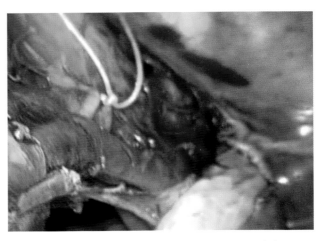

Figure 9.10 The ligated right uterine artery and draining vein are shown

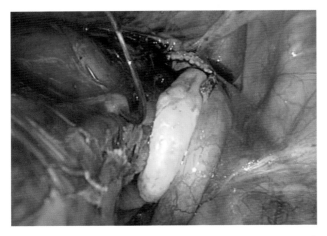

Figure 9.8 A Vicryl 0 suture on a CTB-1 needle is placed around the right uterine artery in preparation for its ligation. The vein is left to drain

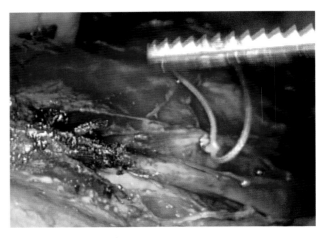

Figure 9.11 After the blood drains out of the uterus, it goes pale and the vein collapses. The vein is then desiccated with bipolar forceps and divided

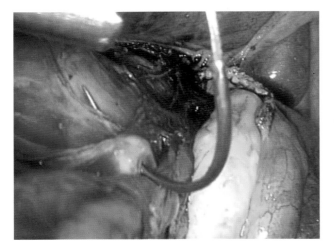

Figure 9.9 Close-up showing same procedure as described in Figure 9.8

by pulling them through a 5-mm incision[18]. The curved needle is placed around the uterine vessel pedicle at the side of the uterus. A short, rotary movement of the needle holder brings the needle around the uterine vessel pedicle. This motion is backhand if done with the left hand from the patient's left side and forward motion if using the right hand from the right side. The uterine artery is a sturdy structure, and can be grasped and elevated carefully to avoid the uterine veins underneath. In some cases, the vessels can be skeletonized completely, and a Vicryl 2-0 free suture ligature passed around them. Sutures are tied extracorporeally using a Clarke–Reich knot pusher.

In large-uterus patients, selective ligation of the uterine artery without its adjacent vein is done to give the uterus a chance to return its blood supply to the general circulation. It also results in a less voluminous uterus for morcellation.

In some cases, the curved needle is inserted on top of the unroofed ureter, where it turns medially toward the previously mobilized bladder. A single suture placed in this manner on each side serves as a 'sentinel stitch', identifying the ureter for the remainder of the procedure.

Division of cervicovaginal attachments and circumferential culdotomy (Figure 9.12)

The cardinal ligaments on each side are divided with the CO_2 laser at high power (80 W), or with an electrode using cutting current. Bipolar forceps are used to coagulate the uterosacral ligaments and are invaluable to control bleeding from vaginal branches. The vagina is entered posteriorly over the uterovaginal manipulator near the cervicovaginal junction. A 4-cm diameter vaginal delineator (Wolf) is placed in the vagina to outline circumferentially the cervicovaginal junction, serve as a backstop for laser work and prevent loss of pneumoperitoneum. First, it identifies the anterior cervicovaginal junction and then the lateral fornices. They are incised using the laser, with the delineator as a backstop to complete the circumferential culdotomy. The uterus is morcellated, if necessary, and pulled out of the vagina.

When the vaginal delineator is not available, a ring forceps is inserted into the anterior vagina above the tenaculum on the anterior cervical lip to identify the anterior cervicovaginal junction. The left anterior vaginal fornix is entered using the laser, so that the aquapurator can be inserted into the anterior vagina above the anterior cervical lip. Following the aquapurator tip or ring forceps, and using this as a backstop, the anterior and lateral vaginal fornices are divided. The aquapurator is inserted from posterior to anterior to delineate the right vaginal fornix, which is divided. The uterus can then be pulled out of the vagina.

Morcellation (laparoscopic and vaginal) (Figures 9.13–9.16)

Morcellation can be done laparoscopically or vaginally. For the laparoscopic technique, a #10 blade on a long handle is introduced gently through the left 5-mm trocar incision after removing the trocar. With care, the uterus and its enclosed large myoma can be bivalved with the blade. The surgeon's fingers in contact with the skin prevent the loss of pneumoperitoneum.

Vaginal morcellation is done in most cases on a uterus free in the peritoneal cavity, but may be considered after securing the ovarian arteries from above and the uterine arteries from above or below. A #10 blade on a long knife handle is used to make a circumferential incision into the fundus of the uterus, while pulling outwards on the cervix

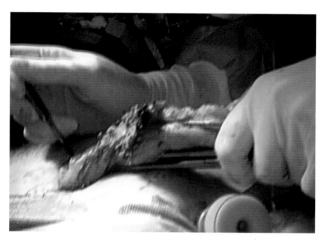

Figure 9.13 A #10 blade is used to morcellate the large fibroid uterus using a coring technique for removal through the left lateral incision

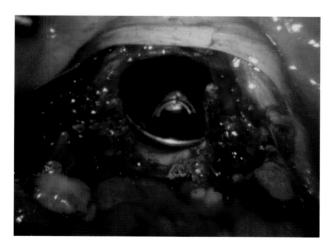

Figure 9.12 The vaginal delineator maintains the pneumoperitoneum, facilitating the vaginal cuff closure

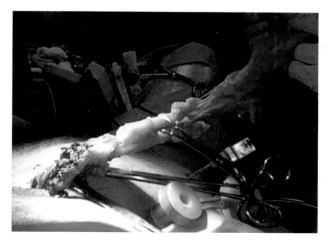

Figure 9.14 Further coring to morcellate the fibroid uterus

and using the cervix as a fulcrum. The myometrium is incised circumferentially parallel to the axis of the uterine cavity with the scalpel's tip always inside the myomatous tissue and pointed centrally, away from the surrounding vagina. The knife is not extended through the serosa of the uterus. The incision is continued around the full circumference of the myometrium in a symmetrical fashion beneath the uterine serosa. Traction is maintained on the cervix, and the avascular myometrium is cut so that the endometrial cavity with a surrounding thick layer of myometrium is delivered with the cervix, bringing the outside of the uterus closer to the operator for further excision by wedge morcellation.

Wedge morcellation is carried out by removing wedges of myoma and myometrium from the anterior and posterior uterine wall, usually in the midline, to reduce the bulk of the uterus. After excision of a large core, the fundus is morcellated with multiple wedge resections, around either a tenaculum or an 11-mm corkscrew device. The remaining fundus, if still too large for removal, can be bivalved so that one half can be pulled out of the peritoneal cavity, followed by the other half.

Morcellation of fibroids through anterior abdominal-wall puncture sites is now practical when vaginal access is limited. The Steiner™ electromechanical morcellator (Storz, Tuttlingen, Germany) is a 10-mm diameter motorized circular saw that uses claw forceps or a tenaculum to grasp the fibroid and pull it into contact with the fibroid. Large pieces of myomatous tissue are removed piecemeal until the myoma can be pulled out through the trocar incision. With practice this instrument can often be inserted through a stretched 5-mm incision without an accompanying trocar. The newer Sawalhe™ morcellator from Karl Storz comes with 12-mm, 15-mm and 20-mm diameter circular saws.

Laparoscopic vaginal vault closure and suspension with McCall culdoplasty (Figures 9.17–9.24)

The vaginal delineator, or a sponge in a glove pack, is placed back into the vagina for closure of the vaginal cuff, occluding it to maintain the pneumoperitoneum. The uterosacral ligaments are identified by bipolar desiccation markings or with the aid of a rectal probe. The first suture is complicated, as it brings the uterosacral and cardinal ligaments as well as the rectovaginal fascia together. The left uterosacral ligament is elevated and a Vicryl 0 suture on a CT-1 needle is placed through it, then through the left cardinal ligament with a few cells of posterolateral vagina

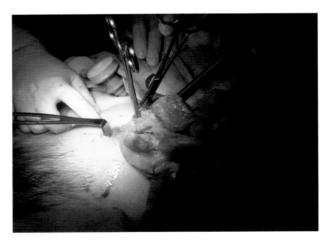

Figure 9.15 Note the blue trocar in the umbilicus. Towel clips and single-tooth tenacula are used to grasp and deliver the fibroid uterus from the 5-mm incision lateral to the left rectus muscle after extending this incision to 12 mm

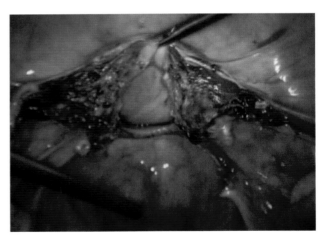

Figure 9.17 Following hemostasis, the vaginal cuff is ready for closure. Each uterosacral ligament has been marked 'white' from bipolar desiccation. Closure is done usually with two sutures to close the vagina and its fascia across the midline. The first suture incorporates both uterosacral ligaments and cardinal ligaments and rectovaginal fascia

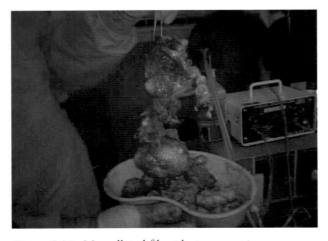

Figure 9.16 Morcellated fibroid uterus specimen

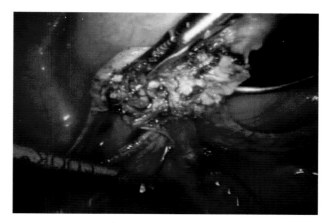

Figure 9.18 Vicryl 0 on a CT-1 needle is placed through the left uterosacral ligament and then the left cardinal ligament just below the uterine vessel pedicle

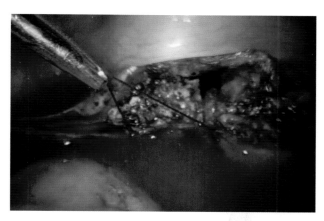

Figure 9.21 The suture is tied extracorporeally and passed down with a Clarke–Reich knot pusher, plicating the uterosacral ligaments, cardinal ligaments and rectovaginal fascia across the midline

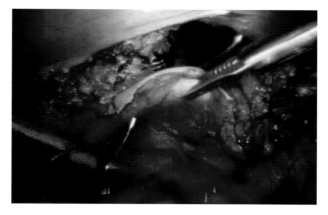

Figure 9.19 The suture continues across the posterior vaginal wall, grasping the rectovaginal fascia

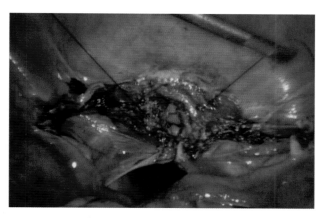

Figure 9.22 The uterosacral ligaments, cardinal ligaments and rectovaginal fascia are together. A second suture is used to close the pubocervicovesicular fascia. This suture is placed just above the uterine vessel pedicles

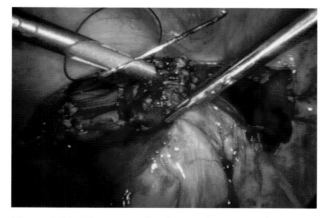

Figure 9.20 The suture finishes with separate bites into first the right cardinal ligament and finally the right uterosacral ligament. A rectal probe is used to help identify the right uterosacral ligament

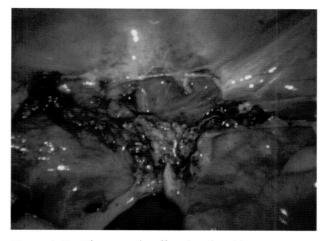

Figure 9.23 The vaginal cuff is closed and hemostatic

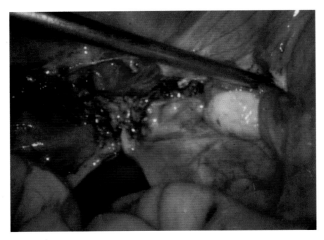

Figure 9.24 The side wall is inspected to follow the course of the ureter and check for hemostasis

just below the uterine vessels, and along the posterior vaginal wall with a few bites over to the right side. Finally, the same suture with needle is put through the right posterolateral vagina and cardinal ligament to the right uterosacral ligament.

This single suture is tied extracorporeally, bringing the uterosacral ligaments cardinal ligaments and posterior vaginal fascia together across the midline. It provides excellent support to the vaginal cuff apex, elevating it superiorly and posteriorly toward the hollow of the sacrum. It also serves to prevent a future enterocele by bringing together the endopelvic fascia from the uterosacral ligaments and rectovaginal fascia.

The rest of the vagina and overlying pubocervicovesicular fascia are closed vertically with one or two Vicryl 0 interrupted sutures. The peritoneum is not closed after TLH, but is closed following supracervical hysterectomy, to cover the cervical stump.

Cystoscopy

Cystoscopy is done after vaginal closure to check for ureteral patency, 10 minutes after intravenous administration of one ampule of indigo carmine dye. This is necessary when the ureter is identified but not dissected, and especially necessary when the ureter has not been identified. Blue dye should be visualized through both ureteral orifices. The bladder wall should also be inspected for suture and thermal defects.

Underwater examination

At the close of each operation, an underwater examination is used to detect bleeding from vessels and viscera tamponaded during the procedure by the increased intraperitoneal pressure of the CO_2 pneumoperitoneum. The CO_2 pneumoperitoneum is displaced with 2–4 l of Ringer's

lactate solution, and the peritoneal cavity is vigorously irrigated and suctioned until the effluent is clear of blood products. Any further bleeding is controlled underwater using microbipolar forceps to coagulate through the electrolyte solution, and at least 2 l of lactated Ringer's solution are left in the peritoneal cavity.

Skin closure

The umbilical incision is closed with a single Vicryl 4-0 suture opposing deep fascia and skin dermis, with the knot buried beneath the fascia. This will prevent the suture from acting as a wick, transmitting bacteria into the soft tissue or peritoneal cavity. The lower quadrant 5-mm incisions are loosely approximated with a Javid vascular clamp (Mueller, McGaw Park, IL) and covered with collodion (AMEND, Irvington, NJ) to allow drainage of excess Ringer's lactate solution.

ENDOMETRIOSIS

Although excision of endometriosis with uterine preservation is almost always possible, hysterectomy should be reserved for women with severe pelvic pain that affects their quality of life, who do not desire fertility preservation. They require extensive counseling regarding alternatives, and may select hysterectomy as their primary procedure if they have persistent or recurrent symptoms after other surgeries, especially when uterine adenomyosis is suspected. Concomitant oophorectomy is elective.

The goal at laparoscopic hysterectomy for endometriosis is the same as for any endometriosis surgery, i.e. to excise all visible and palpable endometriosis implants[8]. The rectovaginal area can be particularly symptomatic, and requires careful evaluation and meticulous, systematic excision. The surgeon must first free the ovaries, then the ureters and finally the rectum from the posterior cervix and vagina to the rectovaginal septum. Deep fibrotic nodular endometriosis involving the cul-de-sac requires excision of the fibrotic tissue from the uterosacral ligaments, posterior cervix, posterior vagina and rectum. Hysterectomy with excision of all visible endometriosis usually results in relief of the patient's pain. Oophorectomy is not usually necessary at hysterectomy for advanced endometriosis if the endometriosis is removed carefully. The most severely affected ovary may be removed, especially if it is on the left, because this ovary frequently becomes adherent to the bowel. Reoperation for recurrent symptoms is necessary in fewer than 5% of the authors' patients in whom one or both ovaries have been preserved. Bilateral oophorectomy is rarely indicated in women younger than 40 years who undergo hysterectomy for endometriosis.

Hysterectomy should not be carried out for extensive endometriosis with extensive cul-de-sac involvement, unless the surgeon has the skill and time to resect all deep fibrotic endometriosis from the posterior vagina, uterosacral ligaments and anterior rectum. In these patients, excision of the uterus using an intrafascial technique leaves the deep fibrotic endometriosis behind to cause future problems. Furthermore, removing deep fibrotic endometriosis may be more difficult when there is no uterus between the anterior rectum and bladder. After hysterectomy, the endometriosis left in the anterior rectum and vaginal cuff frequently becomes densely adherent to, or invades into, the bladder and one or both ureters. In many patients with extensive endometriosis and extensive cul-de-sac obliteration, it is preferable to preserve the uterus to prevent future vaginal cuff, bladder and ureteral problems. Obviously, this approach will not be effective when uterine adenomyosis is present. In these cases, after excision of cul-de-sac endometriosis, persistent pain ultimately requires a hysterectomy.

Endometriosis nodules in the muscularis of the anterior rectum can usually be excised laparoscopically without entering the rectum. Full-thickness penetration of the rectum can occur during hysterectomy surgery, especially when excising rectal endometriosis nodules. Following identification of the nodule or rent in the rectum, a closed circular stapler (Proximate™ ILS curved intraluminal stapler; Ethicon, Stealth) is inserted into the lumen just past the lesion or hole, opened 1–2 cm and held high to avoid the posterior rectal wall. The proximal anvil is positioned just beyond the lesion or hole, which is invaginated into the opening, and the device closed. Circumferential inspection is made to ensure the absence of encroachment of nearby organs and posterior rectum in the staple line and lack of tension in the anastomosis. The instrument is fired, then removed through the anus. The surgeon must inspect and ensure that the fibrotic lesion or a 'donut' of tissue representing the excised hole is contained in the circular stapler. When verified, anastomotic inspection is done laparoscopically under water after filling the rectum with indigo carmine solution or air[13–15].

Surgical technique to excise endometriosis
(Figures 9.25–9.33)

Initially, adhesions from previous surgery are divided until the surgeon can visualize the pelvis. These adhesions frequently involve the omentum and small bowel. When these are all freed from the anterior abdominal wall and pelvis, the pelvic pathological findings are evaluated. Often the rectosigmoid is stuck to the left adnexa and uterus. Each ovary may be stuck to its adjacent pelvic side-wall and uterosacral ligament, often with enclosed endometriomas.

Thus, the steps in endometriosis hysterectomy are to free all pelvic organs, then excise the endometriosis and, finally, remove the uterus. Deep fibrotic nodular endometriosis that involves the cul-de-sac requires cul-de-sac dissection down to the loose areolar tissue of the recto-

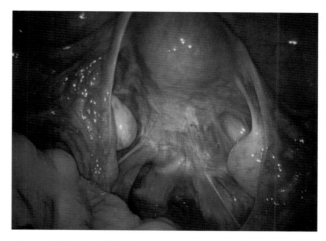

Figure 9.25 A Valtchev uterine manipulator (Conkin Surgical) elevates the uterus anteriorly, stretching out the cul-de-sac. Deep white fibrotic endometriosis is seen, with rectum stuck to posterior vagina and cervix

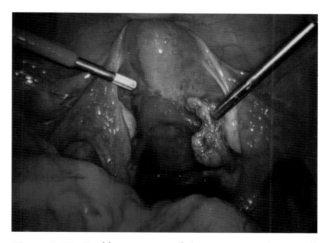

Figure 9.26 *En bloc* excision of the rectovaginal–cervical nodule is done using scissors

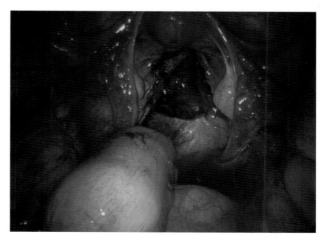

Figure 9.27 The rectal probe is advanced. Hemostasis is seen at the excision site

vaginal septum followed by excision of white fibronodular tissue from the uterosacral ligaments, posterior cervix, posterior vagina and anterior rectum. Less commonly, the sigmoid colon, its mesocolon and lateral rectum are involved[8].

First, rectosigmoid dissection is done starting at the pelvic brim and working downwards. Attention is then directed toward dissection of the anterior rectum from the posterior vagina and cervix throughout its area of attachment until loose areolar tissue in the rectovaginal space is reached. This technique leaves the bulk of the lesion to be excised on the posterior vagina, including some that was more closely associated with the rectum. Using the rectal probe as a guide to rectal location, the rectal serosa is opened at its junction with the cul-de-sac lesion with scissors or the CO_2 laser. Careful sharp and blunt dissection ensues until the rectum, normal or with contained fibrotic endometriosis, is separated from the posterior uterus, cervix and upper vagina. After anterior rectal mobilization is complete, excision of the fibrotic endometriosis from the posterior vagina (the location of which is continually confirmed by a sponge in the posterior fornix), posterior cervix, including its uterosacral ligament insertions, and rectum is done. This procedure is often accomplished *en bloc* as one large specimen, including the insertions of both uterosacral specimens laterally, the anterior rectal component inferiorly and the posterior cervix–vagina superiorly. The blunt scissors is the main instrument used for this excisional dissection, with the tissue to be removed kept on traction using toothed biopsy forceps.

The ureter lies lateral to most cul-de-sac lesions. When the uterosacral ligament is pulled medially, very little risk of ureteral damage exists. When a ureter is close to the lesion, its course is traced starting at the pelvic brim, and when necessary, the peritoneum overlying the ureter is opened to confirm the ureteral position deep in the pelvis.

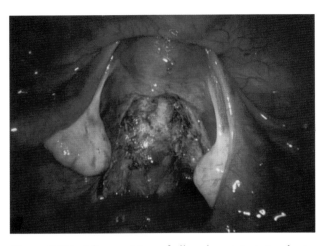

Figure 9.29 After excision of all endometriosis implants, hemostasis is achieved

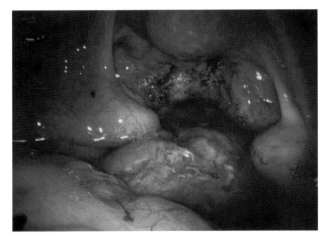

Figure 9.30 Following removal of the rectal stricture, air and dye are instilled via a Foley catheter into the rectum to check for occult perforation and devascularized areas

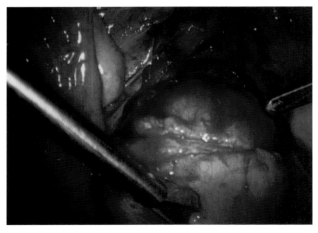

Figure 9.28 A fibrotic band of endometriosis remains across the rectum with resultant early stricture. This will be excised using cold scissors

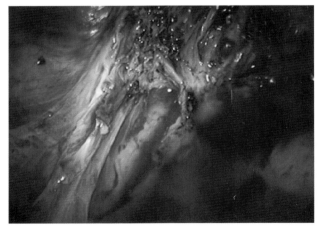

Figure 9.31 The left ureter is inspected and seen traversing the pelvic side wall

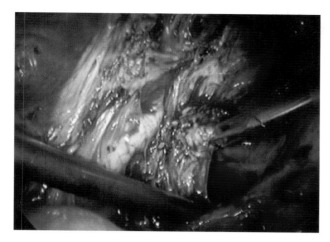

Figure 9.32 An endometriosis nodule just beneath the left ureter is excised

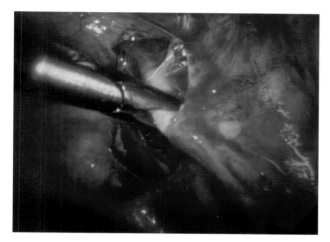

Figure 9.33 The right ureter is grasped and dissected with an atraumatic forceps and endometriosis overlying it excised

Uterosacral fibrotic endometriosis may envelop the ureter, necessitating deep ureteral dissection and excision of the surrounding endometriosis. Microbipolar forceps with irrigation between the tips are used to control arterial and venous bleeding around the ureter.

Uterosacral ligaments infiltrated with endometriosis are removed early in the operation, sometimes before rectal mobilization. They frequently make up a large portion of a rectal nodule. The uterosacral ligament is divided lateral to the rectum where the normal-caliber ligament meets the distended fibrotic ligament and is put on traction. The peritoneum is incised on both sides of the ligament, and the thickened portion of the ligament is excised to, and including, its insertion into the cervix. Soft, loose areolar tissue, adipose tissue, uterine vessels and the ureter are present beneath the ligament. Fibrotic tissue left at the periphery of the excision is coagulated with an irrigating microelectrode, especially at the junction of the cervix with the uterine fundus. Rarely, the ligament will be involved all the way to the sacrum. In these cases, it may be best to divide the middle of the ligament and, with traction on the sacral side of the ligament, pull it away from the rectum, ureter and hypogastric vessels.

Dissection of the fibrotic endometriosis from the thickened vaginal wall proceeds using traction with a biopsy forceps to pull the lesion from one side to the other. Laser, hydrodissection, electrosurgery or scissors are used as needed. Often, with traction and the help of vaginal distension from below using a vaginal sponge pushed forward by a ring forceps, a distinct dissection plane becomes evident above or beneath the rectovaginal fascia, and the lesion can be pulled free from the vaginal wall. Sometimes, an endopelvic rectovaginal fascial layer, infiltrated with endometriosis, is identified, and after this layer is excised, soft, pliable upper posterior vaginal wall is uncovered. Hypertrophied tissue without endometriosis is often present at the cervicovaginal junction between the insertion of the uterosacral ligaments into the cervix, making it difficult to distinguish accurately fibrotic endometriosis from fibromuscular tissue. This inverted 'u' configuration should be excised or at least biopsied.

Bowel surgery (Figures 9.34–9.39)

Endometriosis of the rectum and rectosigmoid may be superficial (serosal or adventitial), in the muscle (muscularis) or full thickness involving both the muscularis and lamina propria of the mucosa; the mucosal surface is rarely broken. The lesions are anterior or lateral. Posterior wall endometriosis is a rarity, but can form a 'napkin ring' deformity. Fibrotic endometriosis nodules infiltrating the anterior rectal wall are most common and may be focal (cicatrixal) or linear (a transverse bar often with associated stricture where the rectum is fused to the posterior vagina). Under the microscope, all these lesions, and those of the uterosacral ligaments, posterior vagina and cervix,

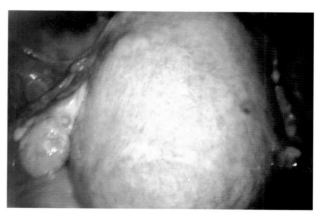

Figure 9.34 A large fibroid uterus fills the pelvis

Complications of laparoscopic hysterectomy are those of hysterectomy and laparoscopy combined: anesthetic accidents, respiratory compromise, thromboembolic phenomena, urinary retention and injury to vessels, ureters, bladder and bowel, as well as infections, especially of the vaginal cuff[21]. Ureteral injury is more common when staplers or bipolar desiccation are used without ureteral identification. Complications unique to laparoscopy include large vessel injury, epigastric vessel laceration, subcutaneous emphysema and trocar site incisional hernias[22]. Port site herniations are a rare event, typically occurring less than 1% of the time, with most occurring at extraumbilical sites following the use of 12-mm trocar sleeves for Endo GIA application.

Some of the above-listed complications that are related more to laparoscopic hysterectomy are discussed separately.

Infection

Febrile morbidity associated with a vaginal hysterectomy is about half that associated with the abdominal procedure. Laparoscopic evacuation of all blood clots and the sealing of all blood vessels after the uterus has been removed should further reduce the infection rate. Morcellation during laparoscopic or vaginal hysterectomy results in a slightly increased risk of fever, especially if prophylactic antibiotics are not used. Experience with serious wound infection after laparoscopic hysterectomy is rare.

Since the introduction of prophylactic antibiotics, vaginal cuff infection is rare. This infection can result in pelvic cellulitis, septicemia, vaginal cuff abscess, adnexal abscesses and pelvic thrombophlebitis. Abdominal trocar wound infection is also rare.

These authors' patients have experience with two cases of pelvic cellulitis and three pelvic abscesses in over 500 laparoscopic hysterectomies.

We now use one dose of a prophylactic antibiotic after induction of anesthesia in all cases. Interestingly, no antibiotic was administered in four of the five cases of infection. All of these cases involved a return to hospital and much patient dissatisfaction.

To decrease postoperative infection, the surgeon should evacuate all large clots, obtain absolute hemostasis and then carry out copious irrigation to dilute fibrin and prostaglandins arising from operated surfaces and bacteria. We believe that leaving 1–2 l of lactated Ringer's solution in the peritoneal cavity dilutes the peritoneal cavity bacterial and blood product counts, and prevents fibrin adherences from forming by separating raw, compromised surfaces during the initial stages of reperitonealization, especially after hysterectomy or bowel resection. No other antiadhesive agents are employed. No drains, antibiotic solutions or heparin are used.

Urinary tract infection, unexplained fever and pneumonia also are rare after LAH. Early cessation of both the Foley catheter and the intravenous line within 2 hours of the end of the operation, followed by early ambulation, may reduce postoperative atelectasis and urinary tract infections.

Hemorrhage

Intraoperative hemorrhage occurs when a previously non-anemic patient loses greater than 1000 ml of blood or requires a blood transfusion. By doing careful laparoscopic dissection, most profuse hemorrhage situations are avoided, or controlled as they occur.

Postoperative hemorrhage is any bleeding event that requires therapy, either conservative or operative. Postoperative hematomas were frequent with the early use of the Multifire Endo GIA 30 (US Surgical, Norwalk, CT) for the upper uterine pedicle during hysterectomy and oophorectomy.

Transfusion rates are often misleading, as they usually include autologous blood, which may be given back to the patient on a routine basis. Currently autologous blood is obtained rarely, because of the reluctance of most anesthesiologists to transfuse it.

Urinary tract complications: prevention and detection

Ureteral and bladder injuries may be expected with complicated cases, but are less suspected in routine operations, and failure to recognize them during these cases or suspect them early postoperatively results in much patient dissatisfaction. These injuries most commonly are associated with laparoscopic ligation of the uterine artery, but surgeons must be aware that both bladder and ureteral injury may occur during the 'easy' vaginal part of a LAVH.

While ureteral protection is advocated by all, how best to achieve it is hotly disputed. These authors remain committed to the prevention of ureteral injury intra-operatively by ureteral identification, often with dissection and by cystoscopy, at the conclusion of the procedure. Isolation by ureteral dissection has been criticized for unnecessarily adding time to the procedure, but this is time well spent if ureteral risk is diminished.

Ureteral stents are not used routinely, although both lighted and infrared catheters are available. Most patients who have stent placement experience postoperative hematuria; anuria from ureteral spasm following surgery with a stent in place has been reported. Ureteral catheters are necessary when ureteral injury occurs during surgical dissection or the release of a ureteral stricture; in these cases the stent is left in place for 6 weeks. Ureteral stricture can be treated by dividing the stricture longitudinally and closing it transversely, or by leaving the resultant uretero-tomy open over a JJ stent connecting the kidney to the bladder.

Cystoscopy is done in all hysterectomy cases after the vaginal cuff is closed, to check for ureteral patency and bladder injury. Failure to see dye through a ureter can result from ureteral ligation (placement of a suture into or around the ureter), kinking from pulling endopelvic ureteral fascia towards the midline during the high McCall culdoplasty or ureteral spasm if a ureteral stent was used. Cystoscopy also confirms bladder wall continuity, and detects intravesicular suture placement and thermal injury that will be seen as a patchy white area. Suture is used instead of staples or bipolar desiccation for uterine artery ligation, as suture can be removed if a ureteral obstruction or a bladder suture is noted on cystoscopy. This has been necessary on more than one occasion[23,24].

The ureters are commonly injured at the level of the infundibulopelvic ligament, uterosacral ligament or pelvic side-wall due to adhesions resulting from endometriosis, pelvic inflammatory disease or previous abdominal surgery. During laparoscopic hysterectomy, ureteral injury may occur while cutting dense adhesions and fibrotic scar tissue, while trying to stop bleeding close to the ureter with bipolar cautery or in the process of ligating the uterine vessels with bipolar electrosurgery, staples or suture. Most ureteral injuries are not identified or even suspected without cystoscopy. Without cystoscopic availability, one can expect problems. This is particularly true during TLH, even if the surgeon is visually able to identify the ureters. Normal peristalsis may occur in the damaged ureter.

In our experience, all but the grossest of ureteral injuries are discovered during the cystoscopic examination near the end of the operation. These injuries cannot usually be identified laparoscopically. If no dye is seen flowing from the ureter, the surgeon should first try to pass a ureteral catheter. If it passes without resistance the ureter is fine. If it does not pass, the surgeon should systematically trace the ureter down into the deep pelvis. Previously ligated vessels must be isolated, skeletonized and released from all ureteral attachments. Sometimes this entails release of the suture followed by religation. Continued attempts to pass the stent should be made while the laparoscopic dissection ensues. The dissection stops when the stent passes.

Careful techniques of bladder dissection are important. In difficult cases, the bladder may invaginate into a cesarean section scar and be surrounded by uterine myometrium. When the bladder location is obscured, the surgeon should fill it intermittently during the procedure to check its position and keep the dissection at its junction with uterine muscle.

Urinary retention is a common undetected complication. Most people who undergo general anesthesia experience some degree of temporary inability to contract their bladder musculature voluntarily. It can take weeks for the bladder to regain normal tone if retention occurs. Postoperative urinary retention is more likely with the use of large amounts of irrigant and hydroflotation, as urine can accumulate rapidly in the bladder of a drowsy patient recovering from anesthesia. The Foley catheter should not be removed at the end of operative procedures lasting longer than 2 hours until the patient is awake and aware that the catheter is in place, usually 1 hour postoperatively. In centers where intravenous fluids are not discontinued soon after the operation, the Foley catheter should be kept in longer. A useful protocol if spontaneous voiding does not occur within 3–4 hours after the catheter is removed is to carry out straight catheterization every 4 hours until spontaneous voiding occurs.

Some endoscopically related injuries to the urinary tract may not become apparent for a few days following surgery. Although the incidence of these complications is low, the surgeon should nevertheless be aware of the risks, and look for signs of such injuries that might have occurred. Unexplained fever, abdominal pain, back pain or abdominal distension may be signs of some injury and should be investigated.

Postoperative recognition of an insult to ureteral integrity is made early by obtaining a single-shot intravenous pyelogram (IVP) in anyone reporting lateralized pain of any kind – abdominal, flank or back. Uncontrollable loss of urine 1–2 weeks postoperatively requires an aggressive work-up to determine whether a ureterovaginal or vesicovaginal fistula is present. Treatment is with a Latzko operation for vesicovaginal fistula, and long-term catheter placement or surgical reimplantation for ureterovaginal fistula.

The bottom line is that an aggressive approach to ureteral protection can reduce but not eliminate ureteral injury. However, prompt recognition and management can prevent multiple surgical procedures and significant patient morbidity, including organ loss.

Bladder injury

Bladder injury can occur during dissection of the bladder off the uterus and cervix or from an inflamed adnexa. In these cases the bladder is repaired using Vicryl 3-0 usually in two layers.

Intravesicular thermal injury can be suspected by cystoscopic visualization of a white patch above the bladder trigone. The area should be reinforced with a laparoscopically placed suture into the bladder musculature surrounding the potential defect.

Bowel injury

Small-bowel injury during laparoscopic hysterectomy is uncommon, and is usually associated with extensive intraperitoneal adhesions. Small-bowel injuries can be suture-repaired. Small-bowel enterotomy may require mobilization from above, delivery through the umbilicus by extending the incision 1 cm and repair or resection. If the hole is confined to the antimesenteric portion, the bowel can be closed with interrupted 3-0 silk or Vicryl. All enterotomies are suture-repaired transversely to reduce the risk of stricture. If the hole involves greater than 50%

of the bowel circumference, resection is done. An extra-corporeal segmental enterectomy with side-to-side stapled anastomosis is preferred.

Rectal injury may occur during rectal endometriosis excision or during vaginal morcellation of a large fibroid uterus. Repair is the same as described above in the 'Endometriosis' hysterectomy section[14].

CONCLUSION

Laparoscopic hysterectomy is clearly beneficial for patients in whom vaginal surgery is contraindicated or cannot be done. When indications for the vaginal approach are equivocal, laparoscopy can be used to determine whether vaginal hysterectomy is possible. With this philosophy, patients avoid an abdominal incision with a resultant decrease in length of hospital stay and recuperation time. The complication of abdominal wound dehiscence can be eliminated and cuff infection reduced. Although laparoscopic hysterectomy is not without complications, the incidence is low, and many intra- and postoperative complications can be managed laparoscopically.

The laparoscopic surgeon should be aware of the risks and how to minimize them, and, when they occur, how to repair them laparoscopically. The participating surgeon's skill and experience with innovative techniques and instruments requires continuous training. All the anticipated advantages of laparoscopic hysterectomy can be lost if the surgeon ventures beyond his level of comfort.

REFERENCES

1. Reich H. Laparoscopic hysterectomy. Surg Laparosc & Endosc 1992; 2: 85–8
2. Liu CY. Laparoscopic hysterectomy: a review of 72 cases. J Reprod Med 1992; 37: 351–4
3. Liu CY. Laparoscopic hysterectomy. Report of 215 cases. Gynaecol Endosc 1992; 1: 73–7
4. Reich H, DeCaprio J, McGlynn F. Laparoscopic hysterectomy. J Gynecol Surg 1989; 5: 213–16
5. Johns DA, Carrera B, Jones J, et al. The medical and economic impact of laparoscopically assisted vaginal hysterectomy in a large, metropolitan, not-for-profit hospital. Am J Obstet Gynecol 1995; 172: 1709–19
6. Lower AM, Hawthorn RJS, Ellis H, et al. The impact of adhesions on hospital readmissions over ten years after 8849 open gynaecological operations. Br J Obstet Gynaecol 2000; 107: 855–62
7. Farquhar CM, Steiner CA. Hysterectomy rates in the United States 1990–1997. Obstet Gynecol 2002; 99: 229–34
8. Reich H, McGlynn F, Sekel L. Total laparoscopic hysterectomy. Gynaecol Endosc 1993; 2: 59–63
9. Kilkku P, Gronroos M, Hirvonen T, Rauramo L. Supravaginal uterine amputation vs. hysterectomy. Effects on libido and orgasm. Acta Obstet Gynecol Scand 1983; 62: 147–52
10. Lyons TL. Laparoscopic supracervical hysterectomy. A comparison of morbidity and mortality results with laparoscopically assisted vaginal hysterectomy. J Reprod Med 1993; 38: 763–7
11. Reich H, McGlynn F, Salvat J. Laparoscopic treatment of cul-de-sac obliteration secondary to retrocervical deep fibrotic endometriosis. J Reprod Med 1991; 36: 516–22
12. Redwine DB, Wright JT. Laparoscopic treatment of complete obliteration of the cul-de-sac associated with endometriosis: long-term follow-up of en bloc resection. Fertil Steril 2001; 76: 358–65
13. Cul-de-sac endometriosis. In Hulka J, Reich H, eds. Textbook of Laparoscopy, 3rd edn. Philadelphia: WB Saunders Company, 1998: 518–19, 405–6
14. Reich H, McGlynn F, Budin R. Laparoscopic repair of full-thickness bowel injury. J Laparoendosc Surg 1991; 1: 119–22
15. Reich H, Wood C, Whittaker M. Laparoscopic anterior resection of the rectum and hysterectomy in a patient with extensive pelvic endometriosis. Gynecol Endosc 1998; 7: 79–83
16. Bridgman SA, Dunn KM. Has endometrial ablation replaced hysterectomy for the treatment of dysfunctional uterine bleeding? National figures. Br J Obstet Gynaecol 2000; 107: 531–4
17. Clarke HC. Laparoscopy – new instruments for suturing and ligation. Fertil Steril 1972; 23: 274–7
18. Reich H, Clarke HC, Sekel L. A simple method for ligating in operative laparoscopy with straight and curved needles. Obstet Gynecol 1992; 79: 143–7
19. Wattiez A, Soriano D, Cohen SB, et al. The learning curve of total laparoscopic hysterectomy: comparative analysis of 1647 cases. J Am Assoc Gynecol Laparosc 2002; 9: 339–45
20. Makinen J, Johansson J, Tomas C, et al. Morbidity of 10,110 hysterectomies by type of approach. Hum Reprod 2001; 13: 431–6
21. Liu CY, Reich H. Complications of total laparoscopic hysterectomy in 518 cases. Gynaecol Endosc 1994; 3: 203–8
22. Kadar N, Reich H, Liu CY, et al. Incisional hernias after major laparoscopic gynecologic procedures. Am J Obstet Gynecol 1993; 168: 1493–5
23. Ribeiro S, Reich H, Rosenberg J. The value of intra-operative cystoscopy at the time of laparoscopic hysterectomy. Hum Reprod 1999; 14: 1727–9
24. Chapron C, Dubisson JB. Ureteral injuries after laparoscopic hysterectomy [Letter]. Hum Reprod 2000; 15: 733–4

Part 2
Tubal pathology and ovarian pathology

Fertiloscopy

A Watrelot

10

INTRODUCTION

The diagnosis of the cause of infertility is not always easy, especially when it is necessary to establish the status of the Fallopian tubes and the relationship between the tubes and the ovaries. Hysterosalpingography (HSG) is very often applied for this purpose, but this examination is of value only when it shows complete tubal blockage. In other cases, the rate of false negatives and even false positives is very high, as shown by laparoscopy. In a meta-analysis, Swart et al.[1] found a point estimate of 0.65 for HSG sensitivity and 0.83 for HSG specificity, and underlined the fact that HSG is not suitable for the evaluation of periadnexal adhesions.

By contrast, laparoscopy is considered the gold standard to explore tuboperitoneal infertility. Nevertheless, laparoscopy is very often performed without discovering any significant pathology.

Unfortunately, laparoscopy presents some risks that can be very serious, as recently shown in the French register of laparoscopic accidents, where six major injuries occurred in diagnostic laparoscopies[2]. The result is either a delay in laparoscopy, which can be detrimental to the patient, for instance if an in vitro fertilization (IVF) procedure is decided on the basis of a wrong diagnosis, or having to conduct a great number of normal laparoscopies, with the potential risks that accompany such procedures.

Other diagnostic procedures, such as hysterosonography or falloposcopy, are not sufficiently accurate to warrant a therapeutic strategy. Culdoscopy could have been an alternative method, but was abandoned in the 1970s in its classic version, in favor of laparoscopy.

More recent improvements have been suggested, such as the use of dorsal decubitus[3], hydroflotation[4] and transvaginal hydrolaparoscopy, which provides very good imaging of the pelvis[5].

Following this initial work, we defined the concept of fertiloscopy[6–8] as the combination of transvaginal hydropelviscopy, a dye test, salpingoscopy, microsalpingoscopy and, finally, hysteroscopy performed under strict local anesthesia (Figure 10.1).

TECHNIQUE

Instrumentation

Single-use introducers

Fertiloscopy uses specific instrumentation of the single-use type. The rest of the equipment is the same as that used for gynecological laparoscopy, even if a special scope is required to exploit all the possibilities afforded by fertiloscopy.

Specially designed disposable introducers are the key to performing fertiloscopy. They come in a kit containing two introducers, one for the uterine cavity and the other for the pouch of Douglas (Figure 10.2).

The uterine introducer (FH 1.29; www.fertiloscopy.com) is fitted with a balloon in order to ensure a good seal during the dye test. It also has a smooth mandrel to allow easy insertion into the uterine cavity. Once in place, the mandrel is removed, and, due to the flexible nature of the introducer, it can be fixed to the patient's thigh with the Velcro® provided.

The Douglas introducer (FTO 1.40; www.fertiloscopy.com) has three channels. The central one is equipped

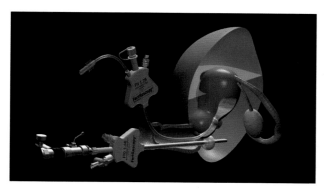

Figure 10.1 Principle of fertiloscopy

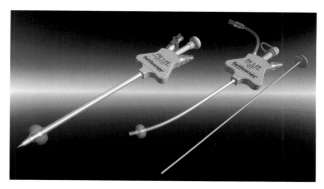

Figure 10.2 Fertiloscopy® introducers

115

with a sharp mandrel to enable insertion into the pouch of Douglas. It is then replaced by the telescope. The second channel allows inflation of the balloon located at the tip of the introducer. The balloon is of paramount importance: first, it prevents the introducer from slipping involuntarily out of the abdominal cavity; second, by pulling on the introducer, the pouch of Douglas can be stretched, providing a better view; third, the balloon acts as a ball-joint from which the telescope can be angled in every direction. The last lumen is an operative channel allowing the use of 5F instrumentation as an outflow channel (Figure 10.3).

Veress needle

A Verres needle is necessary, and it is possible to use either a disposable or a reusable one. The important point is to ensure that the safety mechanism works normally.

Fertiloscope

To perform fertiloscopy, it is necessary for the telescope to have a diameter not greater than 4 mm and a 30° lens. In practice, the use of the Hamou II telescope (Storz, Germany) is strongly recommended for several reasons: its 2.9-mm diameter, 30° foroblique vision and ×120 magnification make it the only telescope capable of performing microsalpingoscopy (Figure 10.4).

Additional instrumentation

The Douglas introducer has an operative channel allowing the use of 5F instrumentation. Biopsy forceps, grasping forceps and scissors are used (Figures 10.5 and 10.6).

Bipolar coagulation (which is the only electrical option with a saline medium) is also useful, by means of electrode or bipolar forceps.

Room set-up

The patient needs to be in the gynecological position. The Trendelenburg position is not required, and slight procubitus is even recommended. Monitors and cold light are installed on a mobile videocart located to the left of the patient. Saline solution is administered from the right by means of a standard infusion set-up.

Technique

The technique of fertiloscopy is rather simple. Nevertheless, it has to be very precise if one is to avoid problems.

Preparation of the patient

Preparation of the colon is useful in order to deflate it and, thus, to increase the safety space in the pouch of Douglas.

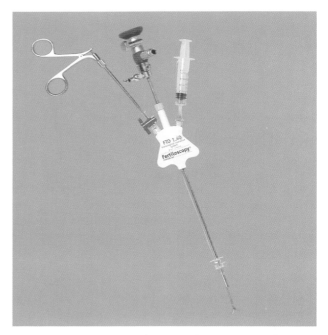

Figure 10.3 FTO 1.40 device with Hamou II telescope, syringe and grasping forceps

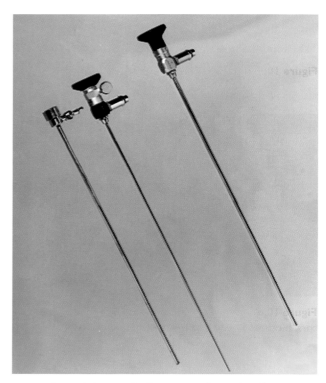

Figure 10.4 Hamou II telescope with its sheath

In practice, a mini-enema such as Normacol® is commonly used.

Careful vaginal examination has to be performed prior to fertiloscopy in order to detect any obstructive Douglas pathology, such as a pelvic mass prolapsed in the cul-de-

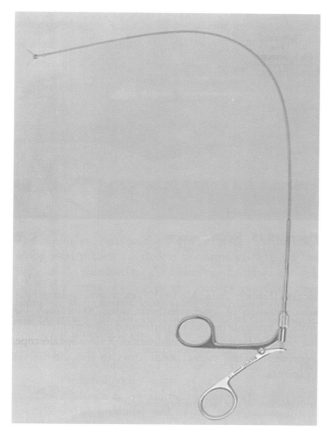

Figure 10.5 Special atraumatic grasping forceps

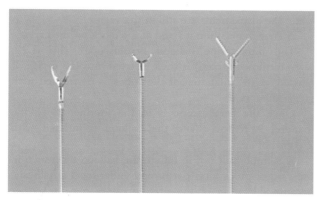

Figure 10.6 5F instrumentation. From left to right: scissors, biopsy forceps, grasping forceps

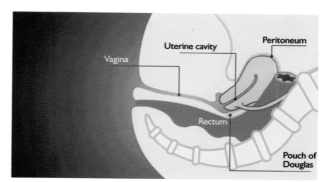

Figure 10.7 Sagittal section of the pelvis

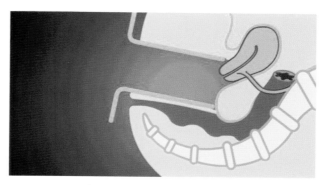

Figure 10.8 The cervix is exposed

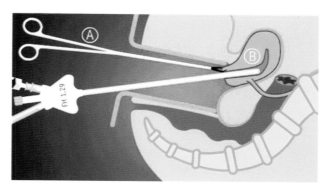

Figure 10.9 (A) Pozzi forceps are attached at 8 o'clock. (B) The uterine introducer is inserted (FH 1.29)

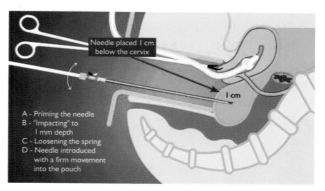

Figure 10.10 Insertion of the Veress needle and creation of a hydroperitoneum with saline solution

sac, or endometriosis of the rectovaginal septum, which are contraindications to the technique (Figures 10.7–10.15).

Anesthesia

Fertiloscopy can be performed either under general anesthesia, or under strict local anesthesia without any general sedation. Here, we describe the technique of local anesthesia. We start by inserting an anesthetic gel into the

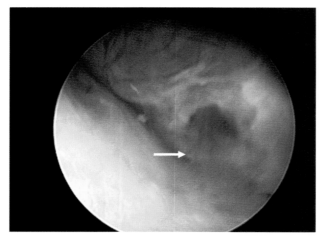

Figure 10.19 Ovulation: note the follicular fluid, indicated by an arrow

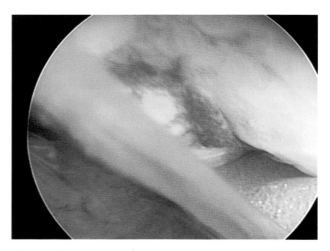

Figure 10.22 Corpus luteum

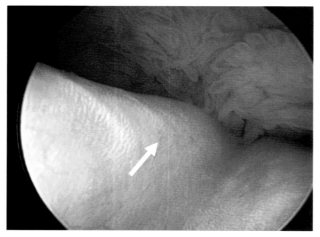

Figure 10.20 Right uterosacral ligament (arrow) and fimbria

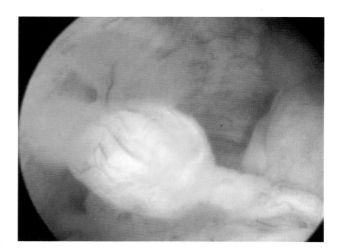

Figure 10.23 Accessory tube

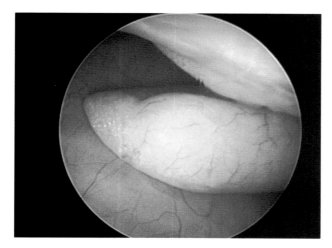

Figure 10.21 Appendix

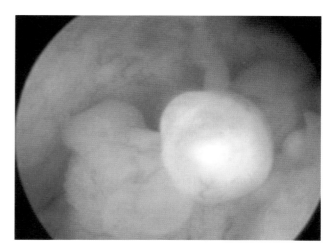

Figure 10.24 Paratubal cyst

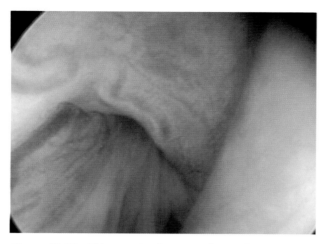

Figure 10.25 Phimosis (under magnification)

telescope, by entering the space between the ovary and the fossa ovarica and rotating the scope on its axis.

The tube can be followed from the isthmus to the ampulla and the fimbria. Due to the inverted view, the tube appears to be located internally to the ovary, which initially can be disorientating.

If visualization of any structure is difficult, it is necessary to wait until more liquid has been instilled, which will improve the view. It is also necessary to move the telescope in all directions, not forgetting forward and backward movements.

The dye test (Figure 10.26)

When all the genital structures have been recognized, the dye test can be performed. Dye is instilled through the appropriate channel of the uterine introducer. A 20-ml syringe is connected, and the dye should be administered gently in order to avoid tubal spasms. The dye is visualized at the fimbria, and it is necessary to move from one side to the other to be sure of bilateral patency.

Salpingoscopy (Figures 10.27–10.36)

Salpingoscopy is known to be a very useful means of investigating the tube[9]. Brosens *et al.*[10], for instance, clearly demonstrated its value in intratubal adhesion pathology. Brosens *et al.*[11] described a salpingoscopic score, which is useful for classifying the findings. Nevertheless, routine salpingoscopy is rarely performed during laparoscopy

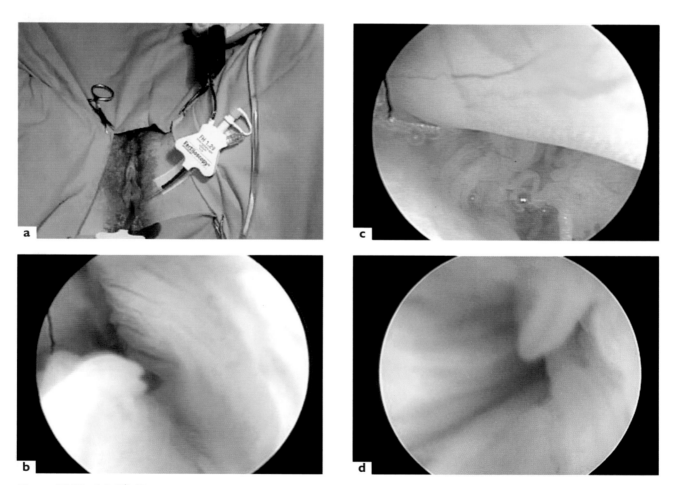

Figure 10.26 (a)–(d) Dye test

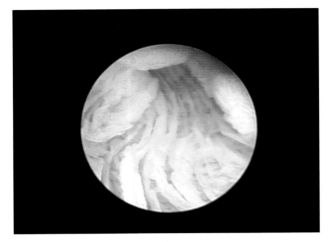

Figure 10.27 Salpingoscopy: panoramic view

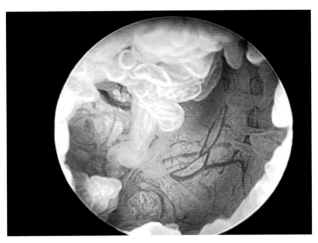

Figure 10.30 Salpingoscopy: flattened folds

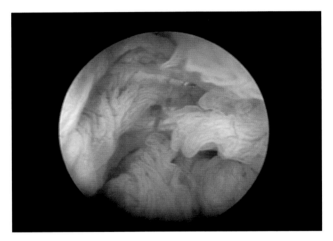

Figure 10.28 Salpingoscopy

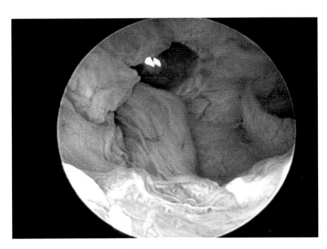

Figure 10.31 Ampulla

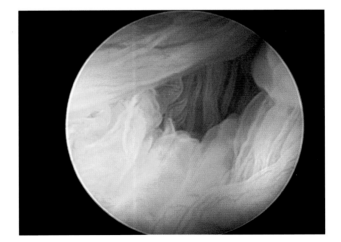

Figure 10.29 Salpingoscopy

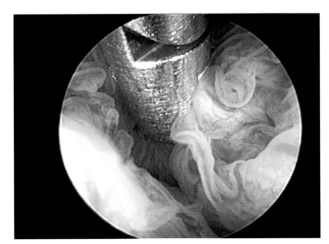

Figure 10.32 Grasping the fimbria

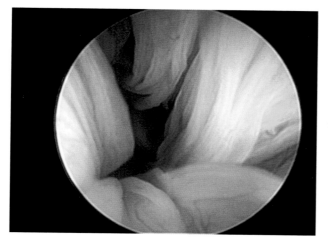

Figure 10.33 Major folds

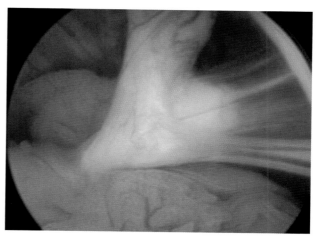

Figure 10.36 Intrafimbrial adhesion

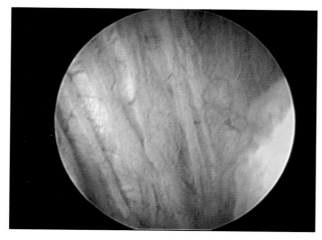

Figure 10.34 Minor folds

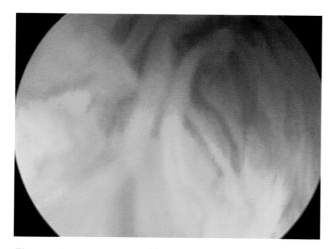

Figure 10.35 Intra-ampullary adhesions

because it is necessary to use a second telescope and an additional cold light source, video camera, monitor and irrigation. In contrast, salpingoscopy is very easily performed during fertiloscopy with the same telescope, due to the position of the fimbria and use of a small telescope. The technique is simple, and involves stabilizing the fimbria by means of grasping forceps introduced into the operative channel. Then, by gently pushing the telescope into the fimbria, it is possible to enter the ampulla and reach the isthmoampullary junction. During the whole procedure, it is necessary to irrigate the tube, through the sheath of the telescope. A tap located on the sheath allows for in-flow adjustment, to avoid too much pressure on the ampulla. By rotating the telescope on its axis, and thanks to the 30° lens, each portion of the ampulla can be examined. All pathological findings can be identified, such as intra-ampullary adhesions or flattened folds. These findings are of great importance when deciding whether surgical repair of a damaged tube is warranted, or whether IVF is a better option.

Microsalpingoscopy (Figures 10.37–10.46)

As we have seen, salpingoscopy is of great value when a tube is blocked, to investigate whether it can be repaired. More often, patent tubes are discovered at the time of fertiloscopy. In these cases, and according to the work of Marconi and Quintana[12], it is interesting to have a more precise evaluation of the tubal epithelium. This can be obtained by performing microsalpingoscopy.

Microsalpingoscopy is possible, owing to the Hamou II telescope (Storz, Germany), which allows a magnification up to ×180 by rotating the wheel near the eyepiece.

Microsalpingoscopy is performed after the dye test, making it possible to examine the number of dye-stained nuclei on the tubal epithelium, which are either intermediary cells on the epithelium or inflammatory cells

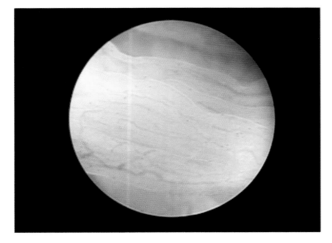

Figure 10.37 Microsalpingoscopy: stage 1

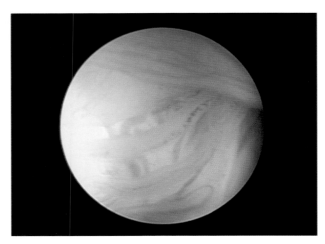

Figure 10.40 Microsalpingoscopy: stage 2

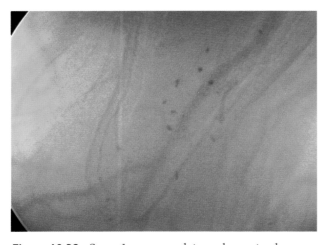

Figure 10.38 Stage 1: some nuclei are dye-stained

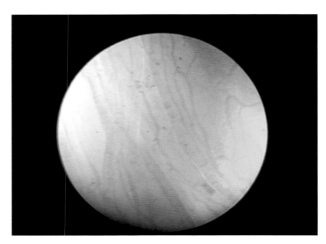

Figure 10.41 Stage 2

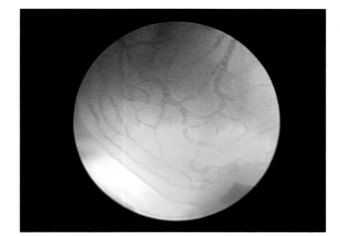

Figure 10.39 Stage 1

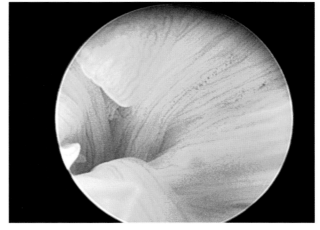

Figure 10.42 Stage 2: dye-stained nuclei are sometimes visible by simple salpingoscopy (without magnification)

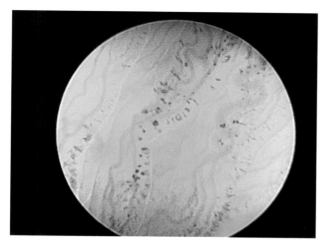

Figure 10.43   Microsalpingoscopy: stage 3

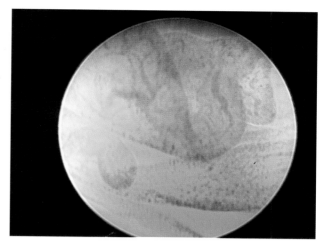

Figure 10.45   Microsalpingoscopy: stage 4: all edges of the folds show many dye-stained nuclei

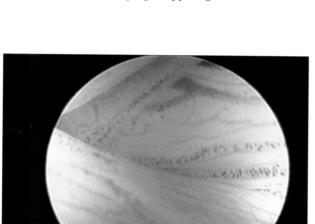

Figure 10.44   Stage 3

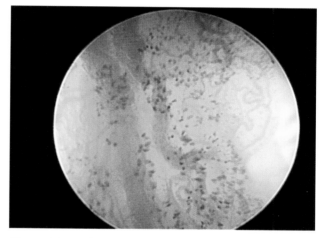

Figure 10.46   Stage 4: mastocytes (between the mucosal folds) and epithelial cells (on edges of the folds) are dye-stained

(mastocytes) in the middle of the tubal folds. According to Marconi and Quintana[12], the number of dye-stained nuclei allows classification of the tubes into four stages, from normal (stage 1) where no nuclei are dye-stained, to pathological (stage 4) where a great number of cells appear to be dye-stained. Such aspects can be confirmed by taking a microbiopsy with 5F biopsy forceps.

Hysteroscopy (Figures 10.47–10.49)

Hysteroscopy is the last step of the procedure. It is carried out using the same scope. Endometrial biopsy is performed at this time if any pathology is suspected.

Operative fertiloscopy

Even if the main aim of fertiloscopy is diagnostic, operative fertiloscopy is a new challenge.

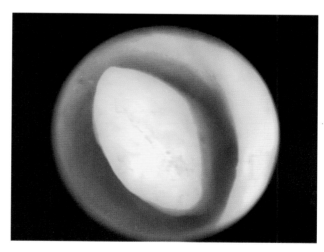

Figure 10.47   Uterine polyp

randomized for the procedure they were to carry out. The procedures were video-recorded and reviewed by two independent investigators. This protocol was submitted for approval by the ethics committee, according to the French Huriet law.

Eighty-two cases were recorded, and the main statistical analysis was a concordance study using the κ score for six sites (both tubes, both ovaries, peritoneum and uterus), leading to a comparison of 492 different sites. The κ score for each site was between 0.75 and 0.91, allowing us to conclude that the concordance between fertiloscopy and laparoscopy was excellent. Thus, the main conclusion of the study was that: 'fertiloscopy should replace diagnostic laparoscopy in infertile patients with no obvious pathology'.

Although it was, to the best of our knowledge, the first time that two endoscopic methods had been evaluated in such a prospective manner, we must underline the fact that salpingoscopy and microsalpingoscopy were not taken into account, due to the difficulties involved in performing salpingoscopy routinely during laparoscopy.

Is fertiloscopy safe and reproducible?

Its reproducibility has already been demonstrated in numerous studies, including our own 1500 consecutive cases.

Safety is a concern, since the risk of bowel injury exists. Insertion of the Verres needle, then the fertiloscope, should be performed between the cervix and the rectum. Safety is, thus, mainly prevention.

In the case of nodules, mucosal attraction or fixed uterine retroversion, fertiloscopy may need to be canceled. The detection of such conditions is essentially clinical; careful vaginal examination before fertiloscopy is critical. Ultrasound scanning may help in some cases, but does not replace clinical evaluation.

If a rectal injury should occur, and if it is of small diameter (less than 5 mm) and located beneath the peritoneum, the treatment is always conservative, using antibiotics for a few days. Indeed, there is absolutely no need to perform a further laparoscopy or a laparotomy, as demonstrated by the study of Gordts et al.[16].

Is fertiloscopy only diagnostic?

It was at the beginning. Today, thanks to the operative channel (see above), we are able to perform proper adhesiolysis, and treatment of minimal endometriosis, which consequently decreases the number of laparoscopic conversions. This is why we increasingly propose performing fertiloscopy under general sedation (similar to oocyte pick-up in IVF) in order to carry out surgery at the same time.

In fact, depending on the health system, fertiloscopy is performed either as a strict office procedure (with local anesthesia), in which case a further operation will be required if pathology is detected, or in an outpatient unit where operative fertiloscopy is possible.

Another possibility is performing ovarian drilling in PCOS patients. Many therapeutic options are already available for PCOS patients, with drugs such as metformin. Nevertheless, the attraction of surgical ovarian drilling is immediate efficacy, lack of ovarian hyperstimulation syndrome (OHSS) and a decrease in miscarriages.

Performed through fertiloscopy, ovarian drilling is very fast and safe, and also allows a thorough evaluation of the pelvic tract at the same time.

Due to the success of IVF, is there still interest in endoscopic evaluation of infertile patients?

Indeed, there is no use in certain circumstances, for instance when infertility is due only to severe sperm deficiency.

In other cases, many IVF doctors claim that HSG is sufficient because, in the end, IVF will be the only option for these couples.

We strongly disagree with this opinion, however. First, HSG is well known for its limitations (around 15% of false positives and 35–40% of false negatives). It is therefore of great interest to detect pelvic abnormalities such as endometriosis or adhesions, as the treatment of these lesions leads to a good pregnancy rate. Furthermore, increasing numbers of young couples are keen to obtain pregnancy in a physiological way.

We believe that, after an era of mainly IVF-focused solutions, it is now time to re-evaluate our practice thanks to new minimally invasive options such as fertiloscopy.

REFERENCES

1. Swart P, Mol BW, Van Beurden M, et al. The accuracy of hysterosalpingography in the diagnosis of tubal pathology: a meta-analysis. Fertil Steril 1995; 64: 486–91

2. Chapron C, Querleu D, Bruhat MA, et al. Surgical complications of diagnostic and operative gynaecologic laparoscopy: a series of 29966 cases. Hum Reprod 1998; 13: 867–72

3. Mintz M. Actualisation de la culdoscopie transvaginale en décubitus dorsal. Un nouvel endoscope à vision directe muni d'une aiguille à ponction incorporée dans l'axe. Contr Fertil Sex 1987; 15: 401–4

4. Odent M. Hydrocolpotomie et hydroculdoscopie. Nouv Press Med 1973; 2: 187

5. Gordts S, Campo R, Rombauts L, Brosens I. Transvaginal hydrolaparoscopy as an outpatient procedure for infertility investigation. Hum Reprod 1998; 13: 99–103

6. Watrelot A, Gordts S, Andine JP, Brosens I. Une nouvelle approche diagnostique: la fertiloscopie. Endomag 1997; 21: 7–8

7. Watrelot A, Dreyfus JM, Andine JP. Fertiloscopy; first results (120 case report). Fertil Steril 1998; 70 (Suppl): S-42

8. Watrelot A, Dreyfus JM, Andine JP. Evaluation of the performance of fertiloscopy in 160 consecutive infertile patients with no obvious pathology. Hum Reprod 1999; 14: 707–11

9. Surrey E. Microendoscopy of the human fallopian tube. J Am Assoc Gynecol Laparosc 1999; 6: 383–90

10. Brosens I, Campo R, Gordts S. Office hydro-laparoscopy for the diagnosis of endometriosis and tubal infertility. Curr Opin Obstet Gynecol 1999; 11: 371–7

11. Brosens I, Boeckx W, Delattin P, et al. Salpingoscopy: a new preoperative diagnosis in tubal infertility. Br J Obstet Gynaecol 1987; 94: 768–73

12. Marconi G, Quintana R. Methylene blue dyeing of cellular nuclei during salpingoscopy, a new in vivo method to evaluate vitality of tubal epithelium. Hum Reprod 1998; 13: 3414–17

13. Fernandez H, Alby JD. De la culdoscopie à la fertilo-scopie opératoire. Endomag 1999; 21: 5–6

14. Watrelot A, Dreyfus JM. Explorations intra-tubaires au cours de la fertiloscopie. Reprod Hum Horm 2000; 12: 39–44

15. Watrelot A, Nisolle M, Hocke C, et al. Is laparoscopy still the gold standard in infertility assessment? A comparison of fertiloscopy versus laparoscopy in infertility. Hum Reprod 2003; 18: 834–9

16. Gordts S, Watrelot A, Campo R, Brosens I. Risks and outcome of bowel injury during transvaginal pelvic endoscopy. Fertil Steril 2001; 76: 1238–41

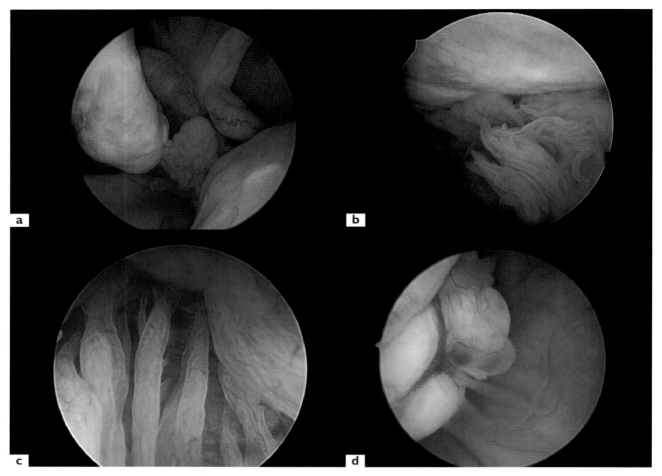

Figure 11.2 The use of Ringer's lactate as distension medium keeps the organs afloat. Without supplementary manipulation, tubo-ovarian structures can be inspected accurately (a) in their normal position. When indicated, a patency test and salpingoscopy can be done (b) and (c). In the absence of high intra-abdominal pressure, subtle lesions on peritoneal and ovarian surfaces can be visualized (d)

FEASIBILITY, ACCURACY AND ACCEPTABILITY

We reported[8], in a consecutive series of 663 patients, no pathology, or pathology of minor clinical significance, in 66.6% of them. In the case of pathology this was mainly endometriosis (33.4%), tubo-ovarian adhesions (28%), hydrosalpinges, benign ovarian cysts, (evaluation of tubal status after) sterilization and subserous myoma.

Some minor complications occurred in this series: inadvertent puncture of the posterior side of the uterus in five patients and bleeding of the vaginal insertion site in one patient. Needle perforation of the rectum occurred in five patients (0.7%) without consequences.

Rectal perforation could be a potentially serious complication of transvaginal access. In a survey of 3667 procedures[9] the incidence of bowel perforation was 0.65%, which decreased after initial experience to 0.25%. However, no delayed diagnosis and sepsis occurred, and all cases except for one were managed conservatively with

antibiotics. Analysis of the occurrence of complications as a function of experience confirmed the importance of the learning curve, with a clear decline of complications and failed access after 50 procedures. Routine vaginal examination and vaginal ultrasound to exclude pathology of the pouch of Douglas are strongly recommended to avoid complications.

Our access failure rate was 3.4% (n = 23), including also our failures in the initial learning period. These findings correspond with the reported experience of others (Table 11.1)[9–15].

In a recently published study of 1000 procedures, Verhoeven et al.[16] reported 32 failures (3.2%), with failed access in 11 patients (1.1%) and absent or poor visualization in 21 patients (2.1%). Bowel perforation occurred in five patients (0.5%).

Acute clinical conditions (bleeding, infection), an obliterated cul-de-sac or a large ovarian cyst are also strict contraindications to the transvaginal approach (Table 11.2).

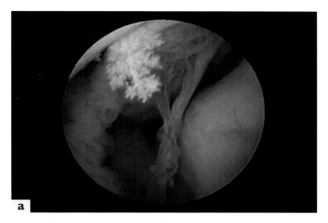
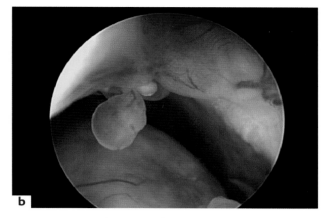

Figure 11.3 In the absence of high intra-abdominal pressure, using prewarmed Ringer's lactate as distension medium enables the visualization of subtle lesions upon the ovarian surface: (a) crystalloid-appearing lesion, diagnosed at histology as a papilloma; (b) small polypoid endometriotic lesion

Table 11.1 Failure of access and complication rates at transvaginal laparoscopy

Authors	n	Access failure (%)	Complications (%)
Gordts et al., 2005[9]	663	3.5	0.9
Watrelot et al., 1999[10]	160	3.8	0.6
Darai et al., 2000[11]	60	10	1.9
Moore et al., 2002[12]	40	0	0
Shibahara et al., 2001[13]	41	7.3	0
Dechaud et al., 2001[14]	23	4.3	0
Moore et al., 2003[15]	109	0.9	0.9
Verhoeven et al., 2004[16]	1000	3.2	0.5

Evaluating the acceptability of the procedure, it has been documented that the procedure was well tolerated by patients[17]. On an analog pain rating scale from 0 to 10 for transvaginal laparoscopy performed in an office setting under local anesthesia, the mean pain score was 2.7 (standard deviation ± 1.5) on a 10-cm visual pain scale. Only five (8%) of the patients marked a score above 5, and 96% of the patients regarded a repeat procedure under the same circumstances as acceptable. Moore and Cohen[18] found, in 17 patients who received conscious sedation, a pain score for cannula insertion, mid-procedure and end of procedure of 2.1, 1.4 and 0.5, respectively.

'One-stop fertility clinic'

With the availability of small, high-quality endoscopes, a complete exploration can now be performed in 1 day. The 'one-stop fertility clinic' is based on transvaginal endoscopy (TVE), and includes a mini-hysteroscopy, transvaginal laparoscopy, chromopertubation test, fimbrioscopy and, when indicated, salpingoscopy[19]. All procedures can

Table 11.2 Contraindications to transvaginal laparoscopy

Narrow vagina
Fixed retroverted uterus
Obliterated pouch of Douglas
Induration of posterior fornix
Acute situation (bleeding, infection)

be performed in the same session under local anesthesia or sedation, in an outpatient setting, using the 2.9-mm endoscope. Prior to attendance, all referred patients receive an information pack, and are asked to complete a detailed medical questionnaire. Non-referred patients are obviously first seen and examined at the routine clinic, and also receive full information and are requested to complete the questionnaire.

On the same day, a sperm examination and the necessary blood analyses can be performed. With the

Herschlag et al.[42], attempting to correlate salpingoscopic findings (including evaluation of the mucosal-fold architecture) with histology, demonstrated a good correlation, but only in cases of mild and severe disease. Our surgical stance depends on a combination of these first two prognostic factors, i.e. the degree of distal occlusion and the preservation of ampullary folds, as assessed by hysterosalpingography[27,43].

Detection of intratubal adhesions

Intratubal adhesions are detected only at falloscopy and/or tuboscopy. The formation of intratubal adhesions is one consequence, among others, of an underlying inflammatory process. It is not recognized specifically as a major prognostic factor, probably because the use of tuboscopy is not generalized. Herschlag et al.[42], however, include this parameter in their tuboscopic score. No intrauterine pregnancy was reported in the presence of intratubal adhesions by De Bruyne et al.[23] in the presence of intratubal adhesions in a series of 17 patients, despite an overall intrauterine pregnancy rate of 59% in their study. Vasquez et al.[30] also clearly addressed this issue; in a multicenter study of 50 patients, it was concluded that mucosal adhesions in thin-walled hydrosalpinges are the most important factor in determining fertility outcome. Indeed, the presence and absence of intratubal adhesions were associated with intrauterine pregnancy rates following surgery of 22% and 58%, respectively, thus differing significantly. The rate of ectopic pregnancy was 11% if adhesions had previously been discovered; this condition is seriously affected by a significant risk of ectopic gestation, as was also stressed by Marana et al.[44].

Evaluation of the tubal mucosa

The tubal mucosa can be assessed endoscopically, and the observations are often included in various scoring classifications[6,27,29,31,39]. Apart from the various features already reviewed above, macroscopic evaluation of the tubal mucosa attempts to determine the tubal wall thickness[31], and also to distinguish areas of normal-appearing mucosa on the tubal wall, the inflammatory aspect of the epithelium and the underlying vascularization. We pointed out[6,10] that the smaller is the area of normal mucosal surface observed under the operative microscope, the lower is the incidence of intrauterine pregnancy. The difference was clearly significant when the cut-off level was determined at 50% of normal-appearing mucosal surface.

Histological data in tubal infertility are available from some authors[10,45], who have studied the histophysiopathological factors of distal tubal occlusions and correlated their findings with pregnancy outcome.

The ciliation index

The ciliation index has proved to be valuable in the prognosis of tubal surgery[3,10,45]. In our original study in which we investigated the prognostic factors of fimbrial microsurgery in 215 patients[27], the ciliated cell percentage, as evaluated on fimbrial microbiopsy, and the pregnancy outcome were significantly decreased in the case of degree III and IV distal occlusion, compared with degree I and II. In our study, the ciliation index was related to the pregnancy rate after microsurgical correction of the distal occlusion.

Fibrosis and the thickness of the tubal wall

Long-standing evolution of hydrosalpinges sometimes leads to invasion of the muscularis by fibrosis, which is responsible for a significant thickening of the tubal wall and ultimately results in so-called thick-walled hydrosalpinx. Vasquez et al.[30] have correlated the incidence of thick-walled hydrosalpinx with histological parameters: in thick-walled hydrosalpinges, the thickness of the tubal wall measures 2–10 mm at the thinnest part and 4–10 mm at the thickest part. Thick-walled hydrosalpinx is usually associated with other unfavorable macro- and microscopic features, explaining the very poor results of fertility-promoting surgery. In our series[27], the intrauterine pregnancy rate for this type of tubal pathology was 0%, as also obtained by some other authors[1–3,30,40]. The recommended approach in this case is to perform a salpingectomy at the time of laparoscopy, in an attempt to enhance the results of IVF[46] and to limit the incidence of tubal gestation, reported to be as high as 11% in tubal infertility patients undergoing IVF[47].

Extratubal factors

Adnexal adhesions and endometriosis are sometimes included in the list of prognostic factors affecting pregnancy rates.

Periadnexal adhesions

The significance of pelvic adhesions is controversial in the prognosis of patients with tubal factors. Studies by several authors[2,28,38,39] suggest that the fertility prognosis correlates with the presence of tubal adhesions and degree of severity. Some investigators[48,49] restrict the negative influence of adhesions to severe cases only; frozen pelvis is still considered as a contraindication to conservative surgery. Nevertheless, it should be noted that microsurgical or laparoscopic adhesiolysis alone has been shown to promote fertility[28,43,50], implicating adhesions in mechanical infertility.

The most recent series, however, appear to challenge the role of adhesions in impairing fertility following surgery. Dubuisson et al.[40], in a series of 90 patients undergoing laparoscopic salpingostomy, failed to show any relationship between adhesion score and pregnancy outcome. Canis *et al.*[9] did not note any significant difference in their group of 87 laparoscopic tuboplasties as far as gross pregnancy and monthly fecundity rates were concerned. The implication of periadnexal adhesions has also recently been questioned by Vasquez *et al.*[30] in a prospectively designed study.

After tubal infections, periadnexal adhesions can be associated with perihepatic adhesions (Fitz–Hugh–Curtis Syndrome; Figure 12.5).

Endometriosis

Endometriosis has rarely been taken into account in the evaluation of the success of tubal surgery. The most recent study in this respect is by Dlugi *et al.*[49], who, on treating 113 patients with tubal factors and comparing pregnancy curves, concluded that endometriosis-related tubal occlusion was less detrimental than post-pelvic inflammatory disease or post-surgical tubal distal occlusion. Obviously, treating any concomitant endometriosis at the time of tubal surgery already improves fertility outcome, and can therefore modulate the actual implication of endometriosis as a prognostic factor for successful tuboplasty.

This finding is corroborated by Nezhat *et al.*[51], who found no significantly abnormal results using tuboscopy in a population of 100 patients with endometriosis. This might suggest a better inner tubal condition in distal tubal occlusion of endometriotic origin, compared with distal tubal occlusion of inflammatory etiology, where mucosal impairment is probably more pronounced.

TECHNIQUES AND RESULTS

Tubal occlusion: degree I

Fimbrioplasty is also carried out during laparoscopy. When fimbrial adhesions are found as the blue dye begins to spill

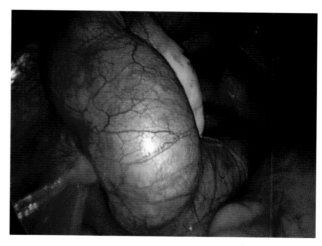

Figure 12.6 Hydrosalpinx: tubal occlusion of degree III; laparoscopic view

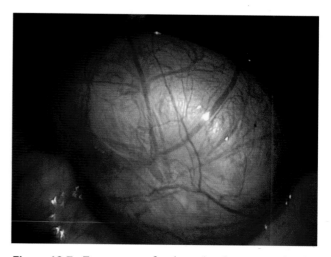

Figure 12.7 Exposure of the distal part of the hydrosalpinx

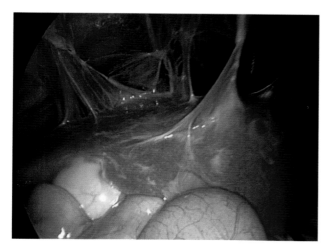

Figure 12.5 Perihepatic adhesions

out through the open tube, these adhesions between the fimbrial folds are carefully grasped by means of a probe with a hook passed through a third-puncture trocar, and cut in a bloodless fashion with the finely focused CO$_2$ beam set at 40 W. Thereafter, a defocused beam (10 W) is used to cause blanching of the serosa.

The SurgiTouch™ is useful for this purpose. It allows adequate eversion of the mucosa and prevents any recurrence of adhesions.

Tubal occlusion: degrees II, III and IV

Salpingostomy can be performed with the CO$_2$ laser, and is indicated in cases of thin-walled hydrosalpinx where both proximal tubal patency and the presence of ampullary folds have been confirmed by a hysterosalpingogram (Figure 12.6).

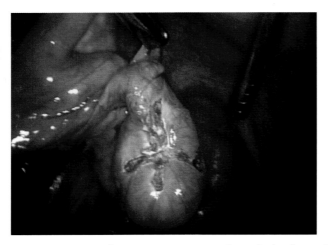

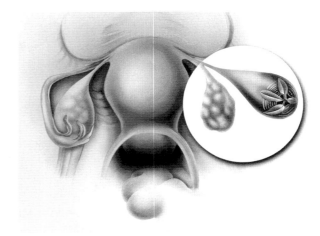

Figure 12.8 Two linear incisions are made with the focused beam

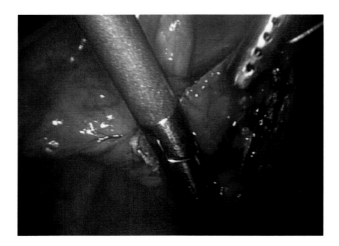

Figure 12.9 The opened tube is gently grasped

Two grasping forceps are introduced for traction and manipulation of the ampullary–fimbrial segment. The blocked tube is held so that the focused laser beam can be aligned at a 90° angle to the dimple (Figure 12.7).

The laser is set to continuous mode (40 W) and two linear incisions are made (Figure 12.8), cutting from the anterior to the posterior part along blood vessels.

As soon as the lumen is entered, the tube collapses; continuous dye injection keeps it distended. Only then is the incision enlarged. At this point, the probes and grasping forceps gently hold the incision edges (Figure 12.9) and a reduced-power (10–15 W), defocused beam (SurgiTouch) is used to evert the serosal aspect of the incised edge (Figure 12.10).

The final aspect of the tube reveals a well-everted fimbria, and, if performed, ampulloscopy reveals the presence of well-vascularized ampullary folds (Figure 12.11). At the end of the procedure, the peritoneal cavity is irrigated with Ringer's solution to remove carbonized particles.

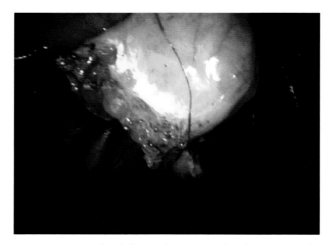

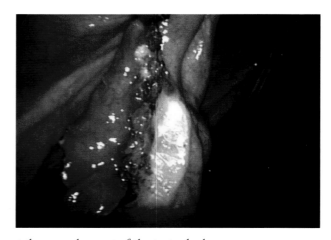

Figure 12.10 The defocused SurgiTouch™ beam is used to evert the serosal aspect of the incised edge

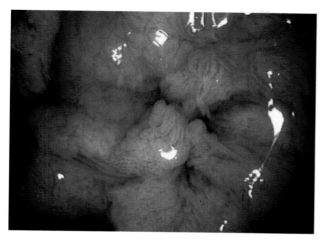

Figure 12.11 Final aspect: well-vascularized ampullary folds

Tubal occlusion: degree V

In the case of thick-walled hydrosalpinx, the ampullary folds are absent. The pregnancy rate after microsurgery[10] is 0%; for this reason, there is no indication for salpingostomy.

We propose laparoscopic salpingectomy to patients before an IVF procedure, in order to avoid the risk of tubal pregnancy after embryo transfer. Table 12.4 reports the results we obtained in a series of 1184 laparoscopic tubal surgery cases[43].

As has been repeatedly reported in the literature, these figures are comparable to results obtained with microsurgery and in other laparoscopic series. Indeed, the pregnancy rates are significantly different after fimbrioplasty for degree I occlusions (60%), and after salpingoneostomy for degree III and IV occlusions. In the case of adhesiolysis, the pregnancy rates are 62% and 51%, according to the type of adhesions (degree I and II, respectively).

Table 12.5 summarizes the results obtained in major series of laparoscopic salpingoneostomies; the intrauterine pregnancy rates range from 19% to 48%, according to the inclusion criteria reported by the authors. These rates remain low and underline the fact that the tubes have probably undergone irreversible damage. The degree of the lesion influences the success of fertility-promoting surgery, so it is essential to rely on prognostic factors, the evaluation of which will help in predicting the success of a surgical approach. We have opted for the technique summarized in Figure 12.12 for the management of distal tubal occlusion.

In degree II–IV distal tubal occlusion, hysterosalpingography is systematically performed 3 months after surgery under antibiotic prophylaxis, in the absence of pregnancy. Reocclusion is, in our opinion, an indication to remove laparoscopically the diseased tube and direct the patient towards IVF, as the presence of hydrosalpinx is thought to impair the success rate of IVF and expose the patient to an increased risk of ectopic gestation[46,47]. In the case of thick-walled hydrosalpinx (degree V, according to Donnez and Casanas-Roux[27]), the ampullary folds are absent. The pregnancy rate after microsurgery is 0%; for this reason, there is no indication for salpingostomy. Since 1991, we have proposed laparoscopic salpingectomy to patients before an IVF procedure, in order to avoid the risk of tubal pregnancy after embryo transfer (ET) and the possibility of embryotoxicity, with subsequently low pregnancy rates.

Table 12.4 Laser laparoscopic management of distal occlusion: 18-month cumulative viable pregnancy rate[43]

Procedure	n	Pregnancies n	%
Fimbrioplasty	380	228	60
Salpingostomy	85	22	27
Adhesiolysis			
degree I	412	255	62
degree II	307	157	51

Table 12.5 Intrauterine pregnancy rate obtained from laparoscopic salpingoneostomies

Authors	n	Intrauterine pregnancy rate (%)
Daniell and Herbert[5] (1984)	21	19
Nezhat* (1984)	33	36
Bouquet[52] (1987)	20	25
Reich[53] (1987)	7	19
Manhes* (1987)	19	48
Donnez et al.[6] (1989)	25	20
Dubuisson et al.[7] (1990)	31	26
Larue[54] (1990)	15	20
Henry-Suchet[55] (1991)	28	32
McComb[56] (1991)	22	22.7
Matvienko* (1991)	50	48
Canis et al.[9] (1991)	87	33.3
Audebert* (1992)	142	20.4
Donnez et al.[43] (1994)	85	27
Total	585	29.03

*Personal communication

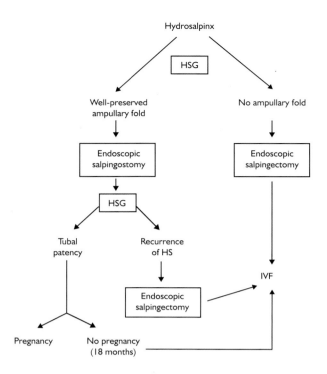

Figure 12.12 Proposed management of hydrosalpinx (HS) in infertility. HSG, hysterosalpingography; IVF, *in vitro* fertilization

HYDROSALPINX AND IN VITRO FERTILIZATION–EMBRYO TRANSFER

In a review, Nackley and Muasher[57] analyzed the effects of hydrosalpinx in IVF–ET.

Sims *et al.*[58] were the first to study the effect of hydrosalpinx on IVF outcome. A retrospective case-controlled study was conducted involving 118 patients with hydrosalpinx undergoing 283 stimulations, and 823 patients with tubal factor infertility without hydrosalpinx undergoing 1431 stimulations. A lower clinical pregnancy rate of 18%, and a higher miscarriage rate of 42% resulting in a lower ongoing pregnancy rate of 10%, were found, compared with the control group. They suggested treatment of hydrosalpinx before IVF by laparoscopic removal or peritransfer antibiotic coverage.

In a retrospective study, Strandell *et al.*[46] concluded that persistent hydrosalpinx was associated with a reduced implantation rate and an increased risk of early pregnancy loss. It was hypothesized that removal of the hydrosalpinx by salpingectomy or salpingostomy would normalize the IVF–ET rates in this group.

Andersen *et al.*[59] reported a marked reduction in implantation rates when hydrosalpinx was visible on ultrasonography. They found the rates of implantation, pregnancy, early pregnancy loss and delivery per aspiration

to be significantly reduced, despite a comparable number of aspirated oocytes and embryos transferred.

Vandromme[60] and Vejtorp[61] and their groups also demonstrated a decreased pregnancy rate after IVF in women with hydrosalpinx. The significant reductions in implantation rate and pregnancy rate per transfer in the hydrosalpinx group suggest an unfavorable uterine environment.

We have suggested[62] that this unfavorable environment could possibly be attributable to hydrosalpingeal fluid drainage into the endometrial cavity. It is conceivable that a connection exists between the hydrosalpinx and the uterine cavity, allowing direct flow of hydrosalpingeal fluid into the uterus, thus exposing the endometrium and the embryo to potentially toxic fluid. It is postulated that the fluid in damaged tubes contains micro-organisms, debris, lymphocytes, macrophages and other toxic agents that flow into the uterus and exert a detrimental effect on the endometrium and developing embryo. There may also be substances, such as cytokines and prostaglandins, interfering with normal endometrial function[46,59].

Freeman *et al.*[63] suggested that not only does hydrosalpinx negatively affect endometrial receptivity during implantation, but it also exerts a negative influence over oocytes early in follicular recruitment. The presence of hydrosalpinx has moreover been shown to affect implantation rates in unstimulated cycles[64].

Hydrosalpinx also predisposes patients to increased ectopic pregnancies after IVF–ET[64–66]. The first human pregnancy after IVF was, indeed, a tubal pregnancy[67].

Zouvres *et al.*[68] suggested prophylactic proximal tubal occlusion to prevent tubal pregnancy after IVF. This recommendation had previously been suggested by Steptoe[69] and Tucker[70] and Herman[71] and their groups. However, we do not recommend proximal tubal occlusion in a case of distal occlusion because of the risk of subsequent pelvic pain and inflammation due to increased intratubal pressure[62]. We advocate prophylactic salpingectomy instead of prophylactic proximal occlusion.

A study by Schenk *et al.*[72] and one by Mukherjee *et al.*[73] examined the effect of hydrosalpingeal fluid on embryogenesis. All samples demonstrated significant embryotoxic effects.

Although the exact mechanism by which hydrosalpinx alters intrauterine receptivity remains unclear, a marker of uterine receptivity has been established. Integrins are adhesion molecules that participate in cell–cell interactions and are present on all human cells. Lessey *et al.*[74] conducted an interesting study that examined endometrial integrin expression to evaluate the effects of hydrosalpinges on uterine receptivity. The expression of β-integrin, measured by immunohistochemical assays of endometrial biopsies, was assessed. Women with hydrosalpinges expressed significantly lower levels than those without hydrosalpinges[74].

REMOVAL OF HYDROSALPINX BEFORE *IN VITRO* FERTILIZATION–EMBRYO TRANSFER

The benefits of salpingectomy before IVF–ET in patients with hydrosalpinx have been debated by Puttemans and Brosens[75]. They believe that preventive salpingectomy should not be performed without demonstration by salpingoscopy of severe pathology, specifically chronic inflammation.

On the other hand, the study by Vandromme *et al.*[64] sought to determine whether surgical treatment would benefit patients with hydrosalpinx attempting IVF–ET. The ongoing pregnancy rate before surgery was 10.1%, whereas the postoperative group had an ongoing pregnancy rate of 31%. In the control group, the rate was 21.3%. The results revealed that surgical correction by ablation of the diseased tubes restored normal chances of success for patients with hydrosalpinges. Shelton *et al.*[76] were the first to conduct a prospective study that demonstrated the positive impact on pregnancy rates of removing hydrosalpinges in patients with repeated IVF failures. Fifteen patients with unilateral or bilateral hydrosalpinges with a history of repeated IVF failures underwent laparoscopic excision of the affected tubes. Because the patients undergoing surgical excision served as their own controls, the ongoing pregnancy rate per transfer was 0% pre-salpingectomy. After salpingectomy, the ongoing pregnancy rate per transfer was 25%. Improved pregnancy rates were noted for both fresh and frozen embryo transfers after surgery.

Lessey *et al.*[74] were also successful in demonstrating an improvement in integrin status, and consequently uterine receptivity, after correction of hydrosalpinx.

It is unclear whether salpingectomy has a detrimental effect on ovarian blood supply and neural linkage, thus affecting folliculogenesis and hormone production.

Studies by Vandromme[60], Shelton[76] and Kassabji[77] and their groups showed no difference in ovarian response, oocyte retrieval or fertilization rates after salpingectomy.

Nevertheless, other authors[78–80] have addressed the importance of maintaining the integrity of the anastomotic vessels between the ovary and the tube. McComb and Delbelke[80] evaluated the relationship between the ovary and oviduct using microsurgery to alter the structure of the Fallopian tube. The number of ovulations was reduced by ablating the vasculature conveyed through the mesosalpinx. Preservation of the anastomotic ovarian blood supply at the time of salpingectomy must be emphasized, to decrease the possible effects of radical surgery on ovarian function[79]. The risk of interstitial pregnancy is not eliminated, and the remote chance of uterine rupture at the site of salpingectomy exists[47,81]. Pavic *et al.*[82] were the first to report an interstitial pregnancy after bilateral salpingectomy for hydrosalpinx and IVF. Cornual resection at the time of salpingectomy does not prevent interstitial pregnancies.

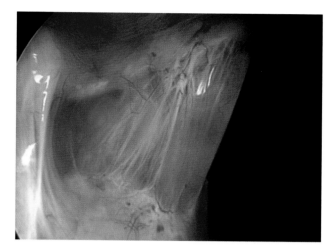

Figure 12.13   Filmy, avascular adhesion

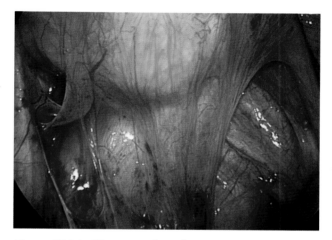

Figure 12.14   Filmy, vascular adhesion

ADHESIONS

Three types of adhesions must be defined:

- Type I (Figure 12.13): filmy, avascular adhesions

- Type II (Figure 12.14): filmy, vascular adhesions

- Type III (Figure 12.15): dense, fibrous, vascular adhesions

Adhesiolysis

In many patients, postoperative or postinfectious adhesions are amenable to vaporization by laser laparoscopy[6,10,27]. When compared with the standard technique using cautery and laparoscopic scissors (Figure 12.16) or blunt dissection, there is probably no difference in the outcome when the adhesions are small and avascular. With more vascular adhesions or particularly thick tubo-ovarian adhesions, however, the CO₂ laser

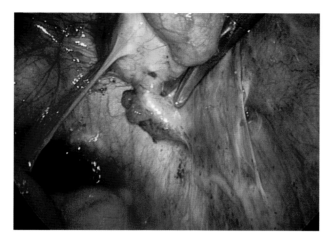

Figure 12.15 Dense, fibrous, vascular adhesion

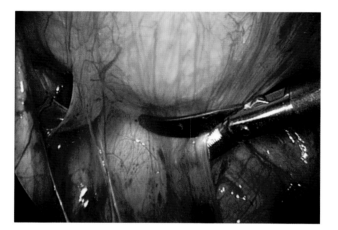

Figure 12.16 Adhesiolysis using scissors

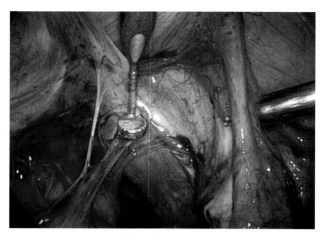

Figure 12.17 The adhesiolysis probe with its backstop should be used to make the procedure safer

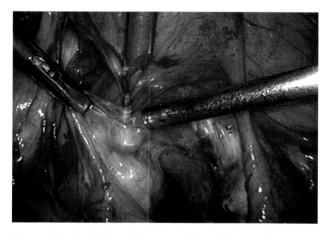

Figure 12.18 Salpingolysis is performed by applying traction to the adhesions with suprapubic atraumatic grasping forceps and another probe

allows more precise destruction of the adhesions with minimal injury to adjacent normal tissue. Filmy peritubal and periovarian adhesions are easily vaporized with the operative laser laparoscope. The adhesiolysis probe with its backstop should be used to make the procedure safer (Figure 12.17).

Traction to adhesions must be applied by two atraumatic forceps. The adhesion is positioned across the 'firing' platform when the laser is activated, to prevent damage to any tissue distal to the adhesion. Using a power output of 40 W, adhesions can be both coagulated and incised. For beginners, single or repeat pulse modes should be used for laser vaporization of the adhesions until confidence in the technique is gained. Great care should be taken when dividing adhesions between the tube and the ovary, because this area is very vascular. Adhesions of types I (filmy and avascular) and II (filmy and vascular, but not very thick) are easily vaporized with the operative laser laparoscope.

Salpingolysis is performed by applying traction to the adhesions with suprapubic atraumatic grasping forceps and another probe (smooth manipulating probe, hook or probe with its backstop) (Figure 12.18).

The probe with a backstop can be used to facilitate the procedure. When this probe is used, the adhesion is placed across the 'firing' platform and the laser is fired to vaporize the band. The use of a probe with a backstop eliminates the risk of inadvertent injury to intraperitoneal structures. Using a power output of 40 W, the adhesions are coagulated and incised. Short exposure times are adequate to vaporize adhesions around the Fallopian tubes and ovaries, and will prevent the laser beam from penetrating more than 100–200 μm. In the hands of more experienced laparoscopists, the continuous mode is easily used.

Ovariolysis is performed by applying torsion to the utero-ovarian ligaments with atraumatic tubal forceps. Elevation and rotation of the ovary are performed while continuing traction and torsion. Adhesions can easily be dissected from the ovarian surface by superficial vaporization. Care must be taken not to apply too much traction for fear of tearing the ovarian ligament from its attachment, which can result in copious bleeding that can only be stopped by hemostatic clips or coagulation. During adhesiolysis, use of the probe with a backstop eliminates the risk of inadvertent injury to other intraperitoneal structures, particularly the bowel.

Irrigation fluid can be introduced into the pelvis as an aqueous backstop to protect the bowel from any damage from diffusion of the laser beam.

CONCLUSION

In conclusion, the list of prognostic factors for tubal infertility is long[83]. It underlines the major role of the investigational examinations performed preoperatively on infertile patients, particularly the hysterosalpingogram and laparoscopy, when exploration of the tubal mucosa must be meticulous. Direct visual investigation of the tube, whether preoperative (falloscopy) or intraoperative (tuboscopy), enables clear documentation of all the endosalpingeal features. Failure to recognize these prognostic factors, and subsequent poor selection of patients for conservative surgery, could lead to an unacceptable loss of time and disillusionment for our patients.

REFERENCES

1. Swolin K. Electromicrosurgery and salpingostomy: long-term results. Am J Obstet Gynecol 1975; 121: 418–19
2. Gomel V. Salpingostomy by microsurgery. Fertil Steril 1978; 34: 380–5
3. Winston RML. Microsurgery of the fallopian tube: from fantasy to reality. Fertil Steril 1980; 46: 521–30
4. Gomel V. Salpingostomy by laparoscopy. J Reprod Med 1977; 18: 265–7
5. Daniell JF, Herbert CM. Laparoscopic salpingostomy utilizing the CO₂ laser. Fertil Steril 1984; 41: 558–63
6. Donnez J, Nisolle M, Casanas-Roux F. CO₂ laser laparoscopy in infertile women with adnexal adhesions and women with tubal occlusion. J Gynecol Surg 1989; 5: 47–53
7. Dubuisson JB, de Jolinière JB, Aubriot FX, et al. Terminal tuboplasties by laparoscopy: 65 consecutive cases. Fertil Steril 1990; 54: 401–3
8. Mettler LR, Irani S, Kapamadzija A, et al. Pelviscopic tubal surgery: the acceptable vogue. Hum Reprod 1990; 5: 971–4
9. Canis M, Mage G, Pouly JL, et al. Laparoscopic distal tuboplasties: reports of 87 cases and a 4-year experience. Fertil Steril 1991; 56: 616–21
10. Donnez J. La Trompe de Fallope: Hystopathologie Normale et Pathologique. Leuven, Belgium: Nauwelaerts Printing, 1984
11. Afzelius BA, Camner P, Mossberg B. On the function of the cilia in the female reproductive tract. Fertil Steril 1978; 29: 72
12. Donnez J, Caprasse J, Casanas-Roux F, et al. Loss of adrenergic innervation in rabbit-induced hydrosalpinx. Gynecol Obstet Invest 1986; 21: 213–16
13. Mol BWJ, Swart P, Bossuyt PMM, et al. Reproducibility of the interpretation of hysterosalpingography in the diagnosis of tubal pathology. Hum Reprod 1996; 11: 1204–8
14. Swart P, Mol BWJ, van der Veen F, et al. The accuracy of hysterosalpingography in the diagnosis of tubal pathology: a meta-analysis. Fertil Steril 1995; 64: 486–91
15. Atri M, Tran CN, Bret PT, et al. Accuracy of endovaginal sonography for the detection of fallopian tube blockage. Ultrasound Med 1994; 13: 429–34
16. Schiller VL, Tsuchiyama K. Development of hydrosalpinx during ovulation induction. J Ultrasound Med 1995; 14: 799–803
17. Friberg B, Joergensen C. Tubal patency studied by ultrasonography. A pilot study. Acta Obstet Gynecol Scand 1994; 73: 53–5
18. Heikkinen H, Tekay A, Volpi E, et al. Transvaginal salpingosonography for the assessment of tubal patency in infertile women: methodological and clinical experiences. Fertil Steril 1995; 64: 293–8
19. Volpi E, Piermatteo M, Zuccaro G, et al. The role of transvaginal sonosalpingography in the evaluation of tubal patency. Minvera Ginecol 1996; 48: 1–3
20. Allahbadia GN. Fallopian tubal patency using color Doppler. Int J Gynaecol Obstet 1996; 40: 241–4
21. Yarali H, Gurgan T, Erden A, et al. Colour Doppler hysterosalpingo-sonography: a simple and potentially useful method to evaluate fallopian tube patency. Hum Reprod 1994; 9: 64–6
22. Brosens I, Boeckx W, Delattin P, et al. Salpingoscopy: a new pre-operative diagnostic tool in tubal infertility. Br J Obstet Gynaecol 1987; 94: 768–73
23. De Bruyne F, Puttemans P, Boeckx W, et al. The clinical value of salpingoscopy in tubal infertility. Fertil Steril 1989; 51: 339–40
24. Kerin J, Daykhovsky L, Grundfest W, et al. Falloscopy. A microendoscopic transvaginal technique for diagnosing and treating endotubal disease incorporating guide wire cannulation and direct balloon tuboplasty. J Reprod Med 1990; 35: 606–12
25. Gomel V, Taylor PJ. In vitro fertilization versus reconstructive tubal surgery. J Assist Reprod Genet 1992; 9: 306–9
26. Gomel V, Yarali H. Infertility surgery: microsurgery. Curr Opin Obstet Gynecol 1992; 4: 390–9
27. Donnez J, Casanas-Roux F. Prognostic factors of fimbrial microsurgery. Fertil Steril 1986; 46: 200–4
28. Singhal V, Li TC, Cooke ID. An analysis of factors influencing the outcome of 232 consecutive tubal microsurgery cases. Br J Obstet Gynaecol 1991; 98: 628–36
29. American Fertility Society. The American Fertility Society: classifications of adnexal adhesions, distal tubal occlusion, tubal occlusion secondary to tubal ligation, tubal pregnancies, Müllerian abnormalities

and intrauterine adhesions. Fertil Steril 1988; 49: 944–55

30. Vasquez G, Boeckx W, Brosens I. Prospective study of tubal mucosal lesions and fertility in hydrosalpinges. Hum Reprod 1995; 10: 1075–8

31. Mage G, Pouly JL, Bouquet de Jolinière J, et al. A preoperative classification to predict the intrauterine and ectopic pregnancy rates after distal microsurgery. Fertil Steril 1986; 46: 807–10

32. Schlief R, Deichert U. Hysterosalpingo-contrast sonography of the uterus and fallopian tube: results of a clinical trial of a new contrast medium in 120 patients. Radiology 1991; 178: 213–15

33. Peters AJ, Coulam CB. Hysterosalpingography with color Doppler ultrasonography. Am J Obstet Gynecol 1991; 164: 1530–4

34. Stern J, Peters AJ, Coulam CB. Color Doppler ultrasonography assessment of tubal patency: a comparison study with traditional techniques. Fertil Steril 1992; 58: 897–900

35. Dunphy BC. Office falloscopic assessment in proximal tubal occlusive disease. Fertil Steril 1994; 61: 168–70

36. Kerin JF, Williams DB, San Roman GA, et al. Falloscopic classification and treatment of Fallopian tube lumen disease. Fertil Steril 1992; 57: 731–41

37. Cornier E, Feintuch MJ, Bouccara L. Ampullafibrotuboscopy. J Gynecol Obstet Biol Reprod 1985; 14: 459–66

38. Schlaff WD, Hassiakos DK, Damewood MD, et al. Neosalpingostomy for distal tubal obstruction: prognostic factors and impact of surgical technique. Fertil Steril 1990; 54: 984–90

39. Boer-Meisel ME, Te Velde ER, Habbema JDF, et al. Predicting the pregnancy outcome in patients treated for hydrosalpinx: a prospective study. Fertil Steril 1986; 45: 23–9

40. Dubuisson JB, Chapron C, Morice P, et al. Laparoscopic salpingostomy: fertility results according to the tubal mucosal appearance. Hum Reprod 1994; 9: 334–9

41. Marana R, Muscatello P, Muzii L, et al. Perlaparoscopic salpingoscopy in the evaluation of the tubal factor in infertile women. Int J Fertil 1990; 35: 211–14

42. Herschlag A, Seifer DB, Carcangiu ML, et al. Salpingoscopy: light microscopic and electron microscopic correlations. Obstet Gynecol 1991; 7: 399–405

43. Donnez J, Nisolle M, Casanas-Roux F, et al. CO$_2$ laser laparoscopic surgery: adhesiolysis, salpingostomy and fimbrioplasty. In Donnez J, Nisolle M, eds. Atlas of Laser Operative Laparoscopy and Hysteroscopy. Carnforth, UK: Parthenon Publishing, 1994: 97–112

44. Marana R, Muzii L, Rizzi M, et al. Salpingoscopy in patients with contralateral ectopic pregnancy. Fertil Steril 1991; 55: 838–40

45. Brosens I, Vasquez G. Fimbrial microbiopsy. J Reprod Med 1976; 16: 171

46. Strandell A, Waldenstrom U, Nilsson L, et al. Hydrosalpinx reduces in vitro fertilization/embryo

transfer pregnancy rates. Hum Reprod 1994; 9: 861–3

47. Dubuisson JB, Aubriot FX, Mathieu L, et al. Risk factors for ectopic pregnancy in 556 pregnancies after in vitro fertilization: implications for preventive management. Fertil Steril 1991; 56: 686–90

48. Laatikainen TJ, Tenhumen AK, Venesmaa PK, et al. Factors influencing the success of microsurgery for distal tubal occlusion. Arch Gynecol Obstet 1988; 243: 101–6

49. Dlugi AM, Reddy S, Saleh WA, et al. Pregnancy rates after operative endoscopic treatment of total (neosalpingostomy) or near total (salpingostomy) distal tubal occlusion. Fertil Steril 1994; 62: 913–20

50. Donnez J. CO$_2$ laser laparoscopy in infertile women with endometriosis and women with adnexal adhesions. Fertil Steril 1987; 48: 390

51. Nezhat F, Winer WK, Nehzat C. Fimbrioscopy and salpingoscopy in patients with minimal to moderate pelvic endometriosis. Obstet Gynecol 1990; 75: 15–17

52. Bouquet de Joliniere J, Madelenat P, Seneze J. Plasties tubaires distales: traitement coelioscopique. Apport du laser CO$_2$: techniques, indications, premiers résultats. Gynécologie 1987; 38: 3330–9

53. Reich H. Laparoscopic treatment of extensive pelvic adhesions, including hydrosalpinx. J Reprod Med 1987; 32: 736–42

54. Larue L, Sedbon E, Crequat J, Madelenat P. Percelioscopic surgery of the distal fallopian tube in infertility. J Gynecol Obstet Biol Reprod (Paris) 1990; 19: 34–7

55. Henry-Suchet J, Tesquier L, Boujenah A, et al. [Pregnancy rate after tuboplasty. Comparison between laparoscopic surgery and transparietal surgery]. Presse Med 1991; 20: 1570–1

56. McComb PF, Paleologou A. The intussusception salpingostomy technique for the therapy of distal oviductal occlusion at laparoscopy. Obstet Gynecol 1991; 78: 443–7

57. Nackley AC, Muasher SJ. The significance of hydrosalpinx in in vitro fertilization. Fertil Steril 1998; 69: 373–4

58. Sims JA, Jones D, Butler L, et al. Effect of hydrosalpinx on outcome in in vitro fertilization (IVF). Presented at the 49th Annual Meeting of the American Fertility Society, 1993, Chicago. Program Supplement, American Fertility Society, 1993: S95

59. Andersen A, Yue Z, Meng F, et al. Low implantation rate after in vitro fertilization in patients with hydrosalpinges diagnosed by ultrasonography. Hum Reprod 1994; 9: 1935–8

60. Vandromme J, Chasse E, Lejeune B, et al. Hydrosalpinges in in vitro fertilization: an unfavourable prognostic feature. Hum Reprod 1995; 10: 576–9

61. Vejtorp M, Petersen K, Andersen AN, et al. Fertilization in vitro in the presence of hydrosalpinx and in advanced age. Ugeskr Laeger 1995; 157: 4131–4

62. Donnez J, Polet R, Nisolle M. Prognostic factors of distal tubal occlusion. Ref Gynecol Obstet 1993; 1: 94–102

63. Freeman MR, Whitworth CM, Hill GA. Hydrosalpinx reduces in vitro fertilization–embryo transfer rates and in vitro blastocyst development. Presented at the 52nd Annual Meeting of the American Society, 1996, Washington. Program Supplement, American Fertility Society, 1996: S211

64. Akman MA, Garcia JE, Damewood MD, et al. Hydrosalpinx affects the implantation of previously cryopreserved embryos. Hum Reprod 1996; 11: 1013–14

65. Herman A, Ron-El R, Golan A, et al. The role of tubal pathology and other parameters in ectopic pregnancies occurring in in vitro fertilization and embryo transfer. Fertil Steril 1990; 54: 79–87

66. Martinez F, Trounson A. An analysis of risk factors associated with ectopic pregnancy in a human in vitro fertilization program. Fertil Steril 1986; 45: 79–87

67. Steptoe P, Edwards R. Reimplantation of a human embryo with subsequent tubal pregnancy. Lancet 1976; 1: 880

68. Zouvres C, Erenus M, Gomel V. Tubal ectopic pregnancy after in vitro fertilization and embryo transfer: a role for proximal occlusion or salpingectomy after failed distal tubal surgery. Fertil Steril 1991; 56: 691–5

69. Steptoe PC. Pregnancies following implantation of human embryos grown in culture. Presented at the 45th Annual Meeting of the American Fertility Society, 1989, San Francisco. Program Supplement, American Fertility Society, 1989: S152

70. Tucker M, Smith D, Pike I, et al. Ectopic pregnancy following in vitro fertilization and embryo transfer. Lancet 1981; 2: 1278

71. Herman A, Ron-El R, Golan A, et al. The dilemma of optimal surgical procedure in ectopic pregnancies occurring in in vitro fertilization. Hum Reprod 1991; 6: 1167–79

72. Schenck LM, Ramey JW, Taylor SL, et al. Embryotoxicity of hydrosalpinx fluid. Presented at the 43rd Annual Meeting of the Society of Gynecologic Investigation 1996. J Soc Gynecol Invest 1996; 3 (Suppl): 88A

73. Mukherjee T, Copperman AB, McCaffrey C, et al. Hydrosalpinx fluid has embryotoxic effects on murine embryogenesis: a case for prophylactic salpingectomy. Fertil Steril 1996; 66: 851–3

74. Lessey BA, Castelbaum AJ, Riben M, et al. Effect of hydrosalpinges on markers of uterine receptivity and success in IVF. Presented at the 50th Annual Meeting of the American Fertility Society, 1994, New York. Program Supplement, American Fertility Society, 1994: S45

75. Puttemans PJ, Brosens IA. Preventive salpingectomy of hydrosalpinx prior to IVF. Salpingectomy improves in vitro fertilization outcome in patients with a hydrosalpinx: blind victimization of the Fallopian tube? Hum Reprod 1996; 11: 2079–84

76. Shelton KE, Butler L, Toner JP, et al. Salpingectomy improves the pregnancy rate in in vitro fertilization with hydrosalpinx. Hum Reprod 1996; 11: 523–5

77. Kassabji M, Sims J, Butler L, et al. Reduced pregnancy rates with unilateral or bilateral hydrosalpinx after in vitro fertilization. Eur J Obstet Gynecol Reprod Biol 1994; 56: 129–32

78. Levy MJ, Murray D, Sagoskin A. The adverse effect of hydrosalpinges on IVF success rates are reversed equally well by salpingectomy, proximal tubal occlusion and neosalpingostomy. Presented at the Meeting of the American Society for Reproductive Medicine, 1996. Program Supplement, American Society for Reproductive Medicine, 1996: S64

79. Donnez J, Wauters M, Thomas K. Luteal function after tubal sterilization. Obstet Gynecol 1982; 37: 38

80. McComb P, Delbelke L. Decreasing the number of ovulations in the rabbit with surgical division of the blood vessels between the fallopian tube and ovary. J Reprod Med 1984; 29: 827–9

81. Sharif K, Kaufmann S, Sharma V. Heterotopic pregnancy obtained after in vitro fertilization and embryo transfer following bilateral total salpingectomy: case report. Hum Reprod 1994; 9: 1966–7

82. Pavic N, Neuenschwander E, Gschwind C, et al. Interstitial pregnancy following bilateral salpingectomy and in vitro fertilization–embryo transfer. Fertil Steril 1986; 46: 701–2

83. Donnez J, Nisolle M. Prognostic factors of distal tubal occlusion. In di Zerega GS, ed. Peritoneal Surgery. New York: Springer-Verlag, 2000: 265–74

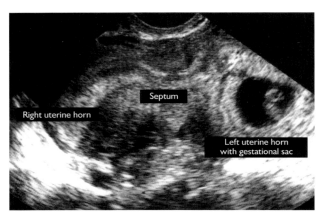

Figure 13.1 Gestational sac in the left uterine horn of an as-yet undiagnosed bicornual uterus

sac was found in the left uterine horn of an as-yet undiagnosed bicornual uterus. In some instances[17] (see later), magnetic resonance imaging (MRI) can confirm a suspected cornual pregnancy.

However, rupture of cornual pregnancies may cause severe bleeding because they are located so close to the uterine blood supply, and, in the literature, some cases of

hysterectomy have been described, because uterine disruption was extensive.

Treatment by surgical management

Laparotomy Cornual ectopic pregnancy is the least common of the four tubal sites for ectopic gestations to be located. These ectopic gestations are most often treated by surgical excision, which at times necessitates the removal of a portion of the myometrium as well. This raises concerns for possible uterine rupture if a subsequent pregnancy is achieved; thus, the mass of tissue excised must be kept to a minimum.

Laparoscopy The possibility of laparoscopic management of cornual gestations has been demonstrated in several case reports (Table 13.1). The initial procedures that were described, however, did not preserve tubal continuity. For example, Hill *et al.*[18] described a patient who presented at 10 weeks' gestation with a large unruptured cornual pregnancy. The authors, after placing an endoloop (Ethicon) around the cornua, were able to evacuate the pregnancy using a unipolar current and blunt removal. In contrast, both Tulandi[19] and Reich[20] and their groups used laparoscopic cornual excision to manage interstitial

Table 13.1 Summary of the reported cases of laparoscopic management of cornual pregnancy

Reference	Operation	β-hCG (mIU/ml)	Diameter (cm)	Rupture	Estimated gestational age (weeks)	Vasopressin
Reich *et al.* (1988)[20]	CE	NA	NA	No	14 (calcified)	Yes
	CE	NA	NA	No	NA	Yes
	CE	NA	NA	No	NA	Yes
Hill *et al.* (1989)[18]	S	NA	NA	No	10	Yes
Reich *et al.* (1990)[21]	CE	16 300	NA	Yes	NA	No
Tulandi *et al.* (1995)[19]	CE	6000	3	No	6	Yes
	CE	14 500	4	No	NA	Yes
	CE	12 000	5	No	10	Yes
	CE	4700	5	No	6	Yes
	S	8000	4	No	6	Yes
Pasic and Wolfe (1990)[22]	S	4400	2	No	6	Yes
Gleicher *et al.* (1994)[24]	S	7704	0	No	NA	Yes
Pansky *et al.* (1995)[23]	S	3000	NA	No	7	Yes
	S	2600	NA	No	9	Yes
Grobman and Milad (2002)[26]	S	32 827	4.5	No	7	Yes
Donnez and Nisolle (1994)[25]	S	6200		No		Yes + MTX
	S	7000		No		Yes + MTX
	S	11 200		No		Yes + MTX
	S + CE	18 250		Yes		Yes + MTX

CE, corneal excision; S, salpingotomy; β-hCG, β-human chorionic gonadotropin; NA, not available; MTX, methotrexate pregnancy. Cornual excision has also been useful for the treatment of ruptured interstitial pregnancy[21].

A less extensive laparoscopic procedure was performed by Pasic and Wolfe[22]. They visualized a small cornual pregnancy which was evacuated through a 1-cm salpingostomy. Subsequent hemostasis was maintained with electrocoagulation. A similar procedure was successfully used by Pansky et al.[23]. Conservative laparoscopic management was also advocated by Gleicher et al.[24]. In their report, a twin gestation visualized on ultrasound, but small enough not to be seen at laparoscopy, was removed from the cornua by salpingostomy. It has been confirmed that conservative laparoscopic surgery can also be used successfully for larger cornual pregnancies[19].

A linear incision is made with monopolar electrosurgery parallel to the axis of the Fallopian tube, in order to minimize bleeding, or perpendicular, in order to minimize extension into the tube. After copious irrigation and suction, removal of the product of conception can be performed by laparoscopy. Cornual injection of diluted vasopressin (5 IU/20 ml saline solution) and coagulation of the implantation site are often necessary to stop the bleeding in this highly vascular region of the uterus. An injection of methotrexate (20 mg) in the implantation site can be administered only in cases of cornual pregnancy where the site of implantation is the distal portion of the intramural tube[25]. The question of sutured closure of the cornual defect is still unresolved. Some authors use electrocoagulation with closure by secondary intention, and others make a sutured closure of the cornual defect.

In our series of ectopic pregnancies, we treated four cases of cornual pregnancy by laparoscopy according to the following technique:

- Injection of diluted vasopressin (2–5 IU/20 ml saline)
- Linear incision (Figure 13.2)
- Removal of trophoblast
- Reduce coagulation to a minimum
- Injection of 20 mg methotrexate in the implantation site

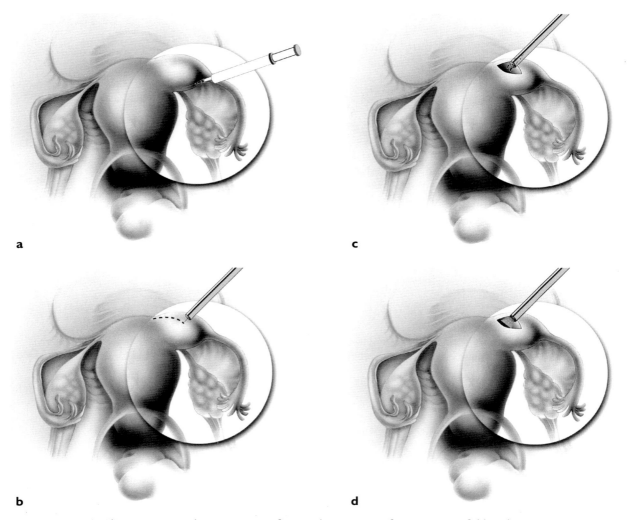

a

b

c

d

Figure 13.2 (a)–(d) Laparoscopic linear incision of cornual pregnancy after injection of diluted vasopressin (2–5 IU/20 ml saline) and subsequent injection of a mixed solution of methotrexate

In one of the four cases, closure of the defect was achieved with one stitch (Vicryl® 2-0).

Some authors have recently published other modalities, which probably do not offer any advantages over the previously described methods. In 1999, Rahimi[27] described the successful management of an interstitial ectopic pregnancy using three endoloops. In 2000, Moon *et al.*[28] reported a new approach to the endoscopic management of interstitial pregnancies (endoloop and encircling suture methods), without the uterine rupture encountered in pregnancies subsequent to these methods of endoscopic management. Laparoscopy-controlled hysteroscopic removal of an interstitial pregnancy and expectant management have also been described[29]. Most authors generally suggest that interstitial pregnancies larger than 4 cm in size may be better managed by cornual excision.

Non-surgical management: methotrexate

Methotrexate is generally preferred, but, as already discussed, in the case of heterotopic pregnancy, KCl injection could also be recommended. Different modalities of treatment with methotrexate exist: systemic, puncture and injection under laparoscopic or ultrasonographic guidance.

In 1996, Fernandez and Benifla[13] reported their experience of the management of cornual pregnancy with methotrexate. Complete resolution was obtained in 13 out of 15 cases (86.6%) with local injection of methotrexate (1 mg/kg) or KCl under transvaginal ultrasound guidance, or during a laparoscopic procedure. In this series, three of the 15 cases were heterotopic pregnancies. However, Agarwal *et al.*[30] reported only one successful methotrexate treatment in a series of four cases of cornual pregnancy. Transvaginal ultrasound-guided puncture has been proposed for the treatment of cornual pregnancy. However, the risks of ectopic rupture and profuse bleeding following needle extraction still exist, even if potentially safer routes for puncture and injection of cornual pregnancies are used, as recommended by Timor-Tritsch *et al.*[31].

In 1997, Batioglu *et al.*[32] reported a case of cornual pregnancy which was successfully treated with two doses of methotrexate under laparoscopic and ultrasonographic guidance.

Anecdotal: triplet cornual pregnancy

We reported a case of triplet cornual pregnancy in a woman who underwent IVF–ET[17]. Transvaginal echography performed 35 days after embryo transfer showed three gestational sacs with heartbeats in a very lateral position in the uterine cavity, and also asymmetric development of the right uterine horn. MRI confirmed the sonographic suspicion of the localization of the three gestational sacs in the right uterine horn (Figure 13.3).

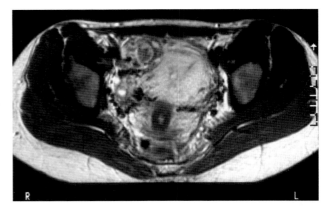

Figure 13.3 Triplet cornual pregnancy: magnetic resonance imaging confirmed the cornual localization of the three gestational sacs in the right uterine 'horn'

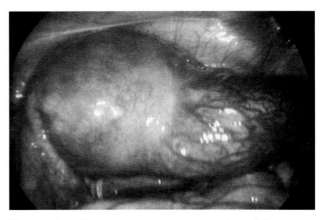

Figure 13.4 Laparoscopic view: very enlarged hypervascularized uterine horn of the case described in Figure 13.3

Laparoscopy confirmed the cornual pregnancy, with a very enlarged hypervascularized uterine horn without rupture (Figure 13.4). Immediate laparotomy permitted conservative treatment and uterine horn reconstruction.

Anecdotal: intramyometrial implantation

We encountered a case of intramyometrial implantation diagnosed after laparoscopy. Indeed, because of a suspected ruptured tubal pregnancy (raised hCG and intraperitoneal hemorrhage), laparoscopy was carried out, which detected a myometrial and serosal defect on the posterolateral side of the uterus. Because the patient had undergone D&C 7 days before, perforation was suspected. Coagulation was performed, and, after the removal of blood clots and peritoneal lavage, methotrexate was injected into this area. There was a substantial decrease in the hCG level. Hysterosalpingography, carried out 2 months later, revealed a diverticulum in the myometrium (Figure 13.5). Two years later, the patient experienced a

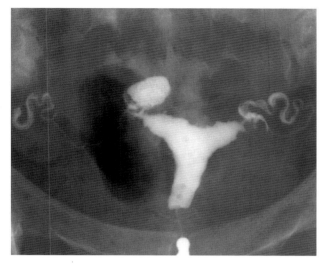

Figure 13.5 After myometrial pregnancy treated by local injection of methotrexate, hysterosalpingography carried out 2 months later revealed a diverticulum in the myometrium

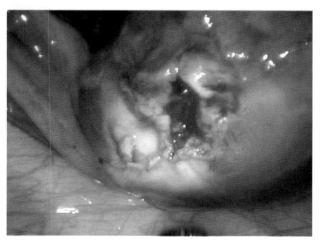

Figure 13.6 Myometrial defect observed at laparoscopy for diagnosis of suspected extrauterine pregnancy. The pregnancy was again located in the myometrial defect

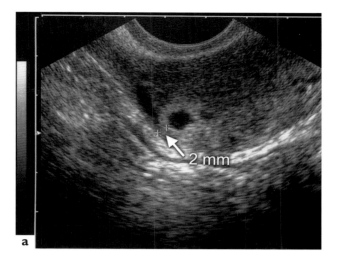

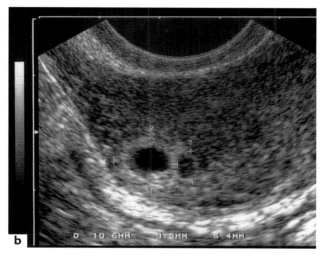

Figure 13.7 Vaginal echography: (a) intramyometrial pregnancy is obvious with only a 2-mm distance between sac and serosa (b)

recurrence of implantation in this 'myometrial' diverticulum. A laparoscopy performed because of hemoperitoneum with an hCG level of 2082 mIU/ml showed a suspected ovarian pregnancy, which was not confirmed according to the criteria of ovarian pregnancy (see section below on 'Ovarian pregnancy'). The myometrial defect was visible (Figure 13.6), but, at the time, intramyometrial pregnancy was not suspected. The hCG levels increased over the following days, and vaginal echography revealed an intramyometrial pregnancy (Figure 13.7) with only a 2-mm distance between the sac and the serosa. This sac was not visible on the day of laparoscopy. Methotrexate (40 mg) was administered, and hCG levels decreased rapidly, proving the efficacy of methotrexate. After an increase to 5648 mIU/ml (day 3 post-methotrexate), hCG levels decreased (Figure 13.8). A second methotrexate injection (40 mg) was then given.

Results from a review

In 1999, Lau and Tulandi[33] carried out a review of 41 patients with interstitial pregnancy who were treated with methotrexate, or by a conservative laparoscopic technique, or with KCl injection (in the case of heterotopic pregnancy). Methotrexate had a success rate of 83%. Conservative laparoscopic techniques had a success rate of 100% ($n = 22$). In the case of heterotopic pregnancy, after treatment (KCl or conservative surgery), 67% of coexisting intrauterine pregnancies resulted in successful deliveries.

There is insufficient evidence to recommend any single treatment modality, and the decision should be based on factors such as clinical presentation, the surgeon's

because fertility after ectopic pregnancy is affected much more by the status of the contralateral tube than by the procedure performed, with fertility rates exceeding 80% after salpingectomy when the opposite tube is normal[58].

REFERENCES

1. Stovall TG, Ling FW, Buster JE. Outpatient chemotherapy of unruptured ectopic pregnancy. Fertil Steril 1989; 51: 535–8

2. Stovall TG, Ling FW, Gray LA, et al. Methotrexate treatment of unruptured ectopic pregnancy: a report of 100 cases. Obstet Gynecol 1991; 77: 749–53

3. Hitara AJ, Soper DE, Bump RC, et al. Ectopic pregnancy in an urban teaching hospital: can tubal rupture be predicted? South Med J 1991; 84: 1467–9

4. Mol BWJ, Hajenius PJ, Engelsbel S, et al. Can noninvasive diagnosis tools predict tubal rupture or active bleeding in patients with tubal pregnancy? Fertil Steril 1999; 71: 167–73

5. Fernandez H, Lelaidier C, Thouvenez V, et al. The use of a pretherapeutic predictive score to determine inclusion criteria for the non-surgical treatment of ectopic pregnancy. Hum Reprod 1991; 6: 995–8

6. Fernandez H, Lelaidier C, Baton C, et al. Return of reproductive performance after expectant management and local treatment for ectopic pregnancy. Hum Reprod 1991; 6: 1474–7

7. Fernandez H, Benifla JL, Lelaidier C, et al. Methotrexate treatment of ectopic pregnancy: 100 cases treated by primary transvaginal injection under sonographic control. Fertil Steril 1993; 59: 773–7

8. Fernandez H, Bourget P, Ville Y, et al. Treatment of unruptured tubal pregnancy with methotrexate: pharmacokinetic analysis of local versus intramuscular administration. Fertil Steril 1994; 62: 943–7

9. Fernandez H, Cappella-Allouc S, Vincent Y, et al. Randomized trial of conservative laparoscopic treatment and methotrexate administration in ectopic pregnancy and subsequent fertility. Hum Reprod 1998; 13: 3239–43

10. Tanaka T, Hayashi H, Kutsuzawa T, et al. Treatment of interstitial ectopic pregnancy with methotrexate: report of a successful case. Fertil Steril 1982; 37: 851–2

11. Pansky M, Bukovsky J, Golan A, et al. Reproductive outcome after laparoscopic local methotrexate injection for tubal pregnancy. Fertil Steril 1993; 60: 85–7

12. Lipscomb GH, McCord ML, Stovall TG, et al. Predictors of success of methotrexate treatment in women with tubal ectopic pregnancy. N Engl J Med 1999; 341: 1974–8

13. Henry MA, Gentry WL. Single-injection of methotrexate for treatment of ectopic pregnancies. Am J Obstet Gynecol 1994; 171: 1584–7

14. Hajenius P, Engelsbel S, Mol B, et al. Randomised trial of systemic methotrexate versus laparoscopic salpingostomy in tubal pregnancy. Lancet 1997; 350: 774–9

15. Thoen LD, Creinin MD. Medical treatment of ectopic pregnancy with methotrexate. Fertil Steril 1997; 68: 727–30

16. Stika CS, Anderson L, Frederiksen MC. Single-dose methotrexate for the treatment of ectopic pregnancy: Northwestern Memorial Hospital three-year experience. Am J Obstet Gynecol 1996; 174: 1840–8

17. Corsan GH, Karacan M, Qasim S, et al. Identification of hormonal parameters for successful systemic single-dose methotrexate therapy in ectopic pregnancy. Hum Reprod 1995; 10: 2719–22

18. Schafer D, Kryss J, Pfuhl J, et al. Systemic treatment of ectopic pregnancies with single-dose methotrexate. J Am Assoc Gynecol Laparosc 1994; 1: 213–18

19. Saraj AJ, Wilcox JG, Najmabadi S, et al. Resolution of hormonal markers of ectopic gestation: a randomized trial comparing single-dose intramuscular methotrexate with salpingostomy. Obstet Gynecol 1998; 92: 989–94

20. Lecuru F, Robin F, Bernard JP, et al. Single-dose methotrexate for unruptured ectopic pregnancy. Int J Gynaecol Obstet 1998; 61: 253–9

21. Glock JL, Johnson JV, Brumsted JR. Efficacy and safety of single-dose systemic methotrexate in the treatment of ectopic pregnancy. Fertil Steril 1994; 62: 716–21

22. Morlock RJ, Lafata JE, Eisenstein D. Cost-effectiveness of single-dose methotrexate compared with laparoscopic treatment of ectopic pregnancy. Obstet Gynecol 2000; 95: 407–12

23. Vermesh M, Silva PD, Rosen GF, et al. Management of unruptured ectopic gestation by linear salpingostomy: a prospective randomized clinical trial of laparoscopy versus laparotomy. Obstet Gynecol 1989; 73: 400–4

24. Yao M, Tulandi T, Falcone T. Treatment of ectopic pregnancy by systemic methotrexate, transvaginal methotrexate, and operative laparoscopy. Int J Fertil 1996; 41: 470–5

25. Tan H, Tay S. Laparoscopic treatment of ectopic pregnancies – a study of 100 cases. Ann Acad Med Singapore 1996; 25: 665–7

26. Shalev E, Peleg D, Bustan M, et al. Limited role for intratubal methotrexate treatment of ectopic pregnancy. Fertil Steril 1995; 63: 20–4

27. Hoppe DE, Bekkar BE, Nager CW. Single-dose systemic methotrexate for the treatment of persistent ectopic pregnancy after conservative surgery. Obstet Gynecol 1994; 83: 51–4

28. Seifer DB, Gutmann JN, Grant WD, et al. Comparison of persistent ectopic pregnancy after laparoscopic salpingostomy versus salpingostomy at laparotomy for ectopic pregnancy. Obstet Gynecol 1993; 81: 378–82

29. Lundorff P, Hahlin M, Sjoblom P, et al. Persistent trophoblast after conservative treatment of tubal pregnancy: prediction and detection. Obstet Gynecol 1991; 77: 129–33

30. Letterie GS, Fasolak WS, Miyazowa K. Laparoscopy and minilaparotomy as operative management of ectopic pregnancy. Mil Med 1990; 155: 305–7

31. Mecke H, Semm K, Lehmann-Willenbrock E. Results of operative pelviscopy in 202 cases of ectopic pregnancy. Int J Fertil 1989; 34: 93–100

32. DeCherney AH, Diamond MP. Laparoscopic salpingostomy for ectopic pregnancy. Obstet Gynecol 1987; 70: 948–50

33. Pouly JL, Manhes H, Mage G, et al. Conservative laparoscopic treatment of 321 ectopic pregnancies. Fertil Steril 1986; 46: 1093–7

34. Bruhat MA, Manhes H, Mage G, et al. Treatment of ectopic pregnancy by means of laparoscopy. Fertil Steril 1980; 33: 411–14

35. Jimenez-Caraballo A, Rodriguez-Donoso G. A 6-year clinical trial of methotrexate therapy in the treatment of ectopic pregnancy. Eur J Obstet Gynecol 1998; 79: 167–71

36. Lipscomb GH, Bran D, McCord ML, et al. Analysis of three hundred and fifteen ectopic pregnancies treated with single-dose methotrexate. Am J Obstet Gynecol 1998; 178: 1354–8

37. Stovall TG, Ling FW. Single-dose methotrexate: an expanded clinical trial. Am J Obstet Gynecol 1993; 168: 1759–65

38. Donnez J, Nisolle M. Postoperative management and reproductive outcome after conservative laparoscopic procedures. In Donnez J, Nisolle M, eds. An Atlas of Laser Operative Laparoscopy and Hysteroscopy. Carnforth, UK: Parthenon Publishing, 1994: 131–44

39. Lipscomb GH, Stovall TG, Ling FW. Nonsurgical treatment of ectopic pregnancy. N Engl J Med 2000; 343: 1325–9

40. Donnez J, Nisolle M. Laparoscopic treatment of ampullary tubal pregnancy. J Gynecol Surg 1989; 5: 19–24

41. Donnez J. Conservative treatment of ectopic pregnancy. A first series of 50 cases. Acta Endosc 1982; 4: 62

42. Rivlin ME, Meeks GR, Cowan BD, et al. Persistent trophoblastic tissue following salpingostomy for unruptured ectopic pregnancy. Fertil Steril 1985; 43: 323–4

43. Rivlin ME. Persistent ectopic pregnancy: complication of conservative surgery. Int J Fertil 1985; 30: 12–14

44. Cartwright PS, Herbert CM, Mawson WS. Operative laparoscopy for the management of tubal pregnancy. J Reprod Med 1986; 31: 589–91

45. DiMarchi JM, Losasa TS, Kobara TY, et al. Persistent ectopic pregnancy. Obstet Gynecol 1987; 70: 555–9

46. Cartwright PS, Etmann SS. Repeat ipsilateral tubal pregnancy following partial salpingectomy: a case report. Fertil Steril 1984; 42: 647–8

47. Spandorfer SD, Sawin SW, Benjamin I, et al. Postoperative day 1 serum human chorionic gonadotropin level as a predictor of persistent ectopic pregnancy after conservative surgical management. Fertil Steril 1997; 63: 430–4

48. Hagstrom HG, Hahlin M, Bennegard-Eden B, et al. Prediction of persistent ectopic pregnancy after laparoscopic salpingostomy. Obstet Gynecol 1994; 84: 798–802

49. Kemmann E, Trout S, Garcia A. Can we predict patients at risk for persistent ectopic pregnancy after laparoscopic salpingotomy? J Am Assoc Gynecol Laparosc 1994; 1: 122–6

50. Graczykowski JW, Mishell DR Jr. Methotrexate prophylaxis for persistent ectopic pregnancy after conservative treatment by salpingostomy. Obstet Gynecol 1997; 89: 118–22

51. Paris FX, Henry-Suchet J, Tesquier L, et al. The value of antiprogesterone steroid in the treatment of extrauterine pregnancy. Preliminary results. Rev Franc Gynecol Obstet 1986; 81: 33–5

52. Perdu M, Camus E, Rozenberg P, et al. Treating ectopic pregnancy with the combination of mifepristone and methotrexate: a phase II non-randomized study. Am J Obstet Gynecol 1998; 179: 640–3

53. Gazvani MR, Baruah DN, Alfirevic Z, Emery SL. Mifepristone in combination with methotrexate for the medical treatment of tubal pregnancy: a randomized, controlled trial. Hum Reprod 1998; 13: 1987–90

54. Rozenberg P, Chevret S, Camus E, et al. Medical treatment of ectopic pregnancies: a randomized clinical trial comparing methotrexate–mifepristone and methotrexate–placebo. Hum Reprod 2003; 18: 1802–8

55. Yao M, Tulandi T. Current status of surgical and nonsurgical management of ectopic pregnancy. Fertil Steril 1997; 67: 421–33

56. Gervaise A, Masson L, de Tayrac R, et al. Reproductive outcome after methotrexate treatment of tubal pregnancies. Fertil Steril 2004; 82: 304–8

57. Job-Spira N, Fernandez H, Bouyer J, et al. Ruptured tubal ectopic pregnancy: risk factors and reproductive outcome: results of a population-based study in France. Am J Obstet Gynecol 1999; 180: 938–44

58. Rulin MC. Is salpingostomy the surgical treatment of choice for unruptured tubal pregnancy? Obstet Gynecol 1995; 86: 1010–13

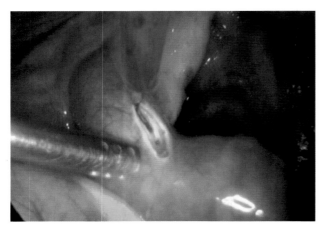

Figure 15.3 The salpingostomy is performed at the proximal part of the hematosalpinx

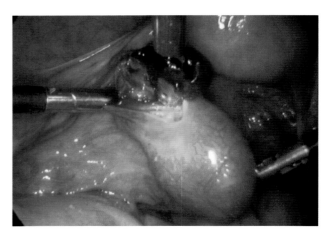

Figure 15.6 The robust, large suction device permits removal of the trophoblast through gentle and progressive traction

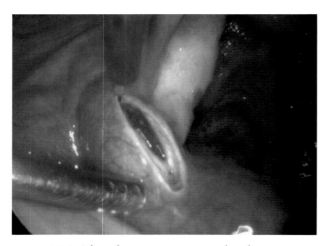

Figure 15.4 The salpingostomy is completed

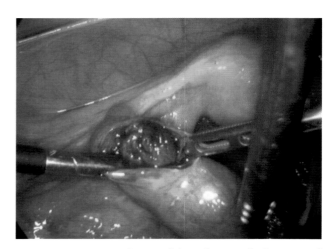

Figure 15.7 Manipulation of the tube reveals that part of the trophoblast is still in place

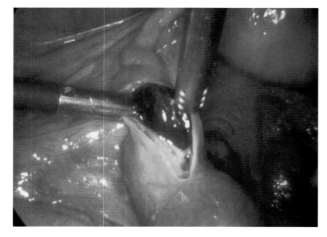

Figure 15.5 The suction device is introduced into the tube

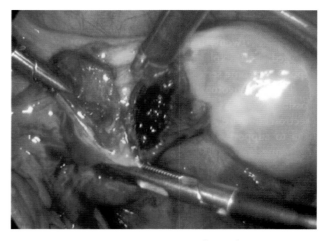

Figure 15.8 A repeat suction is performed

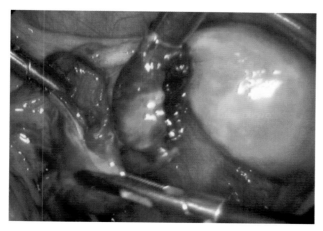

Figure 15.9 The second suction has allowed the trophoblast to be removed completely

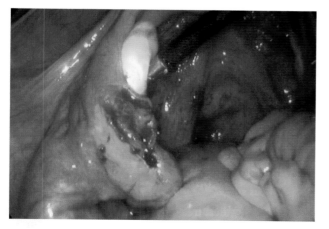

Figure 15.10 This minimal bleeding does not require further hemostasis and coagulation. The abdominal cavity must simply be washed

series is largely explained by the use of inefficient suction devices. Our initial study led to this conclusion, and to the development of a special device (Triton)[3].

The tube must be washed and explored to ensure complete removal of the trophoblast. It appears as a white tissue that can be removed using repeated suction or by grasping it gently with forceps.

Complete hemostasis of the tube is unnecessary or even deleterious. If no vasoconstrictive drugs are used, the bleeding generally comes from the trophoblast implantation area. Bipolar electrocoagulation, used to achieve hemostasis, leads to large destruction of the tube, and is not efficient. Generally, the bleeding stops by itself after 5–10 minutes. In the case of severe bleeding, removal of the tube must be considered, but only after mechanical compres-

sion of the mesosalpinx for at least 5 minutes. A preventive injection of vasoconstrictive drugs (Pitressin®, ornithine-vasopressin) is an elegant and efficient alternative when permitted[3].

The salpingotomy must not be sutured. In the initial study[3], suturing was not performed for technical reasons. Later on, it was proved that suturing the tube increases the risk for obstruction and decreases postoperative fertility[5], and that the tubal scar quality is better without a suture.

Salpingectomy

In the initial study[3], thermocoagulation was used. This has been replaced by bipolar or even monopolar coagulation. No data support a difference in the use of any of these technologies, even though bipolar cautery is generally considered to be less dangerous. There is no difference in the direction of the salpingectomy: it can be carried out from the isthmus to the infundibulopelvic ligament or vice versa.

Extraction of the tubes from the abdominal cavity must be done in an endobag or through a culdotomy, rather than pulling the tube through a trocar incision.

CONTRAINDICATIONS TO LAPAROSCOPIC TREATMENT

There are few contraindications to laparoscopic treatment, but they differ for salpingectomy and salpingostomy.

Salpingectomy

Laparoscopic salpingectomy is rarely contraindicated. Acute bleeding with shock is not a contraindication for experienced personnel. Control of the hemodynamic pattern is as efficient during laparoscopy as during laparotomy. The patient must be quickly insufflated, the trocars set up and the uterus cannulation put in place. As soon as the optic is introduced, the patient is put in an accentuated Trendelenburg position. The tube is located eventually with the help of blood aspiration; then, bipolar coagulation of the tube either at the site of the ectopic pregnancy or away from the ectopic pregnancy is done in order to achieve hemostasis. Thereafter, salpingectomy is carried out normally. This procedure must be performed rapidly by a trained laparoscopist and nurse and an anesthesiologist.

The two main contraindications are interstitial pregnancies and massive adhesions.

In the first case, the ectopic pregnancy cannot be removed through a simple salpingectomy, and medical treatment must be considered, rather than a cornual resection. In the second case, to achieve a salpingectomy can require extensive and potentially dangerous adhesiolysis, and it can be safer to perform a salpingostomy if the hematosalpinx is visible.

Sutures and needles

A more rigid needle is necessary for laparoscopic micro-suturing than for classical microsurgery. Furthermore, it is often easier to insert the needle directly into tissue without the use of a counter-pressing grasper. To achieve this, the needle needs low-force penetration characteristics and superior rigidity. Suitable examples include the BV 175-6 needle swaged to 7-0 and 8-0 Prolene™ or a BV 130-5 needle swaged to 8-0 polypropylene (Ethalloy TruTaper needle; Ethicon). Another excellent needle we have used recently is the Surgipro™ 135-5 needle swaged to 8-0 polypropylene (US Surgical Corporation). Although black nylon would give better discrimination laparoscopically, the needle is not ideal. Plain Vicryl® is the most difficult to see laparoscopically and becomes limp when wet. Monofilament sutures tend not to fray and allow easier intracorporeal suturing.

Other equipment

Trocars

Reusable 3-mm trocars are available with the Ultramicro Series, or 5-mm trocars with rubber valves that allow 3-mm instruments to be used without reducers. Three-millimeter suction irrigators are available and provide a more suitable jet for microsurgery than the 5-mm counterparts.

Stents

These are not used as it can be traumatic to cannulate the distal Fallopian tube.

Uterine manipulator

The Rumi™ uterine manipulator (Cooper Surgical, USA), with its superior anteversion mechanism, is indispensable for tubal anastomosis as multiple permutations of uterine position can be obtained, thereby presenting the proximal tube at a favorable angle for microsuturing. The lateral openings of the Rumi intrauterine tip facilitate retrograde chromopertubation. Uterine manipulators having a terminal opening tend to be lodged in the endometrium and cause intravasation of dye and a false diagnosis of a proximal block.

Energy

A 150-μm microneedle unipolar electrode (Storz 'Koh Ultramicro Series'™) is used for incision and dissection, powered from a low-voltage generator. Power settings of 15–20 W for cutting and 15 W for fulguration are adequate. When the mesenteric vasculature is inadvertently cut, causing more vigorous bleeding, a microbipolar electrode of 1-mm diameter is used.

PREREQUISITES OF THE SURGEON

The aspiring laparoscopic microsurgeon should be highly experienced in classical microsurgery and have highly developed two-handed laparoscopic skills for intra-corporeal knotting. Extracorporeal techniques for 7-0 and 8-0 sutures are impractical and crude and cause 'cutting through', or disruption, of tissue.

TYPES OF ANASTOMOSIS

Isthmic–isthmic anastomosis

Although the lumen may be as small as 500 μm to 1 mm, equivalent luminal size and a thick muscularis allow a technically easier anastomosis, particularly if 8-0 suture is used.

Isthmic–ampullary anastomosis

Luminal disparity is a potential problem. Preliminary dissection of the serosa and visualization of the proximal stump make it possible to create a lumen only slightly larger than the proximal ostium.

Ampullary–ampullary anastomosis

The awkwardness in these cases is due to the thin muscularis and the tendency for prolapse or extrusion of the mucosal folds. The angled probe can be used to delineate the muscularis as well as push the redundant mucosa back into the lumen after tying the muscularis sutures.

Tubo–cornual anastomosis

A linear slit at 12 o'clock is made in the cornual muscularis, using the microneedle electrode after Pitressin® injection. This allows some mobility of the interstitial tube so that it can be aligned to the needle and needleholder to effect suturing.

Selection of cases for the learning curve

The easiest cases for laparoscopic microsurgical anastomosis are mechanical sterilizations. The tissue damage is predictable and there is enough proximal and distal tube available with equivalent luminal sizes. In particular, the availability of proximal tube allows its mobilization to conform with the needle position whereas, with cornual anastomosis, extra steps are needed to mobilize the intra-mural tube and the suture placement may be inaccurate without a considerable amount of experience. Therefore, cases of electrosurgical sterilization, salpingitis isthmica nodosa and failed tubal cannulation are not suitable for anastomosis until the operator has performed more than 50 cases of isthmic anastomosis with good outcome. In this

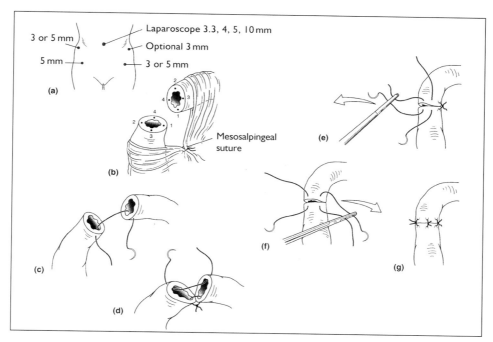

Figure 16.1 Surgical technique for anastomosis. (a) Placement of secondary ports; (b) suturing of the mesosalpinx; (c)–(g) suturing of the proximal tube to the distal tube

regard, a preoperative hysterosalpingogram may provide good prescreening.

SURGICAL TECHNIQUE

After insertion of a Foley catheter, the Rumi uterine manipulator with diagnostic tip is inserted into the uterus for mobilization. The intrauterine balloon is inflated with 3 ml saline. Dilute methylene blue is attached via a syringe to the chromopertubation port. After sterile preparation and draping, the trocars are inserted.

We employ the direct puncture technique using a 10-mm disposable trocar through the umbilical incision. After pneumoperitoneum has been created under direct visualization, the 3- or 5-mm secondary ports are then placed according to the position in the diagram (Figure 16.1a). The surgeon stands on the patient's right side.

Following this, the uterus is mobilized and anteverted and retroverted to inspect the pelvis. The lengths of the proximal and distal tubes are examined, as well as the condition of the fimbria. Any paratubal and periovarian adhesions are treated at this point, using the micro-electrode. If all conditions are satisfactory for anastomosis, the operation proceeds.

The instruments described are all part of the complete Storz 'Koh Ultramicro Series'™ set.

The Pitressin injector is inserted through the right lower port and 1:30 dilute Pitressin is injected into the terminal serosa of the proximal tube, just enough to bulge

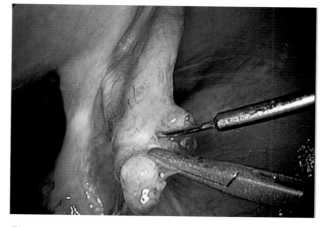

Figure 16.2 A grasper stabilizes the proximal tip of the tube. The surgeon circumscribes the serosa of the proximal tube

the serosa. Next, using the Ultramicro I grasper with his left hand to stabilize the tip of the tube, the operator introduces the microneedle electrode through the right lower port, to circumscribe the serosa of the proximal tube about 5 mm away from the tip (Figure 16.2). If the tubal length is generous and there is obvious bulbous dilatation of the tip, more tube can be sacrificed and the serosal cut would be 1 cm away from the tip. Following this, the microneedle is used to divide the tubal mesentery up to the chosen point for transection. By keeping this incision close to the tube, the mesosalpingeal vessels are not damaged and, therefore, do not require cautery, which may compromise the blood supply to the Fallopian tube (Figure 16.3).

The guillotine is inserted into the right lower port and a right-angled cut is made of the proximal tube (Figure 16.4). Chromopertubation is performed retrogradely by means of the syringe attached to the Rumi uterine manipulator. When dye emerges freely from the proximal tube, the laparoscope is brought to within 1 cm of the tissue to examine the muscularis and the mucosa at 40 times magnification (Figure 16.5). Normal isthmic mucosa stains blue and exhibits three to four folds. The muscularis is found to be circular and non-fibrotic.

The proximal end of the distal tube is now held up and Pitressin is injected, via the right lower port, subserosally. Following this, the microelectrode is used to dissect and expose the proximal stump of the distal tube, which is regrasped using the Ultramicro II grasper at the very tip (Figure 16.6). At this point, the tubal lumen is compared with that of the proximal tube by using the straight chromopertubator, which has 1-mm markings along its tip.

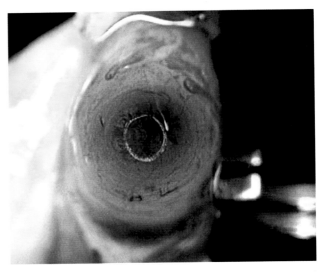

Figure 16.5 The laparoscope is brought to within 1 cm of the tissue to examine the muscularis and the mucosa at 40 times magnification

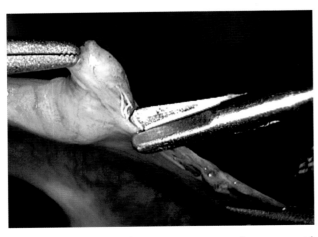

Figure 16.3 During dissection, care is taken to avoid damage to mesosalpingeal vessels

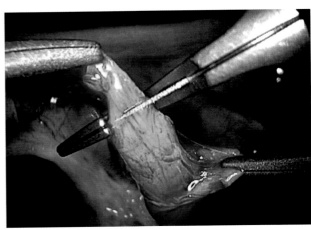

Figure 16.6 Dissection of the proximal end of the distal tube. The guillotine is also used to make a right-angled cut

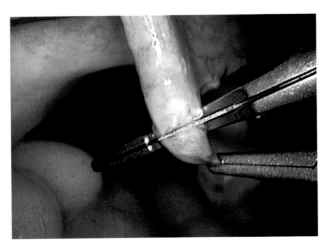

Figure 16.4 By using a guillotine, a right-angled cut is made of the proximal tube

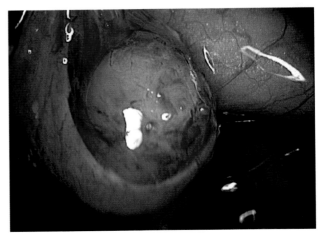

Figure 16.7 The aim is to obtain a distal lumen that is no more than 1 mm larger than the proximal stump

The aim is to obtain a distal lumen that is no more than 1 mm larger than the proximal stump (Figure 16.7).

The guillotine is then reintroduced to cut the distal stump. The curved chromopertubator is introduced to inject methylene blue dye through the proximal lumen, gently, to see that it emerges through the fimbria. When this has been achieved, it confirms patency of the distal tube without the need for cannulation, which is traumatic and difficult to achieve laparoscopically. The lumen is inspected to ensure that the size is adequate and, if not, further cuts are made with the guillotine. Pinpoint hemostasis is performed as necessary. Any redundant segment of Fallopian tube with attached loop or clip may now be removed using the unipolar electrode.

An 8-cm length of 6-0 polydioxanone (PDS) or Prolene is now introduced by holding the suture 2 cm from the needle with the Ultramicro needleholder through the right lower 5-mm port. A grasper (Ultramicro I) is introduced through the right upper quadrant with the operator's left hand. The needle is grasped by the grasper, oriented and then grasped by the needleholder. The mesosalpinx is sutured together using an intracorporeal knot, tying about 5 mm away from the Fallopian tube (Figure 16.8). Care should be taken not to approximate the mesosalpinx too near the tube as it will hinder subsequent anastomosis (Figure 16.1b).

A 6-cm length of 7-0 or 8-0 suture is now introduced in the same way as previously and the needle is positioned on the needleholder similarly. The Ultramicro II grasper is used in the left hand for this suture. Using clockwise rotation of the wrist, the muscularis at 6 o'clock on the distal tube is pierced, including the mucosa (Figure 16.9). The needle is then inserted at 6 o'clock of the proximal tube from mucosa through muscularis, again maintaining the clockwise motion of the wrist (Figure 16.1c). Intracorporeal knot-tying is performed, with three knots thrown (Figure 16.10). Facilitation with intracorporeal

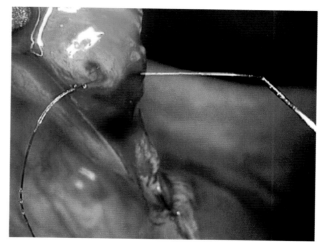

Figure 16.9 Using a 6-cm length of 7-0 or 8-0 suture, the muscularis at 6 o'clock on the distal tube is pierced, including the mucosa

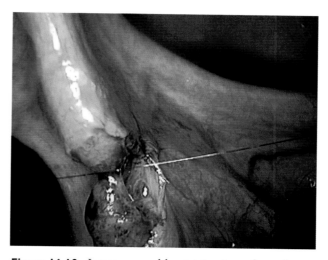

Figure 16.10 Intracorporeal knot-tying is performed

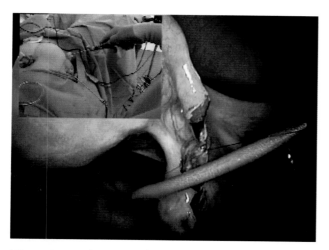

Figure 16.8 The mesosalpinx is sutured together using intracorporeal knot-tying about 5 mm away from the Fallopian tube

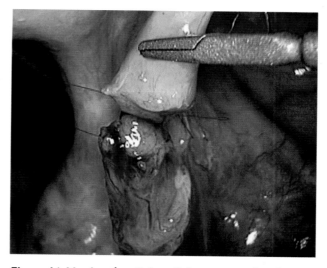

Figure 16.11 Another 7-0 or 8-0 suture is placed at 12 o'clock

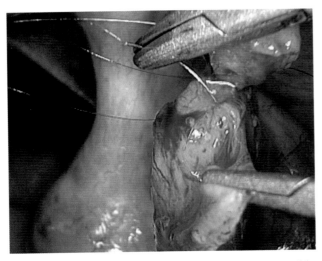

Figure 16.12 Using the Ultramicro II grasper, one is able to rotate the tube so that both the 3 and 9 o'clock positions become available for accurate suture placement

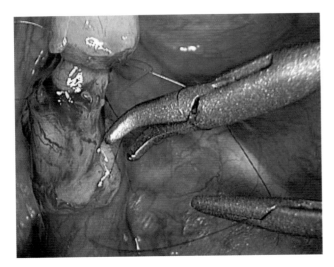

Figure 16.13 The 3 o'clock suture

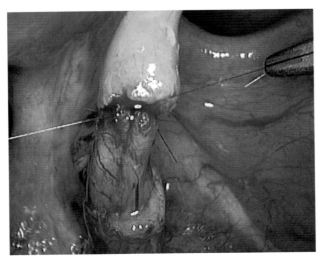

Figure 16.14 Finally, the 12 o'clock suture is tied

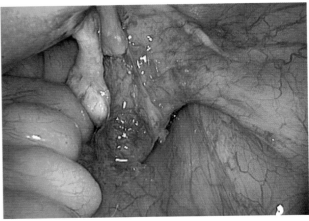

Figure 16.15 The 6-0 Prolene™ is then used to place one or two interrupted serosal sutures which may incorporate the outer muscularis to maintain support of the anastomosis

knotting can be achieved using a curved Ultramicro II grasper. The suture is then cut precisely using the Ultramicro suture scissors. Another 7-0 or 8-0 suture (Figure 16.11) is placed at 12 o'clock of the proximal tube from muscularis to submucosa or mucosa and then to the 12 o'clock position of the distal tube with the needle entering from mucosa/submucosa through muscularis (Figure 16.1d). This suture is now held by the assistant using the Ultramicro II grasper and, together with the use of the uterine manipulator, one is able to rotate the tube so that both the 3 and 9 o'clock positions become available for accurate suture placement (Figures 16.1e and f, 16.12 and 16.13). These are placed next and tied and, finally, the 12 o'clock suture is tied (Figure 16.14). Chromopertubation is performed via the uterine manipulator and the patency of the tube can now be demonstrated. Slight leakage at the anastomotic site is no cause for concern as long as dye emerges from the distal fimbria. The 6-0 or 7-0 Prolene or PDS is then used to place one or two interrupted serosal sutures (Figure 16.15). These sutures may incorporate the outer muscularis to maintain support of the anastomosis (Figure 16.1g). Any gaps evident in the mesosalpinx are similarly closed using 6-0 nylon. The opposite tube is then treated in the same manner (Figure 16.16).

CONCLUSIONS

Laparoscopic microsurgery is an exciting new tool with great promise, like classical microsurgery before it. However, the learning curve is steep, and skill development very intensive. It requires at least 20 midtubal cases before operators begin to develop a fluid rhythm. After 50 cases, one can perform bilateral midtubal anastomosis in 90 min, making it a very efficient procedure.

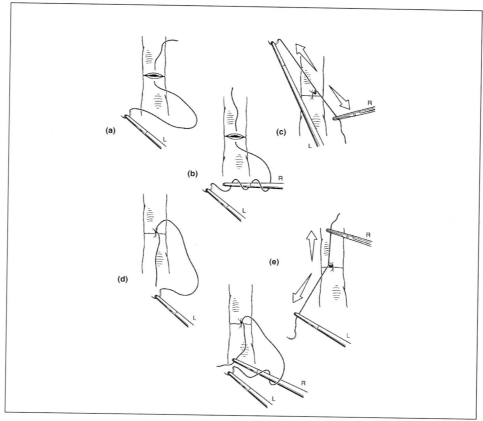

Figure 16.16 Ipsilateral intracorporeal microsuturing using Ultramicro instrumentation with 7-0 and 8-0 Prolene

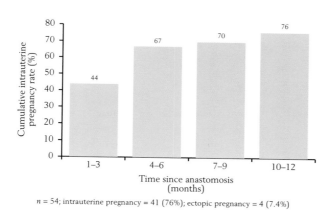

$n = 54$; intrauterine pregnancy = 41 (76%); ectopic pregnancy = 4 (7.4%)

Figure 16.17 Cumulative intrauterine pregnancy rate (%) 1992–1997 (follow-up 6–12 months). Reproductive Specialty Center, Milwaukee, USA

Laparoscopic microsurgery will introduce a new dimension to reproductive surgery and over time will replace laparotomy for microsurgery (Figure 16.17). It is important to realize, however, that the learning curve is considerable and the technique may not be attainable by all, despite their best efforts. The reproductive surgeon of tomorrow will be an expert in microendoscopy and laparoscopic microsurgery, with sufficient numbers of cases to maintain and develop his expertise.

REFERENCE

1. Brosens IA. Risks and benefits of endoscopic surgery in reproductive medicine. In Proceedings of the 15th World Congress on Fertility and Sterility. ASRM 1995; 47: 339–43

Laparoscopic management of ovarian cysts

17

J Donnez, J Squifflet, P Jadoul

In most clinical circumstances, a unilocular ovarian cyst does not require aspiration, but does require medical therapy (such as oral contraceptives) for 3 months. If the cyst does not disappear after a 3-month course of therapy, it requires careful evaluation (echography, CA125 level and, in some instances, computed tomography (CT) and magnetic resonance imaging (MRI)), and, finally, laparoscopic diagnosis and management.

The most frequent types of cysts found in young women are:

- The unilocular clear-fluid cyst (mucous or serous)
- The dermoid cyst
- The endometrial cyst (endometrioma)

Laparoscopic removal of benign ovarian cysts is an effective technique, involving little risk of complications[1,2]. Nevertheless, several criteria must be taken into account before performing this procedure. Various diagnostic methods have been used to discriminate between benign and malignant ovarian tumors: physical examination, transvaginal ultrasound color flow imaging and tumor markers such as CA125.

PREOPERATIVE EVALUATION

Ultrasound examination

Using high-frequency transvaginal sonography, it is possible to detect malignant ovarian tumors more efficiently than by transabdominal echography[3]. The vaginal approach produces greater image resolution than the abdominal, thus allowing a more detailed morphological assessment of ovarian masses (Figure 17.1a and b).

The following criteria must be assessed: size and location, borders of the mass and free pelvic fluid (ascites). The internal structure of a mass is considered to be the most important sonographic criterion for distinguishing benign from malignant disorders. The tumor can be purely cystic, complex (mainly cystic, or mainly solid) or purely solid. Loculations, thick septa, irregular solid parts within a mass, undefined margins, and the presence of ascites are considered as malignant patterns (Figure 17.1c). Such cases certainly require conventional surgery by laparotomy. A sonographic diagnosis of benign disease is generally accurate; indeed, a predictive non-malignant rate of 95.6% was found by Herrmann et al.[4].

Transvaginal Doppler ultrasound with color flow imaging

Transvaginal Doppler ultrasound with color flow imaging is a new technique for the evaluation of ovarian masses[5–7]. It allows positioning of the probe closer to the tumor and reflects visually the state of blood flow of the ovarian tumor (Figure 17.2a and b); it permits the detection of low-resistance intratumoral blood vessels, characteristic of malignant tumors (Figure 17.2c).

The pulsatility index (PI), defined as the difference between the peak systolic and the end-diastolic flow velocity divided by the mean flow velocity, is calculated. Bourne et al.[5] reported that this method can be used to differentiate between primary ovarian cancer and other forms of benign pelvic masses. In their study, low impedance to ovarian blood flow was associated with malignant ovarian tumors (PI < 1).

Weiner et al.[8] made an attempt to compare transvaginal color flow imaging with conventional sonographic findings and other screening procedures to predict ovarian malignancy. They found that suspicious sonographic findings had low specificity, and were inadequate in distinguishing between benign and malignant ovarian tumors. They concluded that transvaginal color flow imaging provided high sensitivity and specificity and was superior to other methods used for the preoperative evaluation of ovarian masses.

A simple measurement of the PI in the newly formed intratumoral blood vessels can discriminate accurately between malignant and non-malignant ovarian tumors. Moreover, because early development of neovascularity may precede tumor growth, screening for ovarian malignancy with transvaginal color flow imaging may detect early ovarian neoplasms before sonography. According to the results of Bourne et al.[5], Fleischer et al.[9] and Kurjak et al.[6], transvaginal color Doppler is a valuable method of differentiating benign from malignant ovarian tumors. However, others[10] have recently been unable to reproduce their results.

CA125

The preoperative evaluation of serum CA125 levels must be made before endoscopic surgery, especially in premenopausal and postmenopausal patients, in order to determine malignant disease preoperatively. Values of CA125 in excess of 65 IU/ml distinguished malignant from benign disease with a specificity of 92% and a sensitivity of

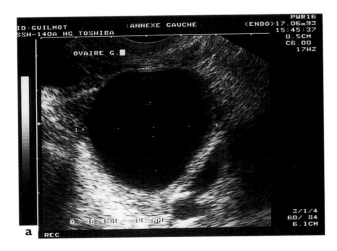

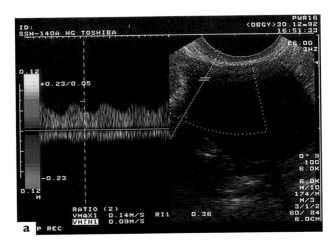

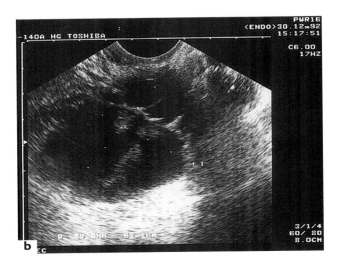

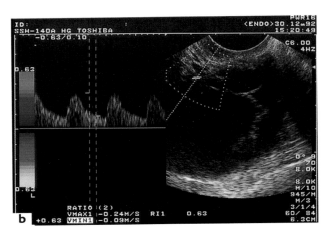

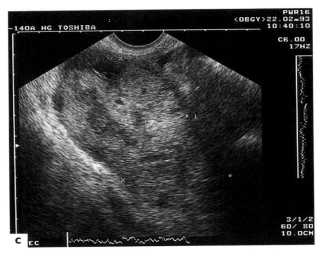

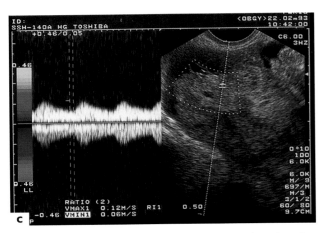

Figure 17.1 Transvaginal sonography: (a) unilocular cyst, without solid structures; (b) multilocular cyst; (c) cyst with thick septa and irregular solid parts suspected to be malignant

Figure 17.2 Transvaginal Doppler ultrasound with color flow imaging (corresponding to the cysts shown in Figure 16.1): (a) unilocular cyst: normal pulsatility index; (b) multilocular cyst: normal pulsatility index; (c) multilocular cyst with hyperechogenic areas. Low-resistance intra-tumoral blood vessels, suggesting malignancy

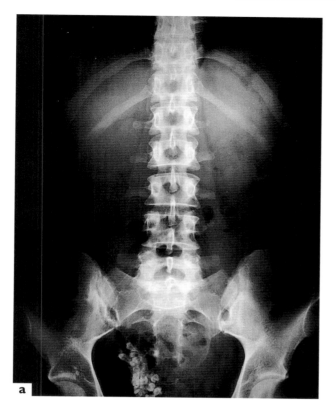

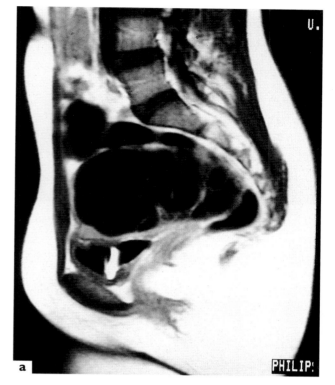

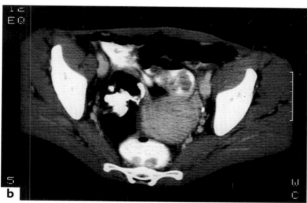

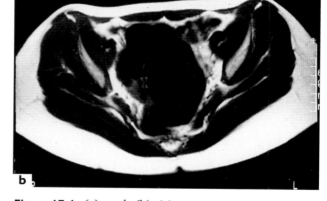

Figure 17.3 (a) and (b) Computed tomography. In the case of dermoid cyst, high-quality images are obtained

Figure 17.4 (a) and (b) Magnetic resonance imaging provides soft tissue contrast and clear pictures of pelvic organs. Multilocular cyst (histology: mucinous cyst)

75% when both premenopausal and postmenopausal patients were studied together[11]. Greater specificity and sensitivity were observed in postmenopausal subjects, in whom the specificity of the assay was 97% and the sensitivity 78%[11].

CT and MRI

CT provides high-quality images of the ovaries but does not give more information than ultrasound, except in cases of dermoid cysts (Figure 17.3). In our experience, CT is less sensitive and less specific than transvaginal echography

in the detection of intracystic structures or septa (Figure 17.3).

MRI provides soft-tissue contrast and clear pictures of pelvic organs (Figure 17.4). This modality is biologically safe and more sensitive than CT in the diagnosis of intracystic structures, and more sensitive and specific than either CT or ultrasound in the evaluation of an ovarian mass.

As a result of the accuracy, convenience, relatively low cost and availability of high-resolution ultrasound equipment, this technique has remained the principal imaging modality in assessing pelvic pathology. In our

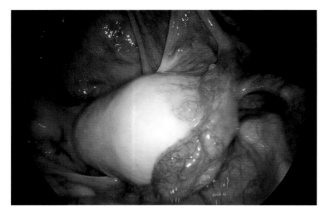

Figure 17.5 Laparoscopic examination of the external cyst wall which must have a smooth appearance

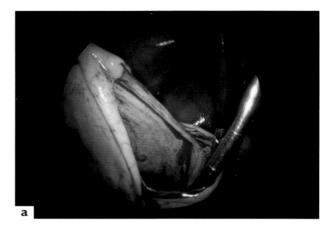

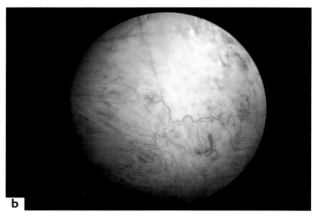

Figure 17.6 (a) Laparoscopic examination of the internal cyst wall; (b) internal view of the cyst. Note the absence of intracystic vegetations (no biopsy required)

department, CT and MRI are indicated in cases of suspected malignant lesions.

INDICATIONS

Indications for laparoscopic cystectomy include serous, mucous, dermoid and endometriotic cysts. The internal wall of the endometriotic cyst, the complete dissection of which from the ovarian cortex could be difficult, can also be vaporized with the CO_2 laser, as previously described[12,13].

The indications for laparoscopic oophorectomy usually include large endometriotic cysts and benign ovarian cysts in patients aged over 40 years.

The laparoscopic aspiration of unilocular, smooth-walled, translucent ovarian cysts remains controversial. The main concern is spillage of malignancy. Thorough preoperative evaluation of the patient, combining ultrasonography of ovarian tumors with the measurement of tumor markers, may greatly improve the accuracy of diagnosis of ovarian malignancy. Moreover, laparoscopy is, in the first place, used as a diagnostic tool whereby the pelvis and the abdominal cavity are thoroughly evaluated.

The ovaries are inspected carefully to ensure that the cyst wall is smooth and that there is no vegetation (Figure 17.5). The interior wall of the cyst can also be carefully examined (Figure 17.6), and a biopsy with frozen histological evaluation can be carried out.

In a retrospective study of 226 patients, Mage *et al.*[14] reported that the diagnosis of malignant tumors by laparoscopy was 100% accurate. The anatomopathological examination of specimens in benign conditions was never wrong. They concluded that laparoscopy is a reliable way of diagnosing the type of ovarian cyst.

According to these data, we have proposed the scheme outlined in Figure 17.7 for the laparoscopic management of ovarian cysts. In patients aged under 35 years, hormonal therapy is first attempted for 3 months if echography

reveals a unilocular, smooth-walled cyst without septa or intracystic structures. If the cyst persists, an ultrasound examination is carried out and the CA125 level is measured, in order to exclude a malignant lesion. In patients under 40 years of age, a cystectomy is usually performed.

In patients aged over 40 years, the preoperative evaluation (echography and CA125) is made directly. If data suggest malignancy, a laparotomy is performed after CT and/or MRI have been performed. Only when a malignant lesion can be excluded is a laparoscopy carried out. If at all possible, the cyst is removed intact. Otherwise, the interior wall of the cyst is examined to exclude the presence of any suspect vegetation, which would require a biopsy and a frozen histological examination. In patients over age 40 years, a cystectomy is rarely performed and a unilateral oophorectomy is the preferred procedure. If the frozen histological examination reveals the presence of malignant cells, a laparotomy and total abdominal hysterectomy are mandatory.

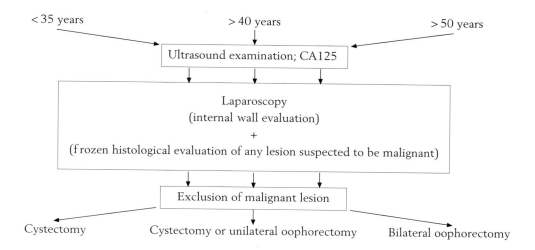

Figure 17.7 Laparoscopic management of ovarian cysts

Table 17.1 Laparoscopic criteria for differentiation between functional and organic cysts. From reference 14

Criterion	Organic cysts	Functional cysts
Utero-ovarian ligament	Lengthened	Normal
Cyst wall	Thick	Thin
Ovarian vessels	Numerous and regular starting from the mesovarium	More scanty, coral-like
Cyst fluid	Clear, dark, brown, or dermoid	Saffron yellow
Internal cyst wall appearance	Smooth or fibrotic with areas of hypervascularization	Retina-like aspect

In patients aged over 50 years, after all the same precautions have been taken, a bilateral oophorectomy is carried out, even if the contralateral ovary is normal.

SURGICAL PROCEDURES

The procedure is performed under general anesthesia. After the induction of a pneumoperitoneum, a 12-mm trocar is inserted subumbilically. The laparoscope is connected to a video camera. Three 5-mm trocars are systematically inserted suprapubically: one in the midline approximately 3 cm above the symphysis pubis, and the other two a few centimeters on either side, taking care to avoid the epigastric vessels.

The initial phase of the laparoscopy is purely diagnostic. First, the abdominal cavity is inspected thoroughly and a peritoneal sampling is sent for cytology. The ovaries are examined carefully in order to exclude the presence of excrescences or other evidence suggesting malignancy.

It is important to differentiate between organic and functional cysts during laparoscopy; 10–20% of functional cysts do not disappear after 3 months of treatment with combination oral contraceptive pills containing 50 µg of ethinylestradiol. According to Mage *et al.*[14], there are five laparoscopic criteria which allow us to distinguish between functional and organic cysts (Table 17.1).

Intraperitoneal cystectomy

The utero-ovarian ligament is grasped with an atraumatic forceps introduced on the side of the tumor, in order to expose the ovary completely (Figure 17.8).

The first step consists of making an incision in the ovarian cortex with the scissors or with the CO_2 laser (Figure 17.9). The incision must be made in the ovarian cortex overlying the cyst, and it must be long enough to permit a straightforward cystectomy. In some cases, the cyst is first aspirated and the liquid examined.

The interior wall of the cyst can be checked by introducing the laparoscope into the ovarian cyst. If there

Table 17.2 Bilateral adnexectomy ($n = 114$ postmenopausal women)

Pathology	n
Serous or mucinous cystadenoma	78
Endometrial cyst	10
'Parovarian' cyst (Wolffian)	8
Dermoid	14
Borderline tumor	4

Table 17.3 Borderline tumors ($n = 4$): preoperative check-up

Case	Echography	CA125 (IU/ml)	Frozen pathology
1	Multilocular	<35	Negative
2	Multilocular	<35	Negative
3	Unilocular	56	Negative
4	Unilocular	<35	Negative

In our department, a colpotomy incision is made through the vagina and the overlying peritoneum using scissors. We have never encountered any complications – no bleeding, rectal injuries or infections – using this technique.

However, Reich[18] suggests that a posterior colpotomy incision using the CO_2 laser or electrosurgery through the cul-de-sac of Douglas into the vagina is preferable to a vaginal incision, because complete hemostasis is obtained while making the colpotomy incision. The anatomic relationship between the rectum and the posterior vagina must be confirmed before making the laparoscopic colpotomy incision, to avoid cutting the rectum. Reich[18,21,22] uses an instrument placed in the uterus for elevation and anteversion. The posterior vaginal fornix is identified by placing a wet sponge in a ring forceps just behind the cervix. A rectal probe can also be used to ensure that the rectum is out of the way.

DISCUSSION

Risk of borderline tumor

The advantages of laparoscopic treatment of ovarian cysts have been described for women under the age of 35 years with simple ovarian cysts, for whom the overall risk of malignancy is only 4.5 per 100 000 cases[14].

The risk is much higher in postmenopausal women. Indeed, a 10-year study[23] suggested that, when a postmenopausal woman undergoes surgery for an ovarian neoplasm, the rate of malignancy may be as high as 45%.

Very often, a malignant tumor is diagnosed or suspected by means of echography, CA125, CT or MRI. We have tried to evaluate the 'true' risk of underdiagnosing an ovarian tumor preoperatively.

In a series of 114 postmenopausal women who underwent bilateral adnexectomy, 78 were found to have a serous or mucinous cystadenoma, ten an endometrial cyst, eight a paraovarian cyst, 14 a dermoid cyst and four (< 4%) a borderline tumor (Table 17.2). In this series, all patients had a preoperative check-up including measurement of the CA125 level and an ultrasound examination. Three of the four borderline-tumor cases presented abnormalities at the preoperative check-up (Table 17.3). Indeed, in two cases, in spite of a normal CA125 level, echography showed a multilocular cyst. In one case, the cyst was unilocular, but the CA125 level was elevated. In the last case, however, there were no evident abnormalities (unilocular cyst, normal CA125 level); therefore, an accurate preoperative diagnosis was impossible (0.9%) (Figure 17.14). In these four borderline cases, the abnormal cells could not be detected on frozen pathology. These four patients underwent hysterectomy 2 weeks later. Peritoneal sampling for cytology did not reveal any abnormal cells, and the histology did not show any residual malignant tissue; to date, no sign of recurrence has been demonstrated.

The preoperative check-up of a mass diagnosed in postmenopausal women is, in most cases, accurate. Indeed, in our series, only one case (< 1%) went undetected preoperatively. However, when an abnormality is observed (Figure 17.15), certain perioperative precautions must be taken to avoid spillage of the intracystic contents.

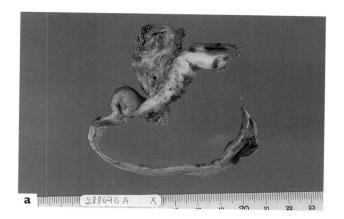

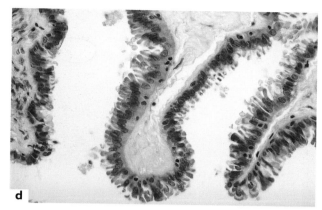

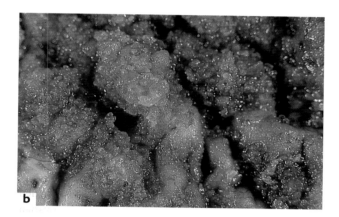

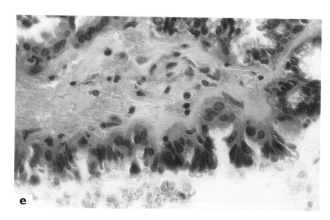

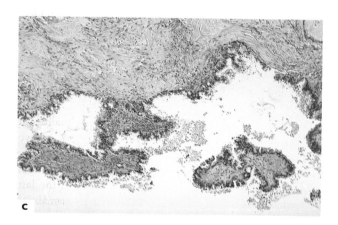

Figure 17.14 Borderline ovarian tumor: (a) unilocular cyst with a normal CA125 level; (b) small (<1 mm) papillary lesions were visible over an area of 1 cm²; (c)–(e) histology reveals the presence of an ovarian borderline tumor

Risk of spillage

Spillage of benign material in cases of benign cystic teratomas or endometriomas can theoretically produce chemical peritonitis. Intraoperative spillage of a mucinous cystadenoma may theoretically initiate pseudomyxoma peritonei. The risk appears to be very low, since pseudomyxoma peritonei, when reported, is usually present at the time of initial surgery[24]. According to several authors, pseudomyxoma peritonei is almost always associated with mucinous cystadenocarcinoma[25]. Furthermore,

pseudomyxoma peritonei does not appear to be a frequent complication of mucinous carcinoma, even when ruptured at laparotomy. To date, Mage *et al.*[1,14] have observed no cases of pseudomyxoma peritonei after laparoscopic treatment of mucinous cystadenoma. Similar results have been reported after laparotomy with cyst rupture. Treatment of the cyst must include careful and copious peritoneal lavage performed immediately, using several liters of Ringer's lactate, with the patient in a reverse Trendelenburg position. Operative spillage should be avoided as much as possible by using 5-mm aspiration systems or a LapSac. In cases of large cysts, the cyst can be punctured before it is placed in the LapSac, which is positioned directly beneath the cyst in order to catch any possible spillage. Moreover, peritoneal lavage and the appropriate surgical treatment, carried out immediately after diagnosis, seem to make the risks of spillage negligible[1,26] (also Donnez and Nisolle, present study). A recent re-evaluation of intraoperative spillage at laparotomy has demonstrated no adverse effect

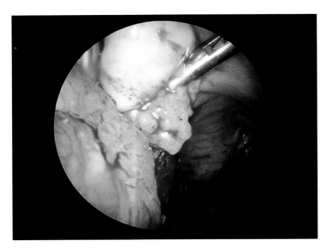

Figure 17.15 Laparoscopic diagnosis of small vegetations on the surface of the ovary. These were not suspected by echography. Frozen histology revealed a 'borderline' tumor. Ovariectomy was carried out. The ovary was removed using a LapSac®

on the prognosis of stage I ovarian cancer[27]. According to this study, the survival term depends primarily on three factors:

- The tumor grading
- The density of adhesions
- Ascites > 250 ml

However, the capsule penetration, the tumor size, the histological type, the age of the patient and the rupture of the tumor were found to have no influence on the prognosis.

It is generally agreed that ovarian cancer should not be managed laparoscopically. One of the drawbacks of operative laparoscopy may be that, in certain cases, malignant cysts cannot be detected.

Risk of postoperative adhesions

What is the risk of postoperative adhesion formation following closure versus non-closure of ovarian defects? It is well known that the ovary is particularly sensitive to surgical trauma, as demonstrated by the high incidence of adhesions after ovarian wedge resection. Buttram and Vaquero[28] performed bilateral ovarian wedge resection for polycystic ovarian disease in 173 patients. Of these, 34% underwent endoscopy or laparotomy at some time after bilateral wedge resection. Although the degree of severity varied, all 59 women were found to have adhesions.

Of nine women of reproductive age who underwent removal of dermoid cysts via laparoscopy without an ovarian suture, Nezhat et al.[15] performed a repeat laparoscopy in four for the evaluation of possible pelvic adhesion formation. Only one had mild periovarian adhesions, and she had experienced no previous spillage of

cyst contents; in the other three women without adhesions at the time of their second laparoscopy, spillage had previously occurred during cystectomy. Because there is little adhesion formation after intraperitoneal cystectomy, most authors consider that no suture is required, and that the ovary can be left open. In our department, ovarian closure is performed only in cases of large endometriotic cysts. Indeed, such cysts are vaporized using the CO_2 laser instead of dissection. Following this type of procedure, the ovarian edges do not approximate spontaneously, and adhesion formation can occur between the vaporized area and the fimbria[12,13]. For this reason, Tissucol® or clips can be used for the ovarian closure[13].

CONCLUSION: THE RIGHT WAY IS THE SELECTION OF PATIENTS

Selection of patients for laparoscopic treatment can be accomplished successfully by excluding those with elevated CA125 levels, suspect ultrasound appearances of cysts containing > 3-mm thick septations, solid components within a cyst, matted loops of bowel or ascites. Large series have demonstrated a reassuringly low incidence of inadvertently encountered malignancy at laparoscopy (0.4%[29,30], 0.9% (Nisolle and Donnez, present study), 1.1%[24], 1.2%[1]), but intraoperative surveillance and numerous biopsies are necessary if unsuspected cancer is to be correctly diagnosed.

We are of the opinion that careful preoperative and perioperative examination will eliminate the high rate of mistakes, published in 1991 by Maiman et al.[31]. For us, this manuscript reveals a lack of experience, or the absence of strict guidelines, for the 29 respondents who took part in a survey concerning the 'laparoscopic management of ovarian neoplasms subsequently found to be malignant'.

REFERENCES

1. Mage G, Canis M, Manhes H, et al. Laparoscopic management of adnexal cystic masses. J Gynecol Surg 1990; 6: 71–9
2. Bruhat MA, Mage G, Chapron C, et al. Present day endoscopic surgery in gynecology. Eur´J Obstet Gynecol Reprod Biol 1991; 41: 4–13
3. Campbell S, Bhan V, Royston P, et al. Transabdominal ultrasound screening for early ovarian cancer. Br Med J 1989; 299: 1363–7
4. Herrmann UJ, Locher GW, Goldhirsch A. Sonographic patterns of ovarian tumors: prediction of malignancy. Obstet Gynecol 1987; 69: 777–81
5. Bourne T, Campbell S, Steer C, et al. Transvaginal colour flow imaging: a possible new screening technique for ovarian cancer. Br Med J 1989; 299: 1367–70
6. Kurjak A, Schulman H, Sosic A, et al. Transvaginal ultrasound, color flow, and Doppler waveform of the

postmenopausal adnexal mass. Obstet Gynecol 1992; 80: 917–21

7. Kawai M, Kano T, Kikkawa F, et al. Transvaginal Doppler ultrasound with color flow imaging in the diagnosis of ovarian cancer. Obstet Gynecol 1992; 79: 163–7

8. Weiner Z, Thaler I, Beck D, et al. Differentiating malignant from benign ovarian tumors with transvaginal color flow imaging. Obstet Gynecol 1992; 79: 159–62

9. Fleischer AC, McKee MS, Gordon AN, et al. Transvaginal sonography of postmenopausal ovaries with pathologic correlation. J Ultrasound Med 1990; 9: 637–44

10. Hata K, Hata T, Manabe A, et al. A critical evaluation of transvaginal Doppler studies, transvaginal sonography, magnetic resonance imaging, and CA-125 in detecting ovarian cancer. Obstet Gynecol 1992; 80: 922–6

11. Malkasian GD, Knapp RC, Lavin PT, et al. Preoperative evaluation of serum CA-125 levels in premenopausal and postmenopausal patients with pelvic masses: discrimination of benign from malignant disease. Am J Obstet Gynecol 1988; 159: 341–6

12. Donnez J, Nisolle M, Karaman Y, et al. CO_2 laser laparoscopy in peritoneal endometriosis and in ovarian cyst. J Gynecol Surg 1990; 5: 391

13. Donnez J, Nisolle M. Laparoscopic management of large ovarian endometrial cysts: use of fibrin sealant. J Gynecol Surg 1991; 7: 163–7

14. Mage G, Canis M, Manhes G, et al. Kystes ovariens et coelioscopie. A propos de 226 observations. J Gynecol Obstet Biol Reprod 1987; 16: 1053–61

15. Nezhat C, Winer WK, Nezhat F. Laparoscopic removal of dermoid cyst. Obstet Gynecol 1989; 73: 278–80

16. Semm K, Mettler L. Technical progress in pelvic surgery via operative laparoscopy. Am J Obstet Gynecol 1980; 138: 121–7

17. Daniell JF, Kurts BR, Lee J. Laparoscopic oophorectomy: comparative study of ligatures, bipolar coagulation, and automatic stapling devices. Obstet Gynecol 1992; 80: 325–8

18. Reich H. Difficulties in removing large masses from the abdomen. In Corfman RS, Diamond MP, DeCherney A, eds. Complications of Laparoscopy and Hysteroscopy. New York: Blackwell Scientific Publications, 1993: 103–7

19. Hsiu JG, Given FT, Kemp GM. Tumor implantation after diagnostic laparoscopic biopsy of serous ovarian tumors of low malignant potential. Obstet Gynecol 1986; 68: 91–3

20. Nisolle M, Donnez J. Laparoscopic ovarian cystectomy. Presented at the Seventh International Symposium on Laser Endoscopic Surgery, Brussels, 1992

21. Reich H. Laparoscopic oophorectomy and salpingoooophorectomy in the treatment of benign tuboovarian disease

22. Reich H. New techniques in advanced laparoscopic surgery. Bailliéres Clin Obstet Gynaecol 1989; 3: 655–82

23. Koonings RP, Campbell K, Mishell DR, et al. Relative frequency of primary ovarian neoplasms: a 10-year review. Obstet Gynecol 1989; 74: 921–6

24. Tasker M, Langley FA. The outlook for women with borderline epithelial tumours of the ovary. Br J Obstet Gynaecol 1985; 92: 969

25. Fernandez RN, Daly JM. Pseudomyxoma peritonei. Arch Surg 1980; 115: 409

26. Lueken RP. Laparoscopic-ovarian surgery. In Lueken RP, Gallinat A, eds. Endoscopic Surgery in Gynecology. Berlin: Demeter Verlag, 1993: 43–7

27. Dembo AJ, Davy M, Stenwig AE, et al. Prognostic factors in patients with stage I epithelial ovarian cancer. Obstet Gynecol 1990; 75: 263–73

28. Buttram VC, Vaquero C. Post-ovarian wedge resection adhesive disease. Fertil Steril 1975; 26: 874

29. Nezhat C, Nezhat F. Complications of laparoscopic ovarian cystectomy. In Corfman RS, Diamond MP, DeCherney A, eds. Complications of Laparoscopy and Hysteroscopy. New York: Blackwell Scientific Publications, 1993: 108–12

30. Nezhat F, Nezhat C, Welander CE, et al. Four ovarian cancers diagnosed during laparoscopic management of 1011 women with adnexal masses. Am J Obstet Gynecol 1992; 167: 790–6

31. Maiman M, Seltzer V, Boyce J. Laparoscopic excision of ovarian neoplasms subsequently found to be malignant. Obstet Gynecol 1991; 77: 563–5

Laparoscopic management of adnexal torsion

18

M Canis, H Manhes, B Rabischong, R Botchorishvili, K Jardon, J L Pouly, G Mage

INTRODUCTION

Adnexal torsion is an infrequent but not rare gynecological disorder. Classical surgical management was adnexectomy without unwinding by laparotomy. As laparoscopy is useful in the diagnosis of adnexal torsion[1,2], we have been performing laparoscopic management since 1978[3,4]. Besides its well known advantages, we think that the main contribution of the laparoscopic approach has been to re-emphasize the value and effectiveness of the conservative treatment of adnexal torsion. This type of management, which was first proposed by Way in 1946[5], is highly desirable, since torsion occurs most often in women of reproductive age. Recently, a review of the literature concluded that the risk of pulmonary embolism after adnexal torsion was 0.2%, and was not increased when the adnexa was untwisted[6]. We report here our experience of 48 cases of conservative management from a series of 72 cases.

PATIENTS AND METHODS

Seventy-two cases of adnexal torsion were diagnosed between June 1978 and December 1994. Only cases with at least a 360° rotation of the pedicle were included in the study. Malignant ovarian tumors and cases of chronic torsion with an axial rotation of <180° and fixed by adhesions were excluded. The mean age was 27.8 years (range 13–55). According to their clinical data, patients were divided into two groups.

Group 1

Fifty-three patients (73.6%) presented with acute pelvic pain. In this group, the preoperative diagnosis was accurate in only 35 cases (66.0%). Other preoperative diagnoses were ectopic pregnancy, salpingitis, hyperstimulation syndrome with sign of acute abdomen[7,8] and corpus luteum hemorrhage.

Group 2

Nineteen patients (26.4%) presented with chronic pelvic pain or were referred for surgical evaluation of an adnexal cyst. The delay between the first visit and surgery ranged from 1 to 3 months. In these cases adnexal torsion was never suspected before laparoscopy.

Method

The laparoscopic technique and the instruments used have been described previously[9]. Two or three 5-mm ancillary trocars were inserted into the suprapubic area. Laparoscopic management involved three steps: diagnosis, management of ischemic lesions and treatment of the etiology (Figures 18.1 and 18.2).

Management of ischemic lesions

As recommended by Way[5] the organs involved were untwisted whenever possible to assess ischemic lesions. To untwist the adnexa, blunt manipulation was preferred to grasping, thus avoiding additional damage and bleeding.

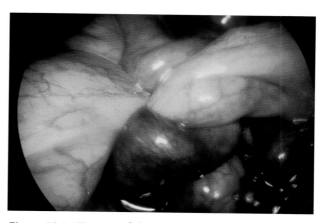

Figure 18.1   Torsion of the right adnexa

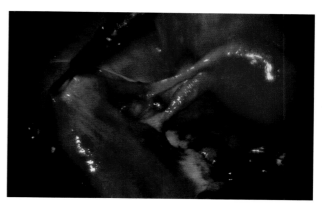

Figure 18.2   Partial ovarian recovery at the end of the laparoscopy

Using an atraumatic forceps or a 5-mm probe, the twisted organs were moved slowly and gently according to 'Kustner's law': Kustner noted that on the left side the pedicle of the twisted organs was rotated in a clockwise direction, whereas it would rotate in a counterclockwise direction on the right side[10]. When adhesions were found on the twisted adnexa, adhesiolysis was the first step of the procedure. Finally, in patients with a very large adnexal cyst, untwisting was sometimes possible after puncture and aspiration of the cyst. According to the initial ischemic lesions and immediate recovery[3,4], the women were assigned to one of the three following groups:

- Group A: no evidence of ischemia or mild lesions with immediate and complete recovery

- Group B: severe ischemia (tube and ovary were dark red or black colored at the time of diagnosis) with partial recovery 10 minutes after the pedicle was untwisted

- Group C: gangrenous adnexa without recovery

In groups A and B, conservative management was chosen whenever it was possible to treat the etiology in this manner. Gangrenous adnexae were removed either by laparotomy or by laparoscopy. In group B a second-look laparoscopy was proposed 6–8 weeks after the initial procedure to assess definitive recovery. Close clinical and sonographic follow-up looking for recurrence of torsion was requested for patients treated conservatively.

Treatment of the etiology

Adnexal cysts were managed as previously described[11], and were treated by laparotomy before 1980 and by laparoscopy in most cases during the last years of this study. Suspicious and/or malignant adnexal cysts were treated by immediate laparotomy. Other causes were managed using previously described laparoscopic procedures[9,11].

RESULTS

Laparoscopy always enabled a definitive diagnosis of adnexal torsion. The right adnexa was involved in 38 cases (52.8%) and the left in 33 cases (45.8%), and one patient had bilateral torsion associated with ovarian hyperstimulation. Laparoscopic unwinding of the torsion was possible in 64 cases (88.9%). In three cases, gentle manipulation of a gangrenous tube resulted in a salpingectomy without any bleeding. In three patients, laparoscopic unwinding of a gangrenous ovary was impossible, and in two patients, adnexectomy was decided upon before the surgical procedure. Indications were a suspicious mass at ultrasound in one case, and the age of the patient in the second case (70 years).

Etiology

Adnexal cysts (72.1%) were the most common cause of torsion. Other causes are listed in Table 18.1. In three cases the etiology was thought to be congenital as we found abnormal ovarian ligaments, either a too-short mesovarium or a too-long utero-ovarian ligament. When the adnexa appeared normal, several punctures were routinely performed to rule out the presence of a small ovarian cyst.

Management

Ischemic lesions were mild in 40 cases (group A, 55.5%), severe in 17 cases (group B, 23.6%) and beyond recovery in 15 cases (group C, 20.8%) (Table 18.2). The incidence of necrosis increased during the last period of the study, as a consequence of the phlegmatic management of torsion by general practitioners who tended to treat acute abdominal syndrome using potent oral anti-inflammatory drugs. All patients with chronic pelvic pain had mild ischemic lesions and were included in group A.

Table 18.1 Etiology encountered ($n = 72$)

	n	%
Ovarian cysts	31	43.1
Functional cysts	11	15.2
Organic ovarian cysts	20	27.8
Para-oophoritic cysts	17	23.6
Ovarian hyperstimulation	5	6.9
Ectopic pregnancy	3	4.2
Hydrosalpinx	3	4.2
Adhesions	3	4.2
Malformation	3	4.2
Normal adnexa	7	9.7

Table 18.2 Treatment according to ischemic lesions ($n = 72$)

Ischemic lesions	n	Conservative	Radical
All patients			
Mild	40	33 (82.5%)	7 (17.5%)
Severe	17	14 (82.3%)	3 (17.7%)
Not gangrenous	57	47 (82.5%)	10 (17.5%)
Gangrenous	15	1 (6.6%)	14 (93.4%)
Total	72	48 (66.6%)	24 (33.3%)
Patients < 40 years old			
Mild	32	28 (87.5%)	4 (12.5%)
Severe	14	14 (100%)	0 (0.0%)
Not gangrenous	46	42 (91.3%)	4 (9.7%)
Gangrenous	6	1 (16.6%)	5 (83.3%)
Total	52	43 (82.7%)	9 (17.3%)

In groups A and B, conservative treatment was achieved for 47 of 57 patients (82.5%) (Table 18.2). Overall, conservative management was achieved in 48 of 72 patients (66.6%) and in 43 of the 52 patients (82.7%) who were less than 40 years old.

The immediate postoperative course was always uneventful. Although heparin was never used, we observed no thromboembolic complications.

In six of the 17 patients included in group B, we found a complete and even surprising recovery at second-look laparoscopy (Figures 18.1–18.3). An ovarian biopsy was obtained in only one case; histological examination showed a thickened ovarian capsule with a normal follicular population. In the seventh second-look laparoscopy, the twisted ovary had disappeared[12,13]. This patient had been treated by unilateral salpingectomy without oophorectomy, despite complete necrosis of the tube. From this case, we assume that the ovary should be removed when the tubal lesions are beyond recovery, i.e. when the tube does not recover within 10 minutes of the detorsion.

Follow-up

Six patients were lost to follow-up 1–2 months after laparoscopic treatment. For the remaining 66 patients, the duration of follow-up ranged from 8 months to 16 years.

We observed five recurrences of torsion.

The first patient had an ovariopexy using a Fallopian ring to treat an overly long utero-ovarian ligament with a normal ovary; 12 months later, another laparoscopy, performed to evaluate a 6-cm diameter ovary, showed a recurrence of torsion without ischemia. A bilateral ovariopexy was performed by laparotomy.

The second recurrence was discovered during laparoscopy performed for chronic pelvic pain, 12 months after a right ovariopexy and ovarian cystectomy. We found

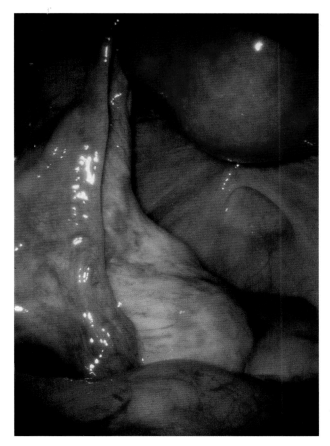

Figure 18.3 Complete recovery at second-look laparoscopy.

torsion of the contralateral ovary, the utero-ovarian ligament was absent and the ovary was fixed by adhesions to the posterior wall of the broad ligament. Conservative management with a left ovariopexy was achieved.

REFERENCES

1. Azoury RS, Chehab RM, Mufarrij IK. The twisted adnexa; a clinical and pathological review. Diagn Gynecol Obstet 1980; 2: 185–91
2. Hibbard LT. Adnexal torsion. Am J Obstet Gynecol 1985; 152: 456–61
3. Manhes H, Canis M, Mage G, et al. Place de la coelioscopie dans le diagnostic et le traitement des torsions d'annexes. J Gynecol Obstet Biol Reprod 1984; 13: 825–9
4. Mage G, Canis M, Manhes H, et al. Laparoscopic management of adnexal torsion. A review of 35 cases. J Reprod Med 1989; 34: 520–4
5. Way S. Ovarian cystectomy of twisted cysts. Lancet 1946; 2: 47–8
6. McGovern PG, Noah R, Koenigsberg R, Little AB. Adnexal torsion and pulmonary embolism: case report and review of the literature. Obstet Gynecol Surv 1999; 54: 601–8
7. Chin NW, Friedman CI, Awadalla SG, et al. Adnexal torsion as a complication of superovulation for ovum retrieval. Fertil Steril 1987; 48: 149–51
8. Hurwitz A, Milwidsky A, Yagel S, et al. Early unwinding of torsion of an ovarian cyst as a result of hyperstimulation syndrome. Fertil Steril 1983; 40: 393–5
9. Bruhat MA, Mage G, Pouly JL, et al. Operative Laparoscopy. New York: McGraw Hill, 1992
10. Kustner O. Das Gesetzmalsige in der torsionspirale torquirter Ovariumtumorstiele. Zentralbl Gynakol 1981; 15: 209–13
11. Canis M, Mage G, Pouly JL, et al. Laparoscopic diagnosis of adnexal cystic masses: a 12-year experience with long-term follow-up. Obstet Gynecol 1994; 83: 707–12
12. Ali V, Lynn S, Schmidt W. Unilateral absence of distal tube and ovary with migratory calcified intraperitoneal mass. Int J Gynaecol Obstet 1980; 17: 328–31
13. Beyth H, Baron E. Tuboovarian autoamputation and infertility. Fertil Steril 1984; 42: 932–4
14. Albayram F, Hamper UM. Ovarian and adnexal torsion: spectrum of sonographic findings with pathologic correlation. J Ultrasound Med 2001; 20: 1083–9
15. Fleischer AC, Brader KR. Sonographic depiction of ovarian vascularity and flow: current improvements and future applications. J Ultrasound Med 2001; 20: 241–50
16. Nichols DH, Julian PJ. Torsion of the adnexa. Clin Obstet Gynecol 1985; 28: 375–80
17. Mashiach R, Canis M, Jardon K, et al. Adnexal torsion after laparoscopic hysterectomy: description of seven cases. J Am Assoc Gynecol Laparosc 2004; 11: 336–9
18. Bider D, Ben-Rafael Z, Goldenberg M, et al. Pregnancy outcome after unwinding of twisted ischemic hemorragic adnexa. Br J Obstet Gynaecol 1989; 96: 428–30
19. MacGowan L. Torsion of cystic or diseased adnexal tissue. Am J Obstet Gynecol 1964; 88: 135–6
20. Reich H, DeCaprio J, McGlynn F, Taylor PJ. Laparoscopic diagnosis and management of acute adnexal torsion. Gynaecol Endosc 1992; 2: 37–8
21. Wagaman R, Williams RS. Conservative therapy for adnexal torsion. A case report. J Reprod Med 1990; 35: 833–4
22. Oelsner G, Cohen SB, Soriano D, et al. Minimal surgery for the twisted ischaemic adnexa can preserve ovarian function. Hum Reprod 2003; 18: 2599–602

Part 3
Uterine and pelvic floor pathology

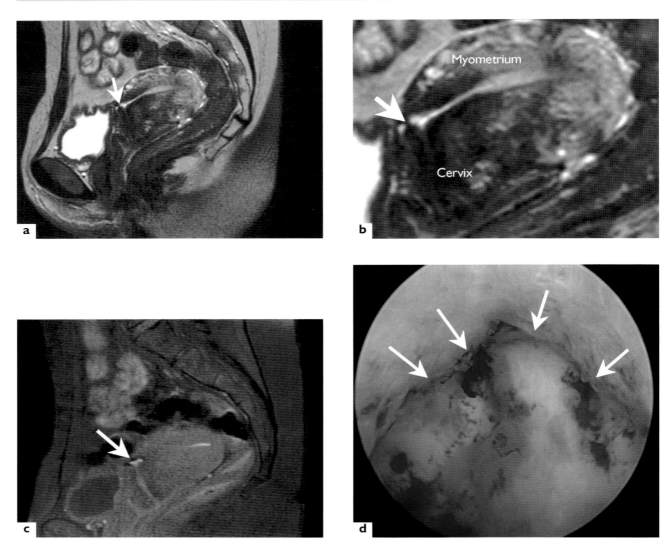

Figure 19.2 (a) and (b) Magnetic resonance imaging (MRI) showing the thickness of the anterior uterine wall (white arrow), highly suggestive of a wide and deep dehiscent cesarean scar. MRI evaluates the residual thickness between the dehiscent scar and the peritoneum at less than 1 mm. (c) Sagittal view of the lower uterine part in T1-weighted image with fatty tissue saturation. Hyperintensive signal (white arrow) is highly suggestive of old blood retention in the cesarean scar dehiscence. (d) Hysteroscopic view of the scar dehiscence (white arrows)

weighted images. As in case 1, a hyperintensive signal on T1-weighted images with saturation of fatty tissue could be seen in the uterine cavity and the cesarean scar (Figure 19.3d). This hyperintensive signal is highly suggestive of old blood retention. Hysteroscopic evaluation of the cervix and the subisthmic area allowed us to evaluate the width of the dehiscence. In Figure 19.3e, we can see the presence of old blood retention in a large scar opened from side to side.

SURGICAL TECHNIQUE

Laparoscopic repair was therefore proposed to the patients, after having explained the risk of uterine rupture

in the case of a subsequent pregnancy if the dehiscent scar was not repaired. A Foley catheter was placed in the bladder in order to ensure an empty bladder throughout surgery. Operative hysteroscopy was then performed in both cases to visualize the dehiscence from the cervix. It allowed us to treat the uterine septum observed in case 1. We used a Nd : YAG (neodymium : yttrium–aluminum–garnet) laser to perform hysteroscopic septoplasty, as previously described[7]. In both cases, laparoscopy revealed a normal-sized uterus associated with normal adnexa. As observed in Figure 19.4a, the cesarean scar was easily distinguishable. A probe was then inserted through the cervix, into the dehiscent scar (Figure 19.4b). The peritoneum was then opened to separate the bladder from the anterior wall

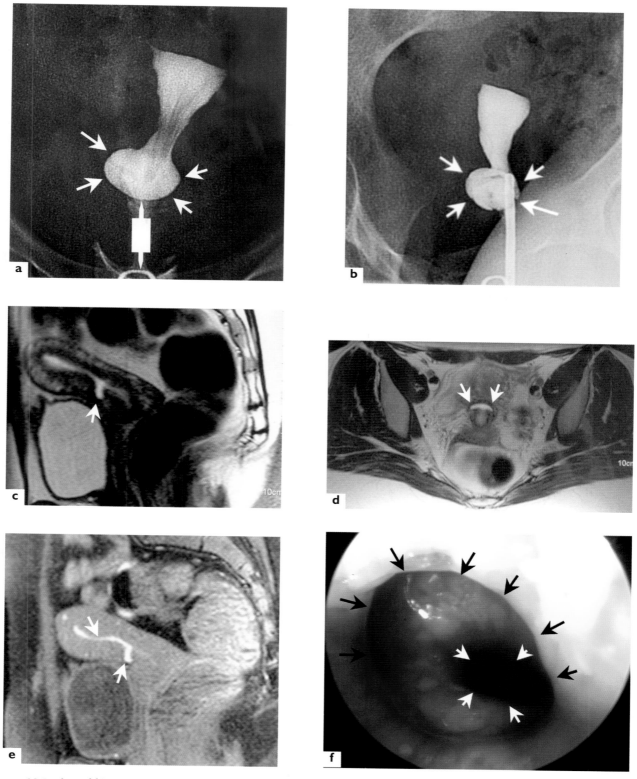

Figure 19.3 (a and b) In case 2, hysterography revealed wide dehiscence (white arrows) at the level of the cesarean scar. (c) and (d) Sagittal and transverse views (T2-weighted images) confirmed the ultrasound findings: the residual myometrium covering the dehiscence was very thin (white arrows). (e) As in case 1, a T1-weighted image with fatty tissue saturation revealed a hyperintensive signal (white arrows), highly suggestive of old blood retention in the dehiscent scar and the uterine cavity. (f) Hysteroscopic view of the subisthmic area confirmed the presence of old blood retention in the scar. The dehiscent scar (black arrows) is visible from side to side in the anterior wall area. The beginning of the uterine cavity can be seen higher than the scar (white arrows)

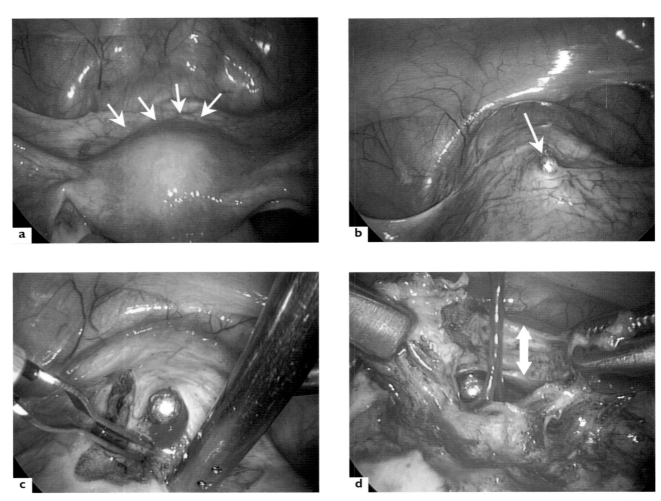

Figure 19.4 (a) The scar (white arrows) could be easily distinguished by a laparoscopic view. (b) A probe (white arrow) was inserted through the cervix into the dehiscent scar. (c) The peritoneum was opened using a CO_2 laser. The laparoscopic approach offered a wide-open view of the vesicovaginal space in order to perform safe dissection of the bladder. (d) The anterior uterine wall (white arrow) was composed of a thin layer of fibrotic tissue covered with peritoneum

safely (Figure 19.4c). The lower uterine segment was composed of only a thin layer of fibrotic tissue covered by peritoneum (Figure 19.4d). A laparoscopic approach gave us wide-open access to the vesicovaginal space, compared with the vaginal approach, and allowed us to avoid bladder injuries during surgery.

Using the CO_2 laser, we completely opened the scar from side to side. The fibrotic tissue was then excised from the edges of the cesarean scar to facilitate further healing. Special care had to be taken on the lateral side of the scar to avoid injury to the uterine blood vessels. The final view of the wide-open scar can be observed in Figure 19.5a. Before closing the scar, a Hegar probe was inserted into the cervix in order to preserve the continuity of the cervical canal to the uterine cavity (Figure 19.5b). Using Vicryl® 2-0 SH+, two separate sutures were first placed on the two lateral sides of the scar (Figure 19.5c and 19.5d). The scar

was finally closed using two more 2-0 sutures, as shown in Figure 19.5e. The scar was then covered with peritoneum. The final view of the repair can be seen in Figure 19.5f. At the end of surgery, we performed hysteroscopy to visualize the repair from the cervical canal (Figure 19.6). It showed complete correction of the defect and normal permeability of the cervix. During these two surgical procedures, no complications occurred. The Foley catheter was removed the day after surgery and the two patients were discharged from hospital on day 1. We recommend waiting 3 months before attempting pregnancy. In the case of pregnancy, the lower uterine segment must be carefully monitored and cesarean section should be performed at 38 weeks of pregnancy to avoid the risk of uterine rupture.

Three months after surgery, hysterosalpingography revealed a uterine cavity with a normal supraisthmic area at the level of the cesarean section in both cases. The resec-

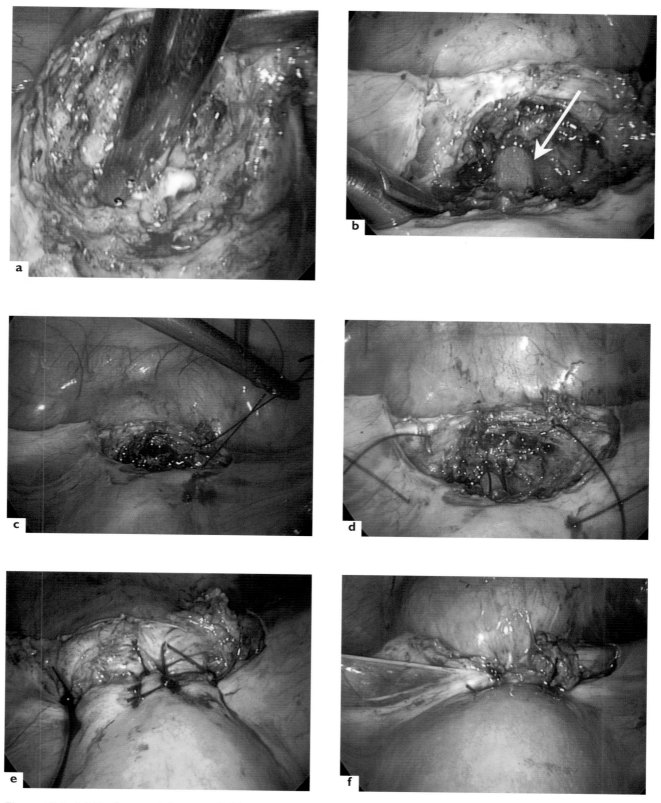

Figure 19.5 (a) Final view of the opened dehiscent scar after resection of the fibrotic tissue with use of the CO_2 laser. (b) A Hegar probe (white arrow) was inserted through the cervix to preserve the permeability of the cervical canal before performing the suture. (c) and (d) Two separate sutures were placed on each side of the scar. (e) The scar was finally closed with two more sutures. (f) A separate suture completed closure of the scar. Final view of the scar after covering it with peritoneum

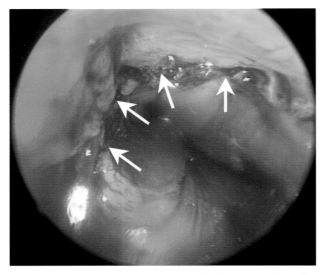

Figure 19.6 Hysteroscopic view of the scar after the suture was completed

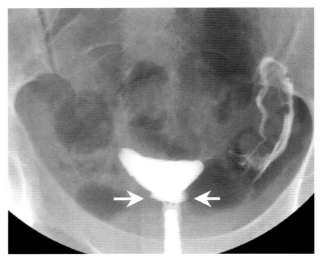

Figure 19.7 Three months after surgery, hysterography was performed in case 1. Resection of the septum and the depth of the cesarean scar were easily assessed and found to be wholly acceptable compared with the preoperative investigations. The uterine cavity was found to be normal and the dehiscence had disappeared

tion of the septum and depth of the cesarean scar were easily assessed in case 1, and found to be wholly acceptable compared with the preoperative investigations (Figure 19.7). The uterine cavity was found to be normal and the dehiscence had disappeared. Ultrasonographic evaluation of the lower uterine segment confirmed the integrity of the anterior uterine wall.

DISCUSSION

Uterine rupture remains the most feared complication of pregnancy and labor in women with previous cesarean delivery. Different imaging modalities, from hysterography to ultrasonographic evaluation, have been used to evaluate the integrity of the anterior uterine wall. Even if hysterography has not proved especially useful[8,9], we found that it provided good visualization of the depth and width of dehiscence at the level of the cesarean scar.

In the literature, ultrasonographic monitoring of the lower uterine segment during pregnancy has been described. The critical cut-off value for lower uterine segment thickness that allows trials of labor is 2.5 mm[10]. Ultrasonographic evaluation of a 1.5-mm lower uterine segment during pregnancy has a sensitivity of 88.9% and a negative predictive value of 96.2% in predicting a dehiscent lower uterine segment, suggesting that ultrasonography can potentially be used to predict the risk of uterine rupture during labor[11].

In these cases, the patients were not pregnant, and the lower uterine segment thickness was less than 1 mm using transvaginal ultrasonography in both women. MRI confirmed the thickness of the anterior wall and the presence of old blood (hematometra) in the scar dehiscence, correlating with the hysteroscopic findings. In the literature, there is a lack of information on the ability of MRI to detect cesarean scar dehiscence. In our cases, ultrasonographic and MRI findings were found to concur with respect to lower uterine segment thickness, which was less than 1 mm. These findings were confirmed by laparoscopy, which revealed the presence of a very thin layer of fibrotic tissue covering the cesarean scar.

Schneider *et al.*[6] used combined laparoscopic/vaginal as well as purely vaginal approaches to repair defects due to dehiscent cesarean scars in five patients. We report a hitherto undescribed laparoscopic technique. The laparoscopic approach offers an optimal view during dissection of the vesicovaginal space to separate the bladder from the anterior uterine wall safely and thereby avoid bladder injuries. Compared with laparotomy, the time to recovery is now widely recognized to be shorter with the laparoscopic technique. Hospital stay is also shorter. CO_2 laser was used to excise the fibrotic tissue in order to restore normal tissue to the edges of the wound. Then, a one-layer laparoscopic suture could be easily placed. The advantage of this technique is recovering the integrity of the anterior uterine wall, as confirmed by further ultrasonographic and hysterographic evaluation. In the case of subsequent pregnancy, special care has to be proposed to follow closely the measurement of the anterior uterine wall in order to prevent uterine rupture. cesarean section at 38 weeks should also be proposed.

CONCLUSION

Ultrasonographic evaluation of the anterior uterine wall is mandatory to evaluate the thickness of the lower uterine segment in a case of previous cesarean section, but, in the cases we describe, MRI provided an objective evaluation of the dehiscent scar. In the case of deep cesarean scar dehiscence with residual myometrial thickness of less than 2.5 mm, laparoscopic surgical repair may be proposed. We report a laparoscopic technique involving resection of the fibrotic tissue in order to restore normal tissue to the edges of the scar. After laparoscopic suture, evaluation of the repaired scar can be performed by ultrasonography and hysterosalpingography. In the present cases, no further dehiscence was visible. However, investigations such as follow-up of pregnancy and evolution of the anterior uterine wall are mandatory to evaluate the strength of the new scar tissue.

REFERENCES

1. Seffah JD. Re-laparotomy after cesarean section. Int J Gynaecol Obstet 2005; 88: 253–7
2. Benbow A, Semple D, Maresh M. Effective Procedures in Maternity Care Suitable for Audit. London: Royal College of Obstetricians and Gynaecologists, 1997: 34
3. Kayani SI, Alfirevic Z. Uterine rupture after induction of labour in women with previous cesarean section. Br J Obstet Gynaecol 2005; 112: 451–5
4. Godin PA, Bassil S, Donnez J. An ectopic pregnancy developing in a previous cesarean section scar. Fertil Steril 1997; 67: 398–400
5. Ito M, Nawa T, Mikamo H, Tamaya T. Lower segment uterine rupture related to early pregnancy by in vitro fertilization and embryo transfer after previous cesarean delivery. J Med 1998; 29: 85–91
6. Klemm P, Koehler C, Mangler M, et al. Laparoscopic and vaginal repair of uterine scar dehiscence following cesarean section as detected by ultrasound. J Perinat Med 2005; 33: 324–31
7. Donnez J, Nisolle M. Endoscopic laser treatment of uterine malformations. Hum Reprod 1997; 12: 1381–7
8. Poidevin L, Bockner V. A hysterographic study of uteri after caesarean section. J Obstet Gynaecol Br Emp 1958; 65: 278–83
9. Bockner V. Hysterography and ruptured uterus. J Obstet Gynaecol Br Emp 1960; 67: 838–9
10. Sen S, Malik S, Salhan S. Ultrasonographic evaluation of lower uterine segment thickness in patients of previous caesarean section. Int J Gynaecol Obstet 2004; 87: 215–19
11. Cheung VY. Sonographic measurement of the lower uterine segment thickness in women with previous caesarean section. J Obstet Gynaecol Can 2005; 27: 674–81

Laparoscopic myomectomy

J B Dubuisson, A Fauconnier

The indications for operative laparoscopy have expanded greatly over recent decades as its many advantages over laparotomy have been recognized. Myomectomy may be performed by laparoscopy in selected cases, particularly in subserous and interstitial myomas[1-4]. At present, a large number of teams use laparoscopic myomectomy, proving that this technique has many advantages. Nevertheless, it is a difficult operation in some cases.

PREOPERATIVE EVALUATION

Preoperative detection and evaluation of the myomas should be particularly meticulous, because with the laparoscopic approach it is impossible to palpate the myometrium thoroughly. This preoperative work-up must include: abdominal and transvaginal ultrasonography with Doppler, and measurement of preoperative hemoglobin levels. Examination of the uterine cavity is performed by diagnostic hysteroscopy if submucous myomas are suspected at ultrasonography.

Abdominal and transvaginal ultrasound examination must include measurement of the diameters of the entire uterus (length, depth and width), the number of myomas and characteristics of the dominant myomas, i.e. their type (intramural, subserous or pedunculated), size and location (anterior, posterior, fundus, broad ligament or isthmus). It should also include measurement of the distance between the endometrium and the myoma[5], and between the serosa and the myoma. Furthermore, it is important to include a systematic search for adenomyosis. Adenomyosis may modify the indication of myomectomy; also, cleavage of the myoma can be more difficult, with more bleeding[6,7]. It is also fundamental to evaluate the vascularization of the dominant myoma, which may be responsible for abnormal bleeding during enucleation and suture. Doppler examination gives important information concerning the origin of the vessels irrigating the dominant myoma: right or left uterine artery, both uterine arteries or the ovarian arteries. In our experience, a left-side myoma is vascularized by the left uterine artery (or both uterine arteries), a right-side myoma by the right uterine artery (or both) and a fundic myoma may be vascularized by the uterine arteries but also by the ovarian arteries. A hypervascularized myoma will grow rapidly. Such information may play a role in determination of the operative strategy.

Diagnosic hysteroscopy must be performed in selected cases: menometrorrhagia, multiple myomas, suspected intrauterine abnormalities at ultrasound and in infertile patients. Hysteroscopy allows the surgeon to differentiate between a deep interstitial myoma and a submucous myoma or a polyp. Comparison of the results of ultrasound and hysteroscopy is important to determine the operative strategy.

Magnetic resonance imaging (MRI) is mandatory when the ultrasound examination is difficult to analyze and in cases of associated adnexal pathology, e.g. a suspected ovarian cyst. Hysterosonography might be useful for evaluating the relationship between the myomas and the uterine cavity[8].

In all cases, it is important to obtain good information with the minimum of exploration for both psychological and economic reasons.

In infertile patients, the investigation should be completed by including a hysterosalpingogram, a study of ovarian function (monthly temperature curve; levels of anti-Müllerian hormone, follicle stimulating hormone, luteinizing hormone and estradiol) and analysis of the partner's semen. In the presence of an associated male or ovulatory factor, the postoperative fertility results are poor[9], and in these cases the perioperative and postoperative strategy should be carefully discussed.

A blood count and serum ferritin test provide information regarding whether to give oral iron (see section below on 'Preoperative treatment'), particularly in patients with menometrorrhagia.

PREOPERATIVE TREATMENT

The correction of sideropenic anemia by giving oral iron is essential in order to reduce the risk of blood transfusion. In some cases it is necessary to postpone laparoscopic myomectomy, until the blood count has been normalized.

Gonadotropin-releasing hormone agonists (GnRH) agonists cause myoma shrinkage by reducing the circulating estrogen levels[10]. The maximal reduction of myoma size is achieved by 12 weeks of therapy, with no further change observed after 24 weeks of treatment[11]. Matta et al.[12] observed that GnRH agonists reduce uterine blood flow.

In patients undergoing laparoscopic myomectomy, preoperative treatment with GnRH agonists may have controversial effects. A marked reduction in blood loss during laparotomic myomectomy has been demonstrated[13]. During laparoscopic myomectomy, the preoperative use of GnRH agonists also had the advantage of

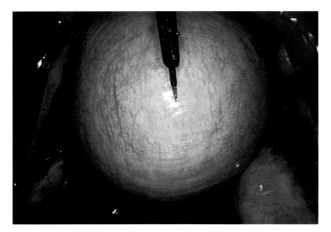

Figure 20.1 Hysterotomy of a posterior intramural myoma

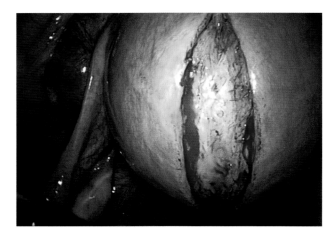

Figure 20.2 Visualization of the myoma after opening of the pseudocapsule

Incision of the myometrium and exposure of the myoma

The hysterotomy is direct, lined up with the myoma. In the case of a posterior myoma, we use sagittal hysterotomies. In the case of an anterior myoma, we tend to use oblique hysterotomies because they are easier to suture. The myometrium is incised with a laparoscopic needle using a low-voltage monopolar current in cutting mode in order to safeguard the myometrium as far as possible (Figure 20.1). Hemostasis of the intramyometrial vessels is carried out progressively, using a bipolar forceps. The myoma is easy to recognize by its smooth appearance and pearly white color, which contrasts with the adjacent myometrium (Figure 20.2).

Enucleation (Figure 20.3)

Dissection of the myoma should run inside the avascular plane surrounding the myoma, leaving the pseudocapsule around the outside and the uterine vessels pushed back. Identification of this avascular plane is assisted by the magnifying effect of the laparoscopic images (Figure 20.3). The myoma is grasped with a strong 10-mm grasping forceps designed specifically for myomas (with claw or tenaculum), and pulled hard towards the anterior abdominal wall or upwards; at the same time the surgeon or his assistant exerts traction in the opposite direction using the endouterine cannula, or by pushing on the edges of the hysterotomy with an instrument. This dissection proceeds from the superficial areas inwards, and always under visual control in order to identify the fine tracti adhering to the myoma (Figure 20.4). The tip of a blunt instrument is used to press against the myoma. The tracti adhering to the myoma are coagulated, then sectioned. The bed of the myomectomy is most often free from hemorrhage at the end of dissection, if care has been taken to follow the avascular cleavage plane, and there is no need to take further steps for hemostasis.

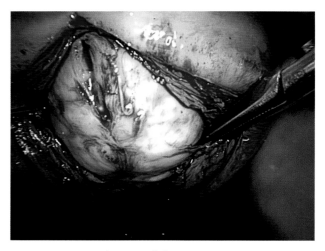

Figure 20.3 Enucleation of the myoma

Hysterotomy suture (Figures 20.5 and 20.6)

We use fine resorbable suture, diameter 00 or 0 gauge, mounted on a curved needle with an atraumatic tip (Vicryl® (polyglactin 910); Ethicon). In the case of a subserosal myoma, the suture is usually carried out in a single plane. We use single, separate intracorporeal knots. The stitches go through the whole thickness of the edges of the hysterotomy, and through the uterine serosa. They are placed sufficiently close for the edges to be approximated completely, yet far enough apart to avoid making the myometrium too fragile (Figure 20.6). When the myomectomy is located deeply, or the uterine cavity has been opened, two planes are performed. We suture along a deep plane with a few single stitches deep in the myometrium, and along a superficial plane taking in the serosa and the superficial part of the myometrium. The superficial plane can be dealt with using a running suture or with individual stitches. When suturing the deep plane,

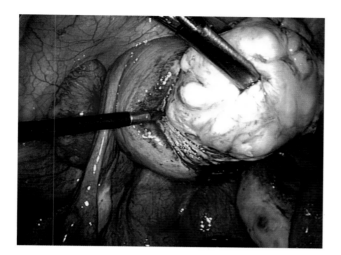

Figure 20.4 End of the myomectomy

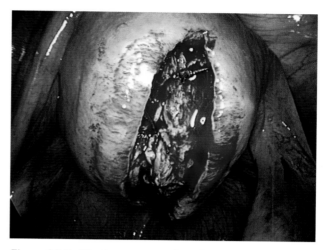

Figure 20.5 Uterine suture: first layer using separate stiches

it can sometimes be difficult to take the needle through the thickness of the defect. In this case it can be an advantage to use Vicryl 1 with a large curved needle, and to perform a U-shaped transfixing stitch[27], running through the uterine serosa and taking in the whole thickness of the edges of the myomectomy. One or two of these stitches are sufficient to ensure that all the deep part of the hysterotomy is brought into contact. When the uterine suture proves difficult to carry out it is essential to know when to stop and use a minilaparotomy for the suture. We recommend, in particular, its use for large anterior or deep intramural myomas.

Extraction of myomas

There are various methods for extraction: direct suprapubic extraction; electric morcellation; and extraction via posterior colpotomy.

Direct suprapubic extraction is appropriate only for small myomas. Extraction takes place through the midline suprapubic incision which may be enlarged (>2 cm). If needed, a manual morcellation is carried out: with one or two single-tooth tenaculums, the myoma is brought up to the suprapubic incision and held against the peritoneum to prevent loss of CO_2 and then fragmented under laparoscopic control, using a small blade passed through the incision.

Electric morcellation is carried out with the use of an electrical morcellator (see above, 'Instrumentation'). This device is an external rotating cylindrical blade that is introduced via a 12- or 15-mm suprapubic trocar. A forceps with 10-mm jaws is inserted through the morcellator channel to grasp the myoma and cut it progressively, like peeling an orange. The position of the rotating blade must be carefully controlled in order to avoid any risk of damaging any neighboring organs.

Posterior colpotomy also allows large myomas to be extracted[46]. The colpotomy may be performed by

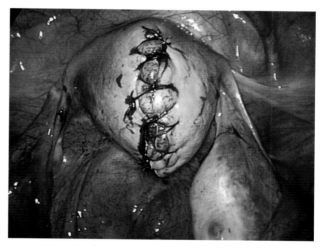

Figure 20.6 Final result

laparoscopy using the monopolar needle, or conventionally through the vagina. The myoma is then grasped with a forceps with 10-mm jaws, inserted through the colpotomy under laparoscopic control. The myoma is extracted vaginally either directly or after morcellation. In the case of large or numerous myomas, the CCL vaginal extractor (Storz, Germany) is useful to prevent leakage of gas.

Preventive uterine artery occlusion combined with laparoscopic myomectomy

In highly vascularized myomas, it is important to limit blood loss during myoma enucleation and myometrium suture. Before 2001, in some cases of excessive bleeding during laparoscopic myomectomy, we had to perform the occlusion of one or two uterine arteries during the procedure to stop the hemorrhage. The decrease in bleeding after uterine artery occlusion was clinically evident. The combined procedure allowed us to carry out

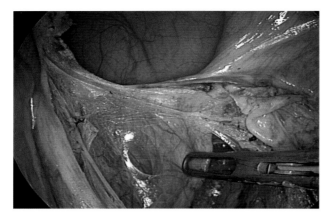

Figure 20.7 Preventive occlusion of the uterine artery before hysterotomy: dissection of the right broad ligament

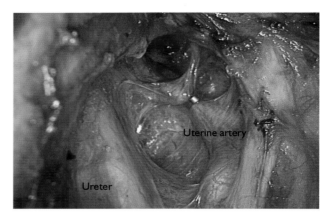

Figure 20.8 Dissection of the right uterine artery after visualization of the right ureter

the end of the myomectomy by laparoscopy without any complication. This prompted us to perform a comparative study in order to demonstrate the advantages of this combined procedure[32]. Now, in the case of a highly vascularized myoma of more than 6 cm, we systematically perform, at the beginning of laparoscopy, uterine artery occlusion on either one or both sides according to the information given by Doppler ultrasonography. This procedure is not indicated when the myoma is poorly vascularized or has a typical aspect of necrobiosis at ultrasonography or at laparoscopy. There is no indication when the myoma is exclusively vascularized with the ovarian vessels. This procedure is not feasible when the myoma is too large and fixed, with no access to the uterine arteries before the myomectomy.

Broad ligament access to the uterine artery (Figures 20.7 and 20.8)   Before the myomectomy, we perform a 3-cm incision of the peritoneum with scissors on the upper part of the broad ligament, behind the round ligament. The umbilical artery is then dissected and followed until the origin of the uterine artery is reached. The origin of the uterine artery is then dissected from the uterine veins. Inside the artery the ureter is also visualized, adherent to the peritoneum. To occlude the artery, one or two non-absorbable clips (titanium Ligaclip™, Storz) are placed at its origin. The hemostasis of small vessels is performed if necessary. A few minutes after the occlusion, the myoma turns white before the uterus (Figure 20.9). At the end of the laparoscopic myomectomy, the peritoneum of the broad ligament is closed using a 00 Vicryl running suture. The same procedure is performed on the other broad ligament if necessary. Then the hysterotomy is performed.

Posterior access to the uterine artery (Figures 20.10–20.15) The occlusion of the uterine artery may be performed using a posterior access (Figures 20.10–20.15). The uterus is pulled hard towards the anterior abdominal wall using the intrauterine cannula. On the chosen side, the uterine artery is visualized under the peritoneum at the inferior

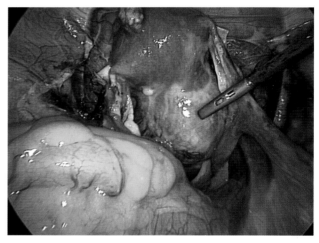

Figure 20.9 Immediate aspect of the uterus after occlusion of the uterine arteries: the myoma turns white before the uterus

area of the posterior leaf of the broad ligament, close to the uterus, just above the origin of the homolateral uterosacral ligament. The ureter is also visualized under the pulsating artery. A 1-cm direct incision of the peritoneum gives immediate access to the uterine artery. One or two clips are then placed, with permanent control of the ureter located under the artery. This second procedure is very quick and easy to perform if access is possible. The peritoneum is then sutured with a 00 Vicryl single suture.

Second-look laparoscopy

A second-look laparoscopy should be proposed to patients desiring pregnancy and who have sutured uterine scars, in order to eliminate adhesions after myomectomy and to assess the strength of the uterine scar[47,48]. The systematic use of second-look laparoscopy could reduce adhesions after myomectomy and consequently enhance fertility[49,50].

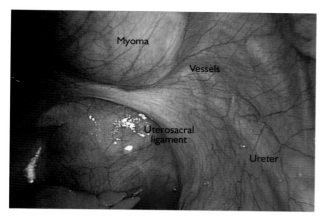

Figure 20.10 Posterior access to perform occlusion of the uterine artery

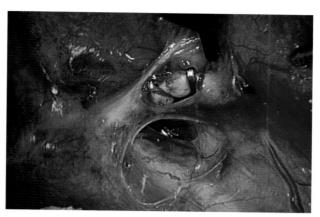

Figure 20.13 Clips are placed, with permanent control of the ureter which is under the artery

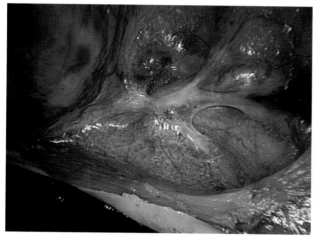

Figure 20.11 Dissection of the right uterine artery, visualized under the peritoneum

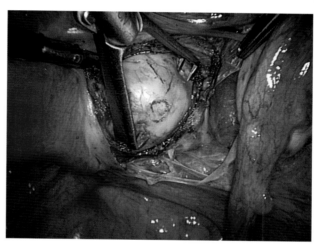

Figure 20.14 The myomectomy is then performed without any bleeding

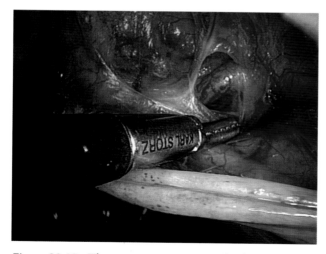

Figure 20.12 The uterine artery is individualized from the ureter

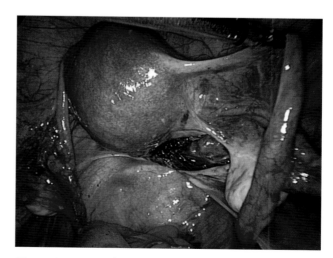

Figure 20.15 Final aspect after myomectomy

Laparoscopic techniques

Laparoscopic myomectomy

Classic laparoscopy is performed using a 12-mm trocar umbilically and three suprapubic trocars of 5, 5 and 10 mm. The 10-mm trocar is useful for introducing strong grasping forceps to apply traction to the myoma.

The surgical procedure starts with incision of the myometrium in line with the myoma. This hysterotomy can be performed with monopolar scissors or with the CO_2 laser (Figure 21.1).

Hemostasis of the intramyometrial vessels is carried out progressively using a bipolar current (Figure 21.2).

The myoma is easily recognizable by its smooth white appearance. Dissection of the myoma should run along the avascular plane around the myoma, leaving the pseudocapsule. The myoma is grasped using strong grasping forceps, and the dissection is carried out with traction and countertraction to the uterus (Figure 21.3). The fine vessels going to the myoma are coagulated and sectioned. The bed of the myoma is often free from hemorrhage at the end of dissection.

Suture of the myometrium is performed in one or two layers depending on the depth of the incision. We use resorbable suture, diameter 1 or 2, to perform single, separate stitches tied intracorporeally (Figure 21.4). The stitches go through the whole thickness of the edges of the hysterotomy, and through the uterine serosa. When the myomectomy is deep or the uterine cavity has been opened, a two-layer suture is performed using single stitches deep in the myometrium, followed by more superficial stitches incorporating the serosa and the superficial part of the myometrium.

To remove the myoma, morcellation is carried out (Figure 21.5).

Myolysis

Laparoscopy is performed transumbilically using a 10-mm endoscope adapted to a video camera. The instruments are introduced through three suprapubic puncture sites (5 mm in diameter). The bare laser fiber (Nd (YAG : neodymium yttrium–aluminum–garnet) laser) is introduced as perpendicularly as possible into the fibroid through a second puncture trocar to a depth depending on the myoma diameter (Figure 21.6). During the application of laser energy, the fiber is inserted, reaching the central part of the fibroid, and is then slowly removed in order to provoke 'strong' coagulation. The power used is 80 W. The procedure is repeated across the entire surface of the myoma in order to coagulate most of the myoma volume. The surface of the myoma is rinsed with 0.9% saline solution during laser application to reduce thermal conduction through the uterine wall. The distance between the holes is about 5–7 mm (Figure 21.7).

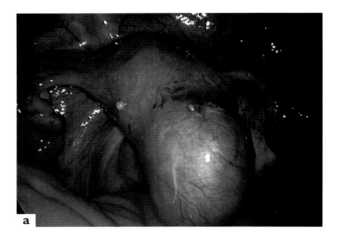

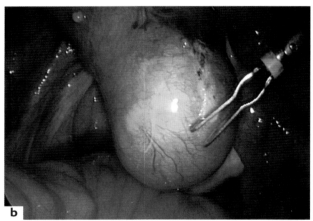

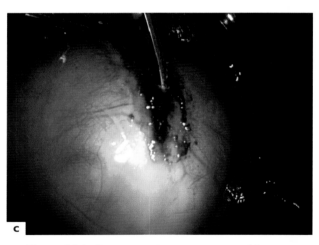

Figure 21.1 Laparoscopic myomectomy: (a) exposure of the myoma; (b) coagulation of the serosa; (c) incision of the myometrium with monopolar scissors

In our series of 48 patients[32], vasopressin (POR8; Sandoz, Brussels, Belgium) was never used to infiltrate the myometrium adjacent to the fibroid to induce temporary myometrial ischemia, reducing blood loss. However, in one case, diluted vasopressin was required to obtain complete uterine hemostasis: 5 IU of vasopressin in 20 ml of saline

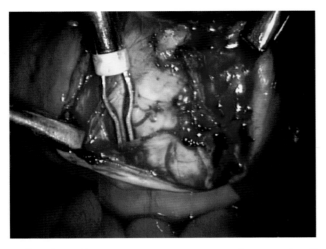

Figure 21.2 Laparoscopic myomectomy: hemostasis of the intramyometrial vessels is carried out progressively using bipolar current

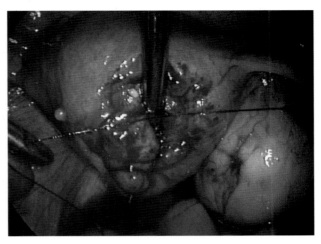

Figure 21.4 Laparoscopic myomectomy: suture of the myometrium

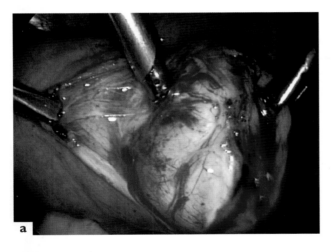

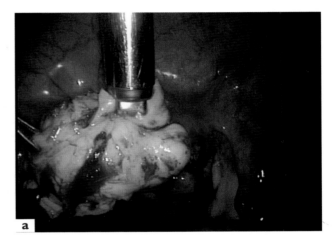

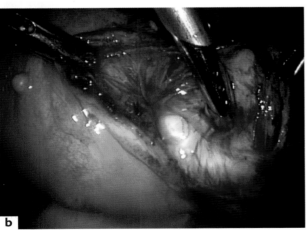

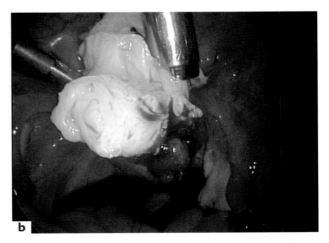

Figure 21.3 (a) and (b) Laparoscopic myomectomy: the myoma is grasped using a strong grasping forceps and the dissection is pursued using traction and countertraction on the uterus

Figure 21.5 (a) and (b) Laparoscopic myomectomy: morcellation of the removed myoma

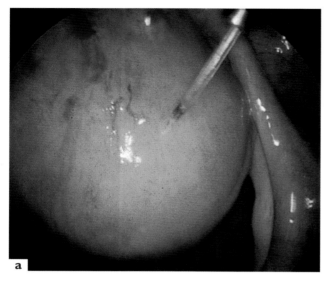 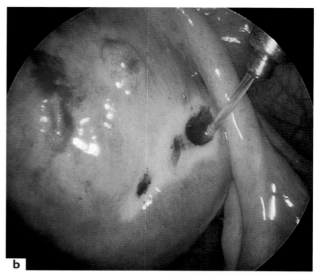

Figure 21.6 (a) and (b) Laparoscopic myolysis: the laser fiber is introduced at an angle perpendicular to the fibroid and removed during the application of energy

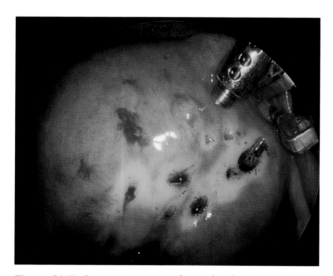

Figure 21.7 Laparoscopic myolysis: the distance between the holes is about 5–7 mm. At the end of the procedure, numerous laser scars are seen. The pale color of the myoma is due to the coagulation

solution was injected around the hemorrhagic site at the end of the procedure.

Immediately following myolysis, many laser scars can be seen on the myoma, which appears paler than normal (Figure 21.7).

In the last ten cases, an Interceed® graft (Johnson & Johnson, New Brunswick, NJ) was used to cover the coagulated area after hemostatic control was obtained, in order to decrease the risk of adhesions (Figure 21.8). Careful aspiration of peritoneal fluid was then carried out and a suction catheter was left in the pouch of Douglas.

In our first series of 48 patients, none required laparotomy for bleeding, and no bladder or bowel injuries

were reported. During surgery, some problems arose because of difficult access to posterior myomas by the laser fiber, introduced through a second puncture. In such cases, the laser fiber can be introduced directly through the laparoscope to achieve better access. The estimated blood loss was minimal (< 50 ml) in all cases but one. The operating time varied from 20 to 45 min, depending on the diameter and number of myomas. All patients were released in good physical condition the following day; none experienced any postoperative infection or hemorrhage.

The number, size and location of the myomas were evaluated by vaginal echography before laparoscopic myolysis and postoperatively at weeks 3, 6 and 12, after 6 months and after 1 year; 15 patients were evaluated after 3 years. Fibroids treated by myolysis ranged from 3 to 8 cm in diameter. The mean decrease in myoma diameter after myolysis was 4% (range 0–6%) at week 6, 12% (range 2–18%) at week 12 and 41% (range 18–62%) after 6 months. The echostructure of the coagulated myoma was such that only experienced echographists could really distinguish its boundaries. The results observed after 1 year were similar to those seen after 6 months; there was neither any further decrease in size nor a regrowth of the myoma.

After 3 years, 15 patients were evaluated by echography. In ten of them, who had two or three myomas (between 3 and 5 cm in diameter), echography revealed only small areas (< 1 cm in diameter) whose echographic structure was slightly different from normal myometrium. Among the five remaining patients, three were stable and two experienced recurrence of myomas in other sites. The last two patients underwent laparoscopic subtotal hysterectomy. Only a few adhesions were present. Failure of treatment, indicated by an absence of any significant decrease in myoma diameter, was never observed.

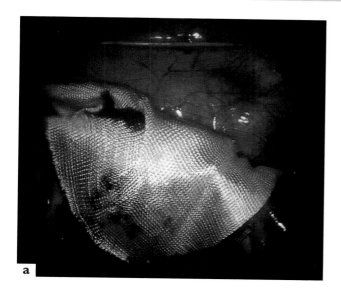

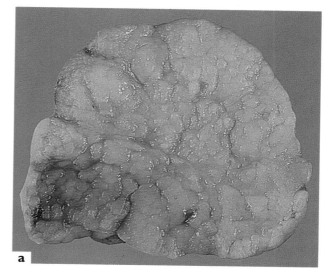

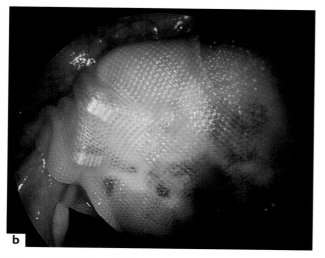

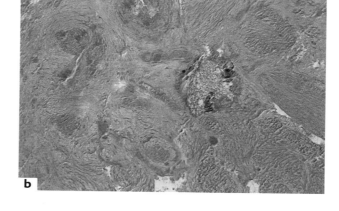

Figure 21.8 (a) and (b) Laparoscopic myolysis: to avoid adhesions, Interceed® is used to cover the laser scars

In 15 patients, second-look laparoscopy was carried out more than 6 months after myolysis for other reasons (ovarian cysts, sterilization, etc.). The appearance of the myoma was noted. In eight cases, dense and fibrous adhesions were observed between the myoma and, most frequently, the small bowel and/or epiploon. After adhesiolysis, the myoma appeared white, without any apparent vessels. In two cases, we decided to remove the myoma. Dissection of myomas from the normal myometrium proved surprisingly easy, and they were removed in order to evaluate histologically the efficacy of myolysis. There was necrosis in most myoma areas, characterized by edema and an absence of viable cells (Figure 21.9). In other areas, giant cells and macrophages containing carbonized particles (Figure 21.10) very close to the necrotic sites suggested that necrosis was actually induced by laser coagulation.

Figure 21.9 Specimen of myoma: (a) 6 months after myolysis; (b) and (c) necrosis characterized by edema and the absence of viable cells

Safety

Three prospective randomized studies have compared abdominal and laparoscopic myomectomy[33–35].

Mais and Seracchioli's groups showed that laparoscopic surgery is associated with shorter hospitalization, faster

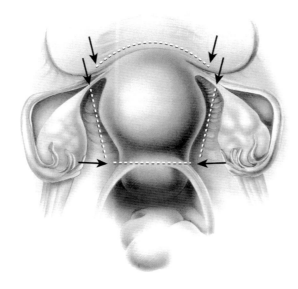

Figure 22.1 Laparoscopic subtotal hysterectomy technique

transection were systematically performed. Bipolar coagulation was used to desiccate the utero-ovarian ligaments and vessels and the isthmic portion of both Fallopian tubes (Figures 22.1–22.4).

Scissors were then used to transect the structures within the coagulated areas. Meticulous hemostasis was achieved by repeated bipolar coagulation of transected vessels. If a bilateral (or unilateral) salpingo-oophorectomy was required, the infundibulopelvic ligaments were similarly coagulated and transected. The round ligaments were treated in the same way.

The anterior leaf and the posterior leaf of the broad ligament were then opened with scissors. Hydrodissection facilitated the procedure and allowed the surgeon to expose the uterine vessels. The vesicouterine peritoneum was then opened with scissors (Figure 22.5). The vesicocervical space was dissected no more than 2 cm below the limit between the cervix and the corpus uteri. After careful identification of the uterine vessels and ureters, the uterine vessels were electrocoagulated with the bipolar coagulation forceps and transected (Figures 22.6 and 22.7). The

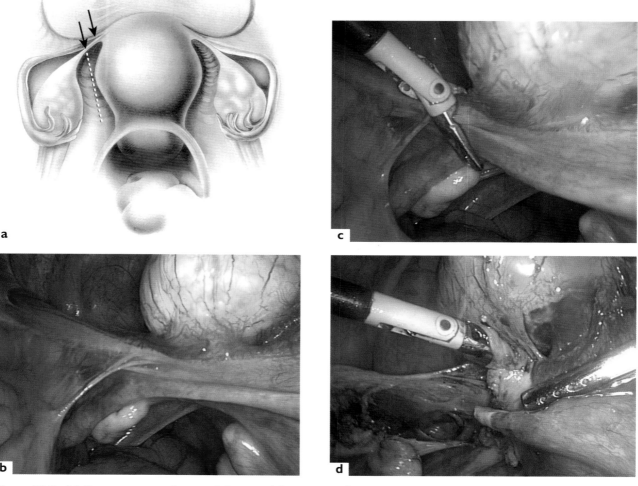

Figure 22.2 (a) First step: coagulation of the round ligament, Fallopian tube and uterolateral ovarian ligament. (b)–(d) Coagulation and section of the round ligament, Fallopian tube and utero-ovarian ligament on the left side

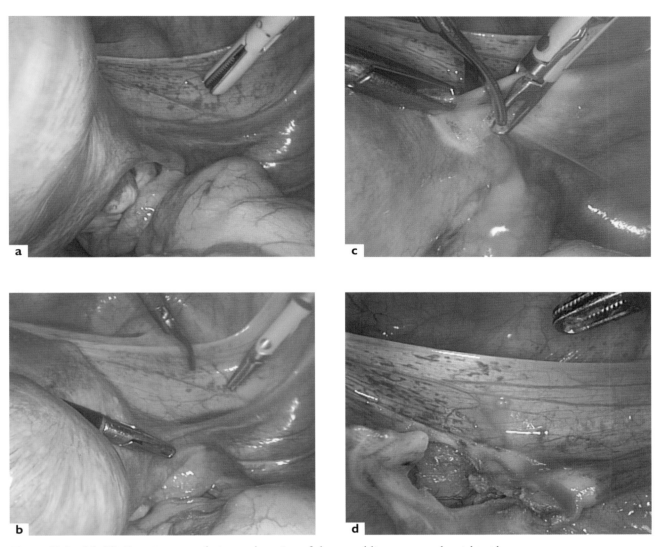

Figure 22.3   (a)–(d) Grasping, coagulation and section of the round ligament on the right side

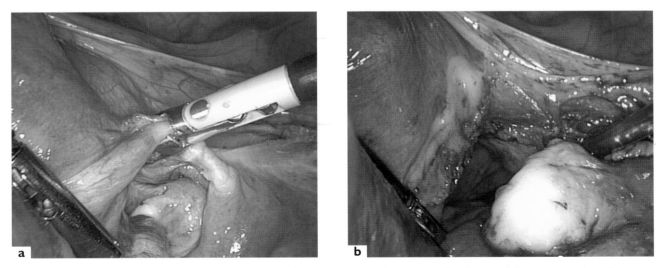

Figure 22.4   (a) and (b) Coagulation and section of the utero-ovarian ligament and Fallopian tube on the right side

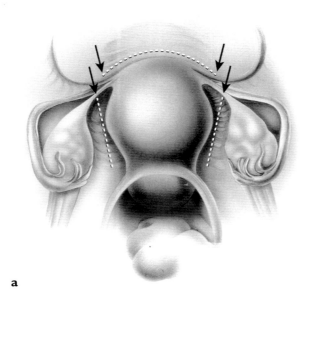

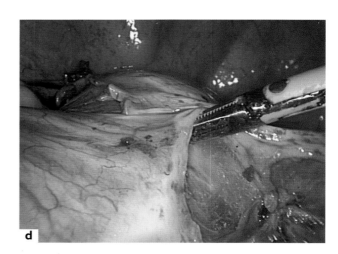

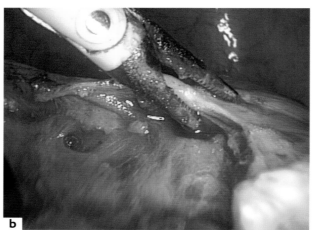

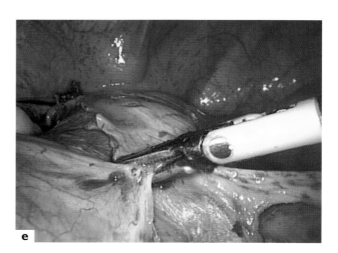

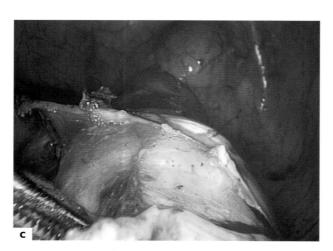

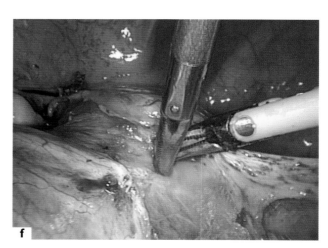

Figure 22.5 (a)–(f) Dissection and section of the vesicouterine peritoneum

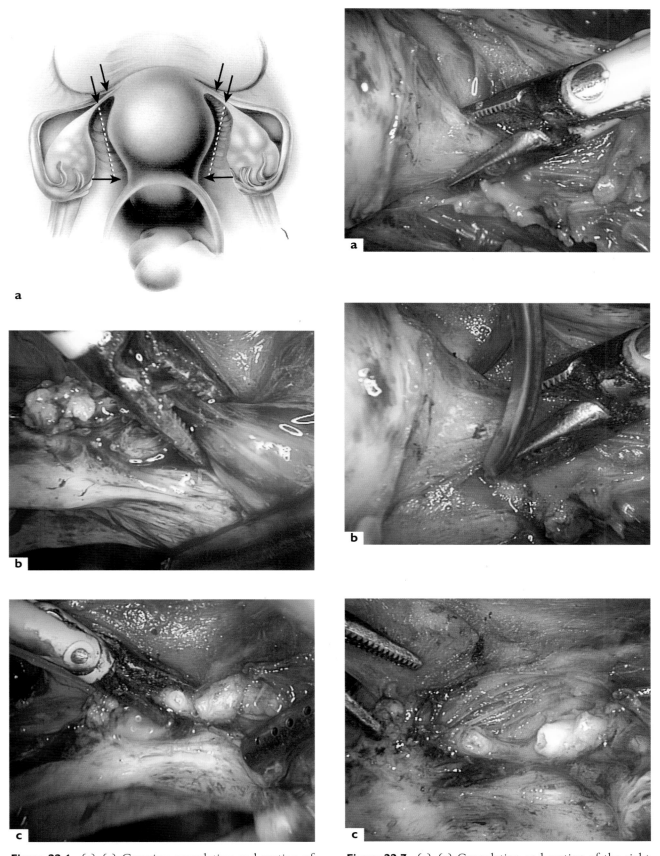

Figure 22.6 (a)–(c) Grasping coagulation and section of the left uterine artery

Figure 22.7 (a)–(c) Coagulation and section of the right uterine artery

unipolar knife or unipolar scissors were then used to cut the cervix below the level of the internal os and separate the cervix from the corpus (Figures 22.8 and 22.9). Hemostasis was achieved by meticulous coagulation.

Until November 1993, longitudinal (vertical or horizontal) posterior colpotomy was performed, either by laparoscopy or through the vagina. Since then, however, the uterus has been removed through a 12-mm trocar after morcellation using Steiner's morcellator[12] (Figures 22.10–22.12). A new morcellator enables the time of morcellation to be reduced (Figure 22.13) (Rotocut™; Storz, Tuttlingen).

Irrigation fluid was instilled into the pelvis and the operative sites were inspected. A titanium clip was then applied to the uterine artery to ensure complete hemostasis.

The cervical stump was never reperitonealized. The instruments were removed from the abdomen and the four incisions were reapproximated with 2-0 nylon suture.

Prophylactic antibiotics (cephalosporin (Zinacef®) 2 g/dl) were administered just before the procedure (5 min before the incision).

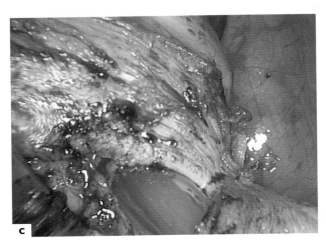

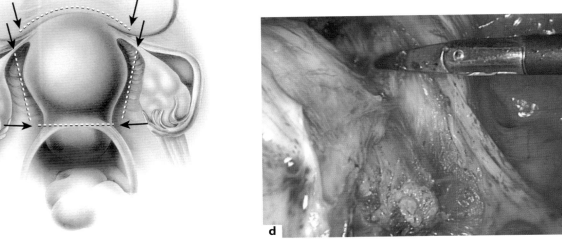

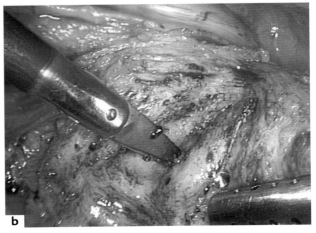

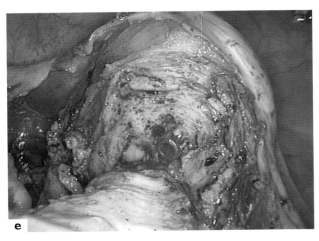

Figure 22.8 (a)–(g) Section of the cervix; the plastic uterine cannula becomes visible

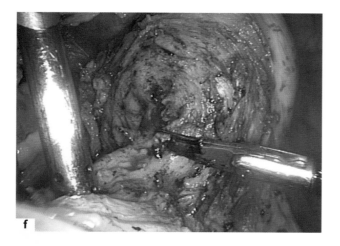

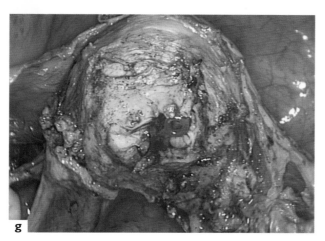

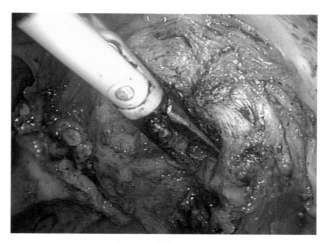

Figure 22.9 Coagulation of the endocervical canal

Figure 22.8 *continued* (a)–(g) Section of the cervix; the plastic uterine cannula becomes visible

RESULTS

All of our LASH procedures were successful. The patients' ages ranged from 34 to 57 years. The mean duration of surgery was 72 min (morcellation included), depending essentially on the uterus weight. In the majority of cases, in experienced hands, the average duration is about 45 min, although in university teaching hospitals the learning curve of registrars leads to an increase in surgery duration. The estimated blood loss was systematically less than 100 ml. There were no intraoperative bowel injuries (Table 22.2). Three ureteral injuries occurred. One ureter was found to be 'blanching' during surgery. A double JJ stent was immediately placed. Two cases of ureteral fistula, caused by thermal damage, were treated by JJ stent. Three patients experienced postoperative fever. All patients were theoretically able to leave the hospital the first day following surgery. Many, however, preferred to stay 2 days, knowing that the Belgian insurance system offers reimbursement for up to 7 days' hospitalization.

In 2000, the length of hospital stay after surgery ranged from 4 to 5 days for vaginal hysterectomy, 3 to 4 days for laparoscopy-assisted vaginal hysterectomy (LAVH) and 5 to 8 days for abdominal hysterectomy (mostly dependent on the age of the patient). Patients who underwent LASH reported much less discomfort than patients who underwent other types of hysterectomy. No patients required major analgesic drugs. Only 8% of patients required analgesic drugs a few hours after surgery, but no patients required drugs the day after surgery.

Patients were able to ambulate very soon after LASH (the same day), similar to patients who underwent laparoscopic adhesiolysis, ovarian cystectomy or salpingo-neostomy.

Sexual intercourse was permitted 2 weeks after surgery. There was only one case of cervical prolapse, and no signs of enterocele were observed in patients reviewed in a 5-year follow-up ($n = 349$). There were no complaints of genuine urinary incontinence except in one case. This patient, however, had already complained of genuine urinary incontinence before LASH, and physiotherapy and biofeedback therapy were proposed at this time. As no improvement was seen after 1 year, surgery was required, and the patient underwent a laparoscopic Burch procedure in 1994.

In seven patients, laparoscopy was performed because of a 'tumor' located in the pouch of Douglas, causing deep dyspareunia. Symptoms were due to iatrogenic 'adenomyomas', specimens of endometrium and myometrium of the morcellated uterus, which had not been removed during the first laparoscopy (LASH). Laparoscopy allowed us to dissect the 'forgotten' specimen, which was covered with peritoneum (submitted for publication).

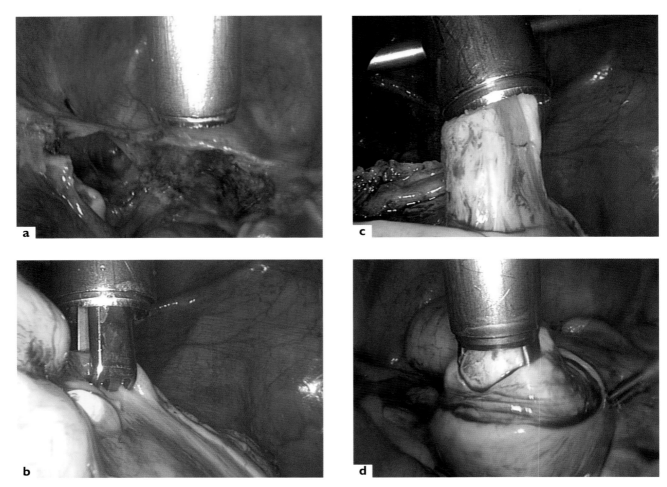

Figure 22.10   (a)–(d) Morcellation of the uterus with a morcellator

COMMENTS

The indications for laparoscopic surgery have expanded greatly over recent decades. An increase has also been seen in the field of hysteroscopic surgery. Endometrial ablation performed endoscopically has been proposed as an alternative to hormonal therapy or hysterectomy in dysfunctional bleeding without intrauterine lesions[13]. Hysteroscopic myomectomy has also been proposed for large submucosal myomas. In our team, the long-term results of hysteroscopic myomectomy were found to be excellent in cases of large submucosal fibroids fewer than three in number. Indeed, in our series, recurrence of menorrhagia did not exceed 5% after a 2-year follow-up. However, in cases of multiple (more than four) submucosal fibroids, recurrence of bleeding due to recurrent myomas was found to be as high as 25%, even when endometrial ablation was performed concomitantly[13–16]. This is why hysteroscopic management of uterine bleeding cannot be systematically proposed, and why an alternative surgical approach was suggested.

In 1990, the LASH technique was not frequently used in our department. Indeed, in a series of 204 hysterectomies carried out in the department in 1990, only four LASH procedures (2%) were performed. At the time, the disadvantage of the technique, which is the remaining cervix, was considered a potential risk factor for cervical cancer. It is obvious that the risk is low in some groups of the population.

Moreover, this question is never asked when endometrial ablation is performed. Subsequently, the incidence of LASH increased from just 2% to 46% of all hysterectomies (Table 22.1). Since the uterus can be removed laparoscopically with the help of Steiner's morcellator or with the new Rotocut (Figure 22.13), LASH must be considered as a strictly laparoscopic approach to hysterectomy. No patients required major analgesics the day after surgery.

Indeed, a serious complication rate of 11% was recently reported after LAVH and LH in two randomized controlled trials in the UK[17]. Ureteral and/or bladder damage occurred at a rate of 2% after LH. Six ureteral and

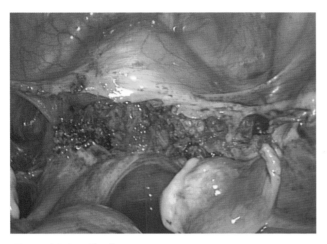

Figure 22.11 Final view

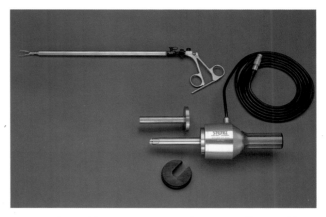

Figure 22.13 New Rotocut™ G1 morcellator allows faster morcellation

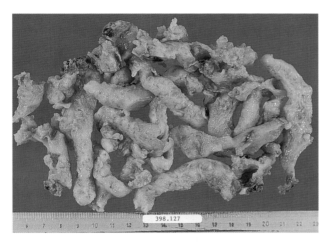

Figure 22.12 Uterus after morcellation

15 bladder injuries occurred in 920 laparoscopic hysterectomies, whereas no ureteral lesions and only five bladder injuries were seen in a series of 460 abdominal or vaginal hysterectomies. This increased risk of urinary tract injuries during laparoscopic hysterectomy compared with abdominal hysterectomy was confirmed in a meta-analysis by Johnson *et al.* in 2005[18].

In this review, 27 trials were included, taking into account that only randomized controlled trials were selected. The increased incidence of urinary tract injury remained the major concern in relation to the laparoscopic surgery. Indeed, ureteral injury occurred in one of 78 women having laparoscopic hysterectomy and one in 492 women having abdominal hysterectomy.

In our series, ureteral injury occurred in two of 1400 women having LASH, thus with a lower incidence than

Table 22.2 Complications in a series of 1363 laparoscopic subtotal hysterectomies

Complication	n
Perioperative	
Hemorrhage*	1 (0.07%)
Bladder incision† (< 1 cm)	3 (0.22%)
Ureteral lesion (blanching treated by JJ stent)	1 (0.07%)
Fever (after second day)	3 (0.22%)
Postoperative	
Urinary tract lesion‡	2 (0.15%)
Colon or rectal perforation	0
Iatrogenic adenomyoma§	7 (0.51%)

*External iliac artery lesion during section of the cervix with monopolar scissors, treated by emergency laparotomy; †sutured laparoscopically (in three patients with previous history of two cesarean sections); ‡fistula caused by thermal damage, treated by JJ stent; §residual specimens of myometrium and endometrium after morcellation

Table 23.3 A series of 3405 hysterectomies for benign diseases

Procedures	1994–1995		1996–1997		1998–1999		2000–2001		2002–2003		2004–2005		Total	
	n	%	*n*	%	*n*	%	*n*	%	*n*	%	*n*	%	*n*	%
LASH	236	46	240	41.5	248	43.5	205	38	179	30	255	41	1363	40
LAVH/LH*	130	26	127	22	177	31	203	37.5	294	50	302	49	1233	36
Vaginal hysterectomy	82	16	159	27.5	111	19.5	102	19	94	16	53	8.5	601	18
Abdominal hysterectomy	60	12	52	9	32	6	31	5.5	24	4	9	1.5	208	6
Total	508		578		568		541		591		619		3405	

*In 2000 we switched from LAVH to LH; LASH, laparoscopic subtotal hysterectomy; LAVH, laparoscopy-assisted vaginal hysterectomy; LH, laparoscopic hysterectomy

Table 23.4 Complications in a series of 1323 laparoscopic hysterectomies

Complication	*n*
Fever > 38.5°C (after second day) requiring 5–7 days of antibiotherapy	9 (0.6%)
Bladder incision (sutured by laparoscopy)	3 (0.2%)
Hemorrhage	1 (0.1%)
Conversion	0 (0%)
Vesicoperitoneal fistula diagnosed by computed tomography (treated by Foley catheter for 14 days) (Figure 23.30)	1 (0.1%)
Urinary tract lesion (two cases treated by JJ stent, one case by ureteral reimplantation (1992))	3 (0.2%)
Rectal perforation (treated by colostomy)	1 (0.1%)

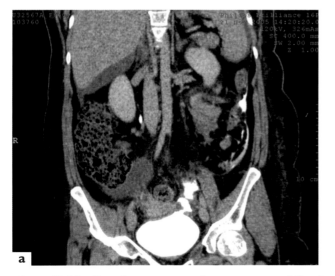 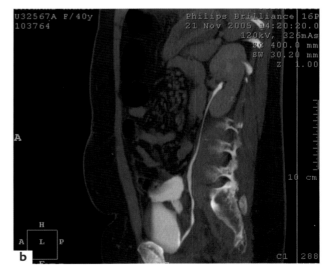

Figure 23.30 Complication: case of vesicoperitoneal fistula. Computed tomography scan (a) and (b). Leakage of contrast medium from the bladder to the peritoneal cavity. The diagnosis was made on day 6 post-op. A Foley catheter was left in place for 14 days

operation, carrying a greater risk of damaging the bladder or ureter, and, once again, we disagree.

Indeed, the experience and skill of the surgeons included in the review (which analyzed randomized trials comparing two surgical approaches to hysterectomy) obviously differed, with some of them still in the learning curve. More experienced laparoscopists would never be associated with such a complication rate, but their rates will never be included in a Cochrane Review, since they are not about to start a randomized study evaluating vaginal hysterectomy, abdominal hysterectomy and laparoscopic hysterectomy at this stage.

We clearly demonstrated, in a paper in the *New England Journal of Medicine*, that laparoscopic hysterectomy was less expensive than any other approach if non-disposable instruments were used[23]. In the United States and in Europe, however, 75% of hysterectomies are performed by an abdominal approach. If laparoscopic hysterectomy is added to our surgical armamentarium, almost all hysterectomies (95%) would be carried out without an abdominal incision. In our department (Table 23.3), the rate of abdominal hysterectomy is less than 5%. The remaining indications for abdominal hysterectomy are myomas >14–15 weeks (unless a GnRH agonist can be administered in order to reduce the volume), malignant (or suspected to be malignant) ovarian masses and cervical cancer stage Ib (Wertheim–Meigs)[24] and frozen pelvis, when a hysterectomy is mandatory.

REFERENCES

1. Findlay S. The health-insurance factor. US News World Rep 1990; 30: 57
2. Kovak SR, Cruikshank SH, Retto HF. Laparoscopic assisted vaginal hysterectomy. J Gynecol Surg 1990; 6: 185–90
3. Isaacs JH. Gynecology and Obstetrics. Clinical Gynecology. Philadelphia: JB Lippincott, 1990; 1: 1–11
4. Smith HO, Thompson JD. Indications and technique for vaginal hysterectomy. Contemp Obstet Gynecol 1986; 27: 125
5. Johns A. Laparoscopic assisted vaginal hysterectomy (LAVH). In Sutton C, Diamond D, eds. Endoscopic Surgery for Gynecologists. London, UK: WB Saunders, 1993: 179–86
6. Reich H. New techniques in advanced laparoscopic surgery. Clin Obstet Gynecol 1989; 3: 655–81
7. Mage G, Wattiez A, Chapron C, et al. Hystérectomie per-coelioscopique: resultats d'une serie de 44 cas. J Gynecol Obstet Biol Reprod 1992; 21: 436–44
8. Donnez J, Nisolle M, Squifflet J, Smets M. Laparoscopy-assisted vaginal hysterectomy and laparoscopic hysterectomy in benign diseases. In Donnez J, Nisolle M, eds. An Atlas of Operative Laparoscopy and Hysteroscopy. Carnforth, UK: Parthenon Publishing, 2001: 251–60
9. Kilkku P. Supravaginal uterine amputation vs hysterectomy: effects on libido and orgasm. Acta Obstet Gynecol Scand 1983; 62: 141–5
10. Donnez J, Nisolle M. LASH: laparoscopic supracervical hysterectomy. J Gynecol Surg 1993; 9: 91–4
11. Querleu D, Leblanc E, Castelain G. Laparoscopic pelvic lymphadenectomy in the staging of early carcinoma of the cervix. Am J Obstet Gynecol 1991; 164: 579–81
12. Reich H, McGlynn F, Wickie W. Laparoscopic management of stage 1 ovarian cancer: a case report. J Reprod Med 1990; 35: 601–4
13. Donnez J, Nisolle M, Anaf V. Place de l'endoscopie dans le cancer de l'endomètre. In Dubuisson JB, Chapron CH, Bouquet de Jolinière J, eds. Coelioscopie et Cancerologie en Gynecologie. Paris: Arnette, 1993: 77–82
14. Reich H. New laparoscopic techniques. In Sutton C, Diamond M, eds. Endoscopic Surgery for Gynaecologists. London, UK: WB Saunders, 1993: 28–39
15. Canis M, Mage G, Wattiez A, et al. Vaginally assisted laparoscopic radical hysterectomy. J Gynecol Surg 1992; 8: 103–5
16. Donnez J, Schrurs B, Gillerot S, et al. Treatment of uterine fibroids with implants of gonadotropin releasing hormone agonist: assessment by hysterography. Fertil Steril 1989; 51: 947–50
17. Donnez J, Gillerot S, Bourgonjon D, et al. Neodymium : YAG laser hysteroscopy in large submucous fibroids. Fertil Steril 1990; 54: 999–1003
18. Garry R, Fountain J, Mason S, et al. The eVALuate study: two parallel randomised trials, one comparing laparoscopic with abdominal hysterectomy, the other comparing laparoscopic with vaginal hysterectomy. Br Med J 2004; 328: 1229–36
19. Donnez J, Squifflet J, Jadoul P, Smets M. High rate of complications need explanation [Letter]. Br Med J 2004; 328: 643
20. Wattiez A, Soriano D, Cohen SB, et al. The learning curve of total laparoscopic hysterectomy: comparative analysis of 1647 cases. J Am Assoc Gynecol Laparosc 2002; 9: 339–45
23. Donnez J, Nisolle M, Smets M, et al. LASH: laparoscopic subtotal hysterectomy. In Donnez J, Nisolle M, eds. An Atlas of Operative Laparoscopy and Hysteroscopy. Carnforth, UK: Parthenon Publishing, 2001: 243–50
22. Johnson N, Barlow D, Lethaby A, et al. Surgical approach to hysterectomy for benign gynaecological disease [Review]. Cochrane Database Syst Rev 2005; (1): CD003677
23. Nisolle M, Donnez J. Alternative techniques of hysterectomy [Letter to the Editor]. N Engl J Med 1997; 336: 291–2
24. Canis M, Mage G, Wattiez A, et al. La chirurgie endoscopique at-elle une place dans la chirurgie radicale du cancer du col utérin? J Gynecol Obstet Biol Reprod 1990; 19: 921

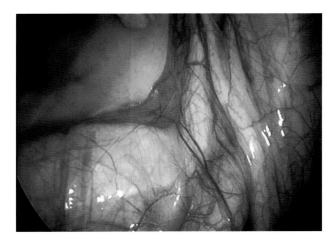

Figure 25.1 The abdominal cavity is explored first. The ureters are traced along the pelvic sidewall and the major iliac vessels are carefully located

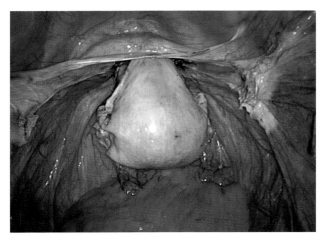

Figure 25.2 Laparoscopic subtotal hysterectomy: the uterus and adnexa have been freed

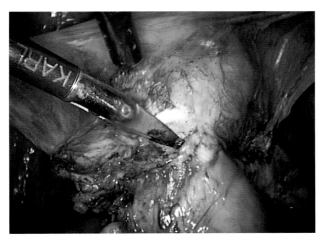

Figure 25.3 Laparoscopic subtotal hysterectomy: section of the cervix

vulsellum holds the posterior lip of the cervix to provide exposure (Figure 25.7). In order to avoid vaginal mesh erosion and to ensure strong fixation, the mesh should be fixed deep in the cervix. The posterior part of the cervix is therefore incised vertically to a depth of approximately 1 cm (Figure 25.8). The polypropylene mesh (Figure 25.9) is then tightly stitched to the posterior part of the cervix with two absorbable stitches (Vicryl® 0 or 1) (Figures 25.10 and 25.11). The mesh is placed in the abdominal cavity. One or two round circumferential sutures are then placed high on the peritoneum in order to carry out a culdoplasty to treat associated enterocele (Figure 25.12).

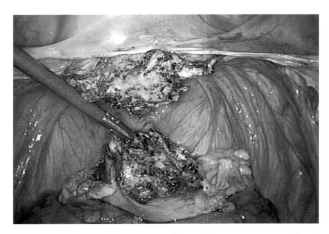

Figure 25.4 Laparoscopic subtotal hysterectomy: final view

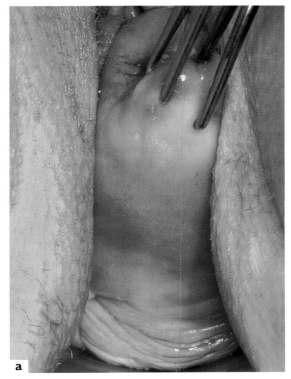

Figure 25.5 (a)–(c) Posterior colpotomy is performed along a sagittal vaginal incision over a length of 4–5 cm

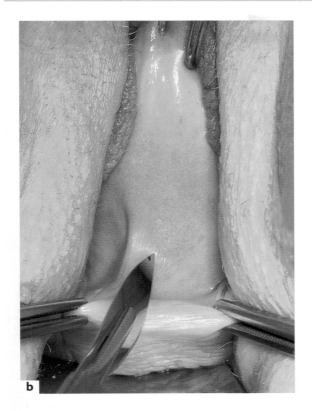

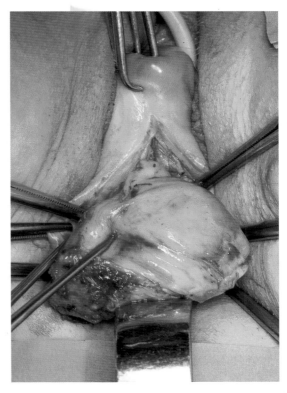

Figure 25.6 The uterus is removed through the colpotomy

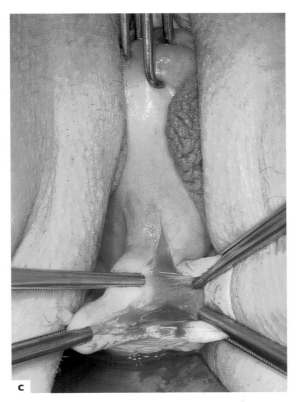

Figure 25.5 *continued*

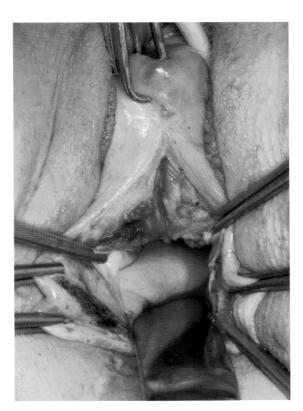

Figure 25.7 A right-angled retractor is placed on the posterior lip of the vagina. Other forceps hold the posterior lip of the cervix to provide exposure

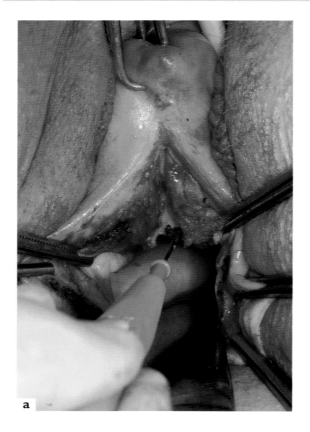

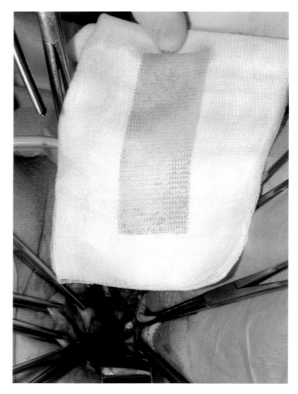

Figure 25.9 Polypropylene mesh

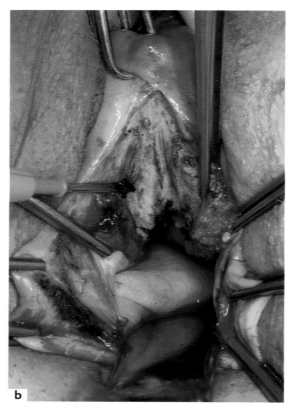

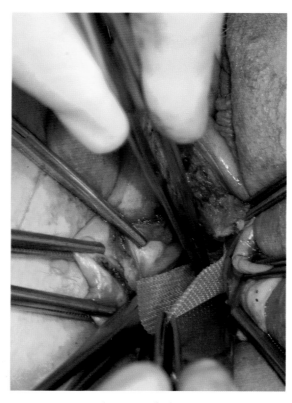

Figure 25.8 (a) and (b) Incision of the posterior part of the cervix

Figure 25.10 Introduction of the polypropylene mesh into the abdominal cavity

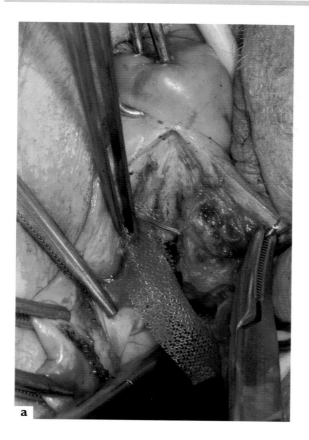

The highest suture brings both uterosacral ligaments to the medial line to prevent any future recurrence. The culdotomy is then closed. Separate points or a running suture are applied to both vaginal lips (Figure 25.13).

Third step: laparoscopic dissection of the presacral tissue

The patient, still in the Trendelenburg position, is placed slightly in left lateral decubitus. After careful coagulation of the peritoneum (Figure 25.14), an opening is made with scissors (Figure 25.15) from the lumbosacral joint towards the cervix. The prevertebral space is opened. The presacral peritoneum is grasped with two atraumatic forceps on the right lateral side of the rectum. The right ureter is situated 1–2 cm from the presacral peritoneal incision and is systematically checked over the length of this incision. The sigmoid is pushed laterally, and careful dissection and hemostasis of the presacral tissue provide exposure of the anterior common vertebral ligament. Coagulation and section of the medial sacral artery and vein are sometimes necessary. The most prominent point of the space is the lumbosacral joint (the mesh must be fixed to either the anterior wall of the corpus of the first sacral vertebra or the fifth lumbar vertebra).

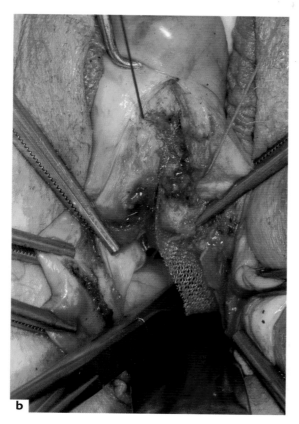

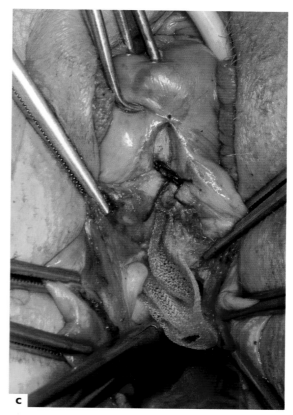

Figure 25.11 (a)–(c) The polypropylene mesh is sutured inside the cervical incision

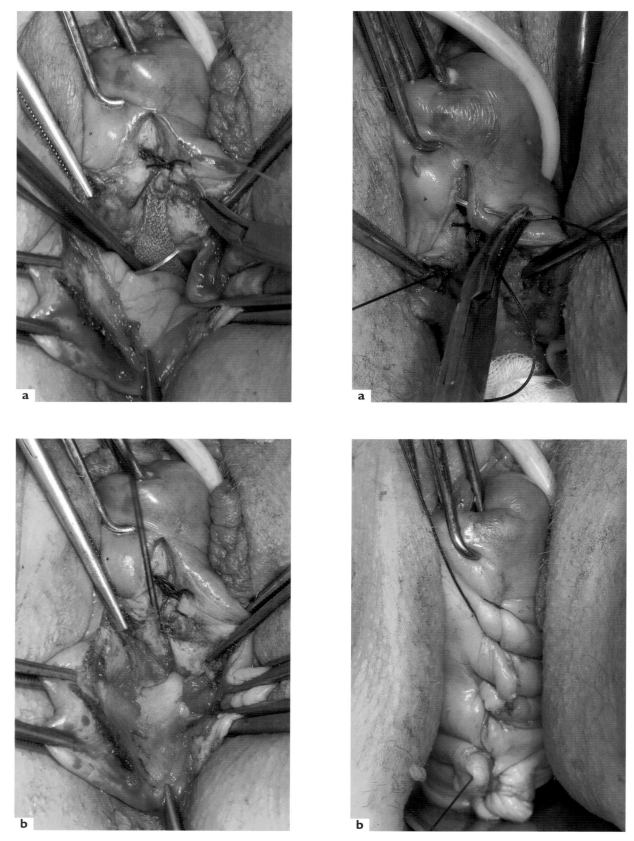

Figure 25.12 (a) and (b) One or two round circumferential sutures are placed high on the peritoneum in order to carry out a culdoplasty to treat associated enterocele

Figure 25.13 (a) and (b) The vagina is closed by a running suture

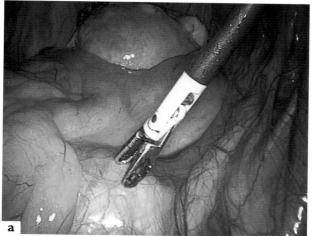

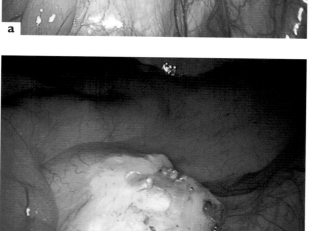

Figure 25.14 (a) and (b) Coagulation and opening of the presacral peritoneum

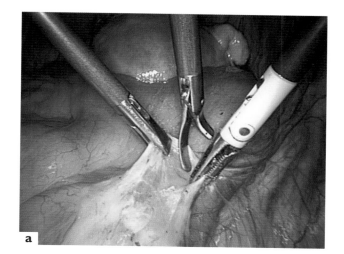

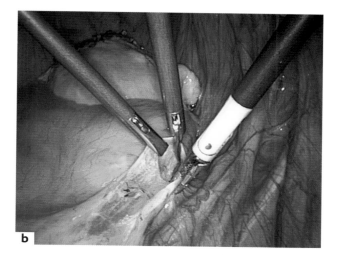

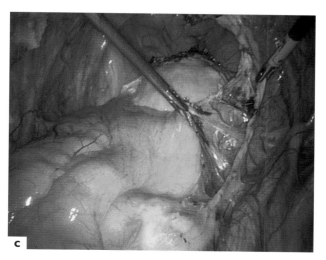

Figure 25.15 (a)–(c) Opening of the peritoneum from the lumbosacral joint towards the cervix

Fourth step: sacral fixation of the polypropylene mesh

Two grasping forceps hold the edges of the parietal posterior peritoneum to give access to the anterior wall of the first sacral vertebra. The Origin Tacker is introduced through the medial suprapubic trocar. This tacking device utilizes a helical coil of 3.9 mm in diameter to achieve secure fixation to the vertebra. Forceps grasp the prosthesis (Figure 25.16), which is then tightened until the cervix or the uterus recovers its anatomic position. The tip of the Tacker is placed on the mesh, in front of the anterior wall of the first sacral vertebra, and several tacks are inserted through the mesh into the periosteum of the vertebra and the common vertebral ligament (Figure 25.17). Excess mesh is cut away and removed (Figure 25.18).

Fifth step: reperitonealization

Both folds of the peritoneum are sutured with resorbable material (Figure 25.19) or stapled with endoscopic staples.

Careful washing of the peritoneal cavity is then performed and an antiseptic solution of Rifocine® (Rifamycin; Merrel Dow, Kansas City, MO) is instilled into the pelvis. Finally, a Douglas catheter is inserted through one of the

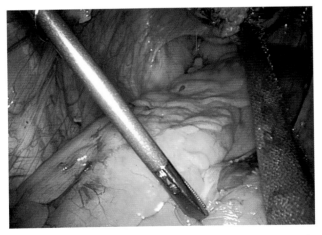

Figure 25.16 Grasping of the polypropylene mesh with forceps

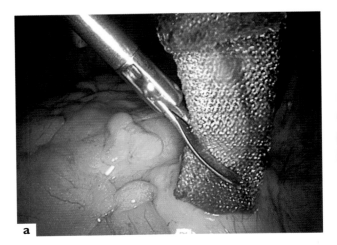

a

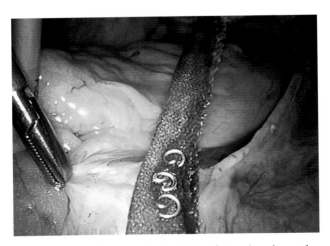

Figure 25.17 The tip of the Tacker® is placed on the mesh, in front of the anterior wall of the first sacral vertebra, and several tacks are inserted through the mesh into the periosteum of the vertebra and the common vertebral ligament

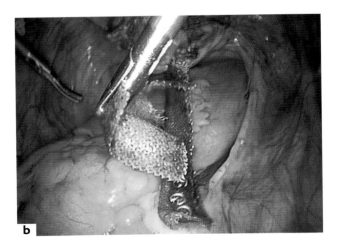

b

Figure 25.18 (a) and (b) Excess mesh is cut away and removed

suprapubic trocars. It is clamped for 2–4 h and removed the day after surgery.

Vaginal vault sacrofixation

Fixation of the mesh to the vagina can be performed either vaginally or laparoscopically using the tacking technique, but the vaginal route may be preferred because it allows quick repair of enteroceles. Using the vaginal route, the vagina is opened along its posterior wall with a 4–5-cm incision, perpendicular to the vaginal vault. Dissection is performed to enter the abdominal cavity. The enterocele is then dissected and excess peritoneum is cut away. The polypropylene mesh is fixed to the vaginal vault through the vaginal incision by two or three absorbable stitches.

The mesh is introduced into the peritoneal cavity. The peritoneum is then closed with two high, continuous, round circumferential sutures to close the pouch of Douglas (Douglasorrhaphy). The vagina is finally closed.

It is important to note that none of the patients underwent a concomitant Burch procedure, or a procedure using tension-free vaginal tape (TVT) or transobturator tape (TOT).

Recently, laparoscopic vaginal vault suspension was carried out by a purely laparoscopic approach. With this technique, the ureters are identified and, if an enterocele defect is observed, the enterocele sac is excised, after a rectal probe is inserted to identify the rectal wall. A sponge is then placed in the vagina (Figure 25.20) and the bladder is dissected from the vagina (Figure 25.21). Using a polypropylene mesh (Figure 25.22), the surgeon places an initial suture through the uterosacral ligaments (Figure 25.23), laterally, 2 cm from the ureters and on the anterior peritoneal leaf of the rectosigmoid (Douglasorrhaphy)

(Figure 25.24). This first suture ensures closure of the enterocele, by attaching it to the posterior part of the vaginal apex (Figure 25.25). No gap is left between the vagina and the uterosacral ligaments. The anterior part of the mesh (U mesh) is then fixed to the anterior part of the vaginal apex (Figure 25.26). The mesh is subsequently fixed to the promontorium (Figure 25.27) and covered with peritoneum closure (Figure 25.28) using a running Vicryl suture. On postoperative day 3, radiography of the sacrum (Figure 25.29) confirms the correct position of the coils.

COMPLICATIONS

We did not observe any intraoperative complications. No bleeding occurred during the procedure among the 146 patients in this study. There was one immediate post-operative complication (Table 25.2). One patient complained of difficulty in moving her left foot straight after leaving the operating room. It was associated with severe pain in the left buttock and in the upper part of the

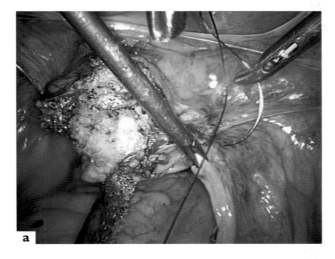
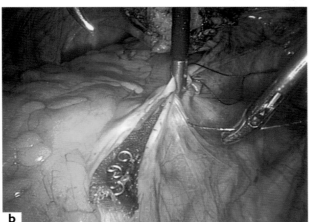
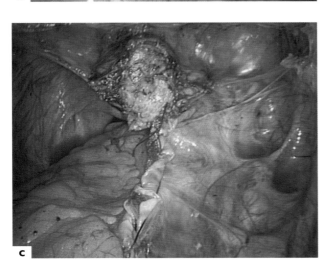

Figure 25.19 (a)–(c) The peritoneum is sutured with resorbable stitches

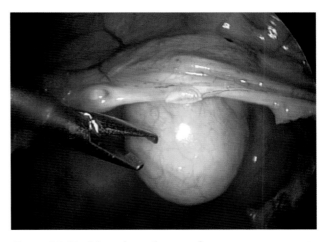

Figure 25.20 Vaginal vault sacrofixation: a sponge is placed in the vagina

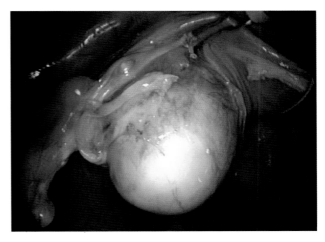

Figure 25.21 The bladder is dissected from the vagina

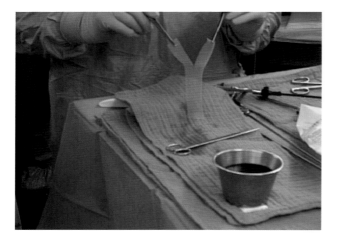

Figure 25.22 Polypropylene mesh

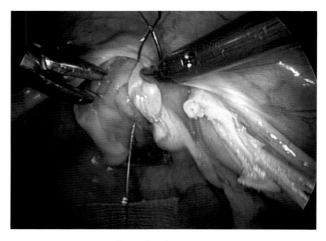

Figure 25.24 Douglasorrhaphy

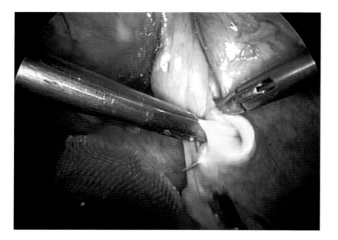

Figure 25.23 Suture of the uterosacral ligaments

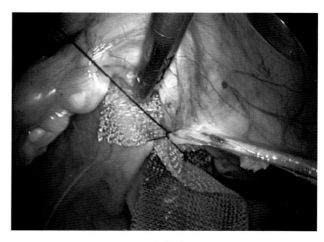

Figure 25.25 No gap is left between the vagina and uterosacral ligaments

left thigh. Electromyography concluded that the fifth left lumbar neural root or one of the first left sacroneural roots was affected. Radiography of the sacrum showed that one coil was too laterally placed on the left, near the neural root (Figure 25.30a). After magnetic resonance imaging (MRI) (Figure 25.30b) confirmed that one spring had been placed in the foramen intervertebrale of the second root, we decided to perform a laparotomy, and the spring was carefully removed. The patient made a rapid recovery and now has only a slight mobility defect of her left foot.

Postoperative discomfort was similar to that observed after any straightforward laparoscopy. Bowel function resumed within 24 h and the patients were able to leave hospital, on average, on day 4 postoperatively. Sexual intercourse was allowed 3 weeks after surgery. Patients were reviewed every 6 months. The average follow-up is now 1–10 years.

Two patients experienced spondylitis, 9 and 12 months postoperatively. The first underwent laparotomy with disc resection and bone transplantation. The second underwent a laparoscopic procedure to remove the mesh and coils from the presacral space. Both patients recovered well without sequelae.

Two cases of mesh erosion with significant symptoms (vaginal discharge, postcoital bleeding) were described, both after vaginal vault suspension. In the first case, resection was carried out to remove the lower part of the mesh, resulting in a recurrence of vaginal vault prolapse, which was treated by laparoscopy with extravaginal suture of the vault. In the second case (Figure 25.31), vaginal examination revealed mesh erosion and the coils were visible. Laparoscopic and vaginal resection of the eroded mesh were carried out and the residual mesh was laparoscopically fixed to the vaginal apex, after 3 cm² of vaginal apex had been removed.

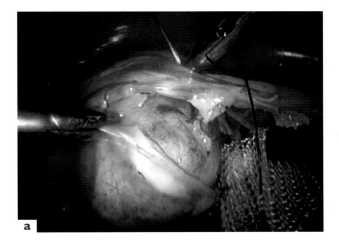

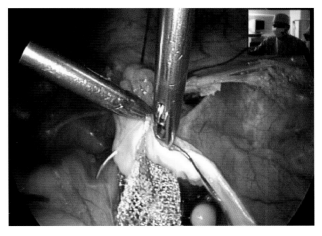

Figure 25.28 The mesh is covered with peritoneum

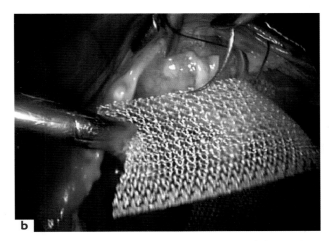

Figure 25.26 (a) and (b) The anterior part of the mesh is fixed to the anterior part of the vagina

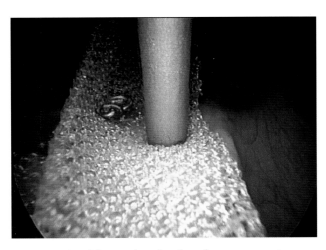

Figure 25.27 The mesh is fixed to the promontorium

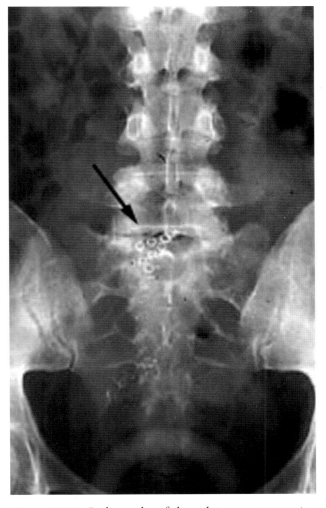

Figure 25.29 Radiography of the pelvis on postoperative day 3 checks the correct position of the coil (arrow) at the level of the first sacral vertebra

Table 25.2 Complications and recurrence after laparoscopic sacrofixation ($n = 146$)

Complications $n = 5$ (3.5%)
    compression of sciatic nerve (wrong insertion): $n = 1$
    spondylodiscitis (9 and 12 months postoperatively) (1.5%): $n = 2$
    mesh erosion (posthysterectomy colpocele) (1.5%): $n = 2$
Recurrence $n = 2$ (1.5%)
    defective application to the cervix: $n = 1$
    enterocele after vaginal vault prolapse without enterocele repair: $n = 1$

We observed two cases of recurrence. The first case was observed 8 months after surgery in one patient from group II. The patient underwent another laparoscopy which showed that the mesh was well fixed to the sacrum but was detached from the cervix. The mesh was separated from the covering peritoneum and then fixed to the cervix with the help of two non-absorbable sutures. The second case was due to incomplete surgery. Indeed, this patient, who had undergone fixation of the vaginal vault, developed a severe enterocele several months later. She underwent surgery a second time, and laparoscopy showed that the vaginal vault was well fixed to the mesh but an enterocele had developed below the point of fixation of the mesh to the vagina. Vaginal surgery of the enterocele was easily carried out. There has been no recurrence in more than 2 years of follow-up.

COMMENTS

The goal of pelvic reconstruction is to restore normal anatomy, maintain or restore normal bladder and bowel function and provide a vagina of normal length to ensure pain-free coitus[29]. A well supported vagina lies on the rectum and levator plate with its axis directed towards the hollow of the sacrum and its apex at or above the ischial spines. It is suspended from the sacrum by the paracolpium. Vaginography[30] and contemporary MRI demonstrate this anatomic fact. Vaginal eversion and

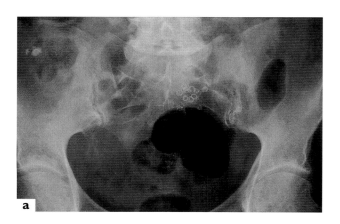

a

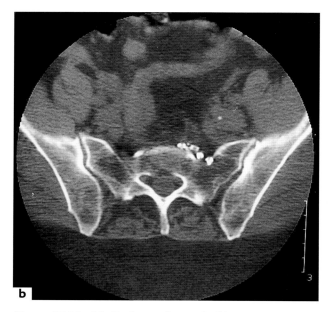

b

Figure 25.30 (a) Radiography and (b) magnetic resonance imaging confirm the presence of a coil in the foramen intervertebrale of the second sacral root

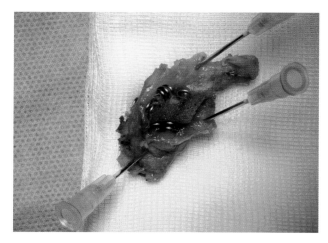

Figure 25.31 Vaginal erosion of the mesh and coils after sacrofixation of the vaginal vault

uterine prolapse are the result of disruption of the upper paracolpium, which includes the fibromuscular tissue of the cardinal and uterosacral ligaments[20]. Many different corrective procedures use this anatomic principle, and anchor the vaginal apex or cervix to the available supporting tissue at this level, including the sacrospinal ligaments, cliococcygeus or coccygeus fascia, uterosacral ligaments or sacrum. Many authors have advocated vaginal surgery as the only approach to this type of pathology. The main problem is that, in the case of severe attenuation of both uterosacral ligaments, which is frequent in vaginal vault prolapse, vaginal repair of cystocele and rectocele often fails[31]. The technique, first proposed by Amreich[32] and later modified by Richter and Albrich[1], involves fixation of the vaginal vault to the sacrospinal ligament. One of the disadvantages of sacrospinal ligament fixation is that the marked vaginal retroversion subsequent to this type of fixation may predispose patients to recurrent support defects in the anterior vagina, resulting in cystocele, urethral hypermobility or both[33,34]. The majority of cases were asymptomatic, however, and only a small number required a subsequent surgical procedure (5.5%).

A second disadvantage of sacrospinal ligament fixation is the possible neuropathy produced by vaginal dissection[35]. Such neuropathy may have an effect on subsequent muscle strength and the integrity of muscular tissue support. It can also be related to dysfunction of the lower urinary tract, and explain the higher incidence of incontinence after sacrospinal ligament fixation than after sacrofixation[36]. In a prospective study comparing the vaginal versus the abdominal approach, Benson et al.[36] demonstrated that the abdominal approach is more effective in treating uterovaginal prolapse, with the probability for an optimal surgical outcome twice as high with an abdominal operation, and the probability for an unsatisfactory surgical outcome twice as high with a vaginal operation. Among the transabdominal approaches described so far, the most frequently published is fixation of the vaginal vault to the midsacrum or sacral promontory using artificial material.

Sacral colpopexy has a high success rate (85–99%) in vault prolapse repair and does not shorten the vagina[5,6,8,17,22,23,25,37,38]. Laparoscopic approaches to sacrofixation[12,20,39] have been described. The advantage of sacrofixation is that it ensures vaginal length with a larger-caliber, normal horizontal vaginal axis and a more anatomic repair[36]. Sacral colpopexy is performed to correct severe vaginal vault eversion by replacing the upper paracolpium with synthetic mesh, which results in stronger fixation than does a simple culdoplasty[20]. According to Ameline and Huguier[40], the only physiological suspension involves placement of suture material into the ligamentous and periosteal fibrous connective tissue in the midline of the anterior sacrum. Although sacral segments 3 and 4 are anatomically ideal, control of the tip of the needle deep in the hollow of the sacrum is difficult, and laceration of presacral veins is an ever-present

risk, leading to life-threatening hemorrhages which are extremely difficult to control[41]. Fixation to the first vertebra (beyond the sacrolumbar joint) or the lower part of the fifth lumbar vertebra restores to the genital tube its triple angulation – postero-ascending vaginal obliquity, anteflexion of the cervix over the uterine corpus and anteversion – and thus correctly restores the anatomy[22]. Like Hoff et al.[42], we believe that, in the great majority of cases, anterior colporrhaphy with sacrofixation is not needed to treat associated cystocele, unless the cystocele is of degree 3 or more. Nevertheless, we believe that posterior colporrhaphy can be helpful in treating even a huge rectocele completely. We performed posterior colporrhaphy only in cases where the rectocele was so large that simple fixation of the cervix or vagina did not yield a sufficient reduction.

Like Smith[6], we believe that osseous anchorage of the prosthesis is stronger than sacrospinal ligament stitching (Tables 25.3 and 25.4). The tacking technique described here allows fixation of the mesh to the vertebra with the same reliability. It is less invasive (no penetration of the bones but only the periosteum), and thus reduces the risk of bone infection. It enables us to avoid difficulties related to a prevertebral suture. The most common complications of sacropexy are intraoperative bleeding and a postoperative temperature. Spondylodiscitis and bleeding due to presacral vessel lesions are rarely observed[41,43,44]. The mesh should be reperitonealized to prevent bowel adhesions[45,46]. Undue tension must be avoided to prevent pain[5].

We observed two prolapse recurrences among the 146 patients who underwent sacrofixation (1.5%) and three cases of recurrence of cystocele, requiring anterior colporrhaphy. It should be noted that, in all cases, the vaginal vault maintained its correct position without prolapse. This rate of recurrent anterior defects led us to repair the anterior compartment either laparoscopically or vaginally at the time of promontofixation in cases of associated cystocele of degree 3 or more.

In contrast to sacrospinal fixation, because of its more anatomic repair, sacrofixation does not favor the development of secondary cystoceles, does not cause vaginal shortening and, providing that particular care is taken to insert the springs into the central part of the body of the vertebra, is without risk for nerves if the prevertebral area dissection is easy and well performed. In overweight women, in whom there is a wide area (with fatty tissue) between the prevertebral peritoneum and the vertebral bone itself, we believe that intraoperative X-rays are indicated in order to determine the exact site of coil insertion.

As stressed by Vancaillie[47], sacrocolpopexy remains a potentially high-morbidity procedure, with invasion of the presacral space. Nevertheless, recent publications reported a low rate of complications; the most frequent complication in these series was vaginal mesh erosion, which

Borderline tumors of the ovary or epithelial ovarian tumors of borderline malignancy

J Donnez, A Münschke, P Jadoul, J Squifflet

26

INTRODUCTION

In 1929, Taylor[1] first described borderline tumors of the ovary (BOT) (Figure 26.1), also known as 'epithelial ovarian tumors of low malignant potential'. These neoplasms occupy a position somewhere between benign and clearly malignant ovarian epithelial tumors. As a consequence of this histological peculiarity, they were recognized as a special clinical entity by the International Federation of Gynecologists and Obstetricians (FIGO) and included in its classification in 1971, with the World Health Organization (WHO) following 2 years later. When compared with the 'classic' malignant ovarian tumor, they are characterized by the following features[2]:

- Younger age at time of diagnosis (approximately 10–15 years earlier)

- Earlier stage when first diagnosed (almost 70% of all borderlines are discovered when still at stage I)

- Infrequent and late recurrence (recurrence possibly up to 20 years after surgery)

- Excellent long-term survival

EPIDEMIOLOGY, PROGNOSIS AND RISK FACTORS

Borderline tumors account for approximately 10–15% of all epithelial ovarian cancers in Caucasian populations. The mean age at the time of diagnosis ranges (according to different studies) from 38 to 56 years, which is approximately 10–15 years younger than for malignant tumors of the ovary[3].

In their review, Link et al.[4] found the following distribution at the time of diagnosis: 69.6% of tumors at stage I, 10.3% at stage II, 19.2% at stage III, and 0.6% at stage IV.

The most important adverse factors are[3,5,6–9]:

- High FIGO stage

- Histological subtype

- Presence of invasive peritoneal implants

- Pseudomyxoma peritonei

- Tumor size

- Patient's age at the time of diagnosis

- Presence of a residual mass after surgery

- High mitotic index

- Cell atypia

- Ploidy of the tumor: aneuploidy

Survival

One of the most important prognostic elements is the FIGO stage. As for most other cancers, it is one of the oldest prognostic tools, and still the most widely used.

A review of more than 1000 cases by Massad et al.[10] showed the following 5-year survival rates: stage I, 98.1%; stage II, 94.1%; stage III/IV, 79.0%; overall survival, 94.6%.

The histological type of the lesion was considered to be of lesser importance until recently. As more epidemic data become available, differences between histological subtypes become increasingly evident. The micropapillary serous subtype in particular is known to be of more prognostic significance. This subtype shows a greater incidence of bilateralism (59–82%), exophytic vegetations are more common (50–65%), stromal microinvasion or invasive peritoneal implants are more frequently encountered (16–91%) and the FIGO stage at the time of diagnosis is significantly higher[5,11]. The recurrence rates are therefore significantly higher too, and the survival rates not as good as for the typical serous form. Deavers et al.[6] found survival rates for stage II and III typical BOT of 85% after 5 years, while the micropapillary form was associated with survival rates of 72%.

Because of the inherent risk of late recurrence with this disease, overall survival at 20 years drops to approximately 80%[4]. It worsens when patients with pseudomyxoma peritonei are taken into account: their 10-year survival

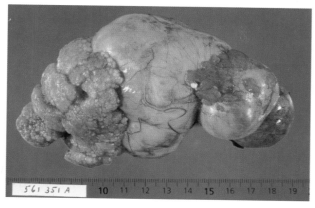

Figure 26.1 A cystic ovary: papillary vegetations and neovascularization can be seen on the outer surface of the ovary

rates are estimated to be as low as 40%. The chances of recurrence or persistent disease depend on the FIGO stage and on the nature of the peritoneal implants[4,10,12]. Massad et al.[10] encountered the following rates: stage I, 2.1% recurrence or persistent disease; stage II, 7.1%; stage III/IV, 14.4%. Lin et al.[12] found 11% recurrence if peritoneal implants were non-invasive and 45% if they were invasive. Deavers et al.[6] compared the recurrence rates for typical and micropapillary serous BOT and reported 31% and 78%, respectively, for stage II and III disease.

Risk factors

The same risk factors as for malignant tumors have been evaluated, but they do not all appear to be equally relevant[13]. No significant relationship has been found with the following parameters:

- Family history
- Hormone replacement therapy (HRT)
- Menstrual history
- Body mass index (BMI)
- Use of an intrauterine device (IUD)

The same protective effects as for invasive cancers have been confirmed[13]:

- Pregnancy and birth (relative risk 0.7)
- Breast-feeding (relative risk 0.5)

The suggested protective effect of oral contraceptives is still a matter of debate[14,15].

Infertility and infertility treatment as risk factors for borderline tumors of the ovary

Borderline tumors are encountered more often in patients who suffer from infertility. As a result of this observation, some authors[16–19] initially blamed infertility treatments. They suggested that the recurrent microtraumas associated with repeatedly induced ovulations might be responsible for the higher risk of malignancies. Nevertheless, evidence[20,21] shows an equal increase in the incidence of BOT in patients suffering from infertility without any treatment, as in those being treated; furthermore, many BOT are discovered during infertility work-ups. It is therefore suggested that an underlying pathology of the ovary itself, and not the attempts to overcome this problem, might be the cause of BOT. Nowadays, many teams consider ovulation-inducing treatment or even in vitro fertilization (IVF) after conservative treatment for BOT in young women wishing to conceive. Several studies have demonstrated the safety of these treatments in carefully chosen cases[22–26].

HISTOLOGY

Histological criteria used to diagnose borderline tumors of the ovary include[12]:

- Epithelial budding
- Multilayered epithelium
- Mitotic activity
- Nuclear atypia
- Absence of signs of stromal invasion

To make sure that this last and most important criterion is met, the thorough investigation of a large number of slides must be carried out by an experienced anatomopathologist. Otherwise, the risk of mistaking BOT for invasive epithelial cancer, or for a benign cystadenoma, is high. Indeed, up to 10% of borderline tumors are upstaged to invasive carcinoma after complete anatomopathological examination. The results of frozen section analysis should therefore be treated with caution until confirmation.

Recently, several authors have been inclined to consider borderline tumors with focal microinvasion of the stroma as ordinary BOT[7,26–28]. Their prognosis seems to be the same as for other BOT, at least in the case of low-stage disease, and in certain carefully selected cases even conservative treatment might be contemplated.

Different subspecies of borderline tumors of the ovary

The most frequent types of tumors of low malignant potential are the serous and mucinous forms. Together, they account for more than 95% of all BOT, and are therefore the most widely studied and understood.

Serous BOT

Fifty-five per cent of all BOT are of the serous subtype (15% of all serous tumors of the ovary being borderline variants). Recently, anatomopathologists divided serous tumors into two different subtypes (Bethesda Workshop[26–28], 2003): the more common typical serous BOT and the more aggressive micropapillary variant. New data subsequently proved the clinical interest of this classification, as several authors confirmed the worse prognosis of these subtypes.

Typical serous BOT This variant accounts for 74% of all serous forms, and may be bilateral (38%)[12] and cystic, and have a mean diameter between 6 and 12 cm (generally smaller than mucinous BOT). At the time of diagnosis, serous BOT are confined to the ovaries in 75% of all cases. Ascites is uncommonly encountered, at least in the early stages of the disease. The most common lesion observed is a unilocular cyst, often filled with clear liquid (Figure 26.2), with small papillary structures bordering the inner walls (Figure 26.3). These structures are generally covered with low-grade proliferative epithelium (Figures 26.4).

Exterior vegetations are found more frequently than in mucinous BOT, but they do not appear to constitute an unfavorable element. Psammomas may be present, even extensively in some cases.

Micropapillary serous BOT This variant is also called the cribriform serous type. These tumors are more commonly bilateral than their typical counterparts (59–89%), and involvement of the surface is more frequently encountered (50–65%). This may be the reason for the significantly higher stage at the time of diagnosis (43–84% stage II or higher). Focal microinvasion of the stroma or invasive peritoneal implants are also more common (16–91%)[6,29–31].

For these reasons, patients with this subtype might be considered as a population at risk, and conservative

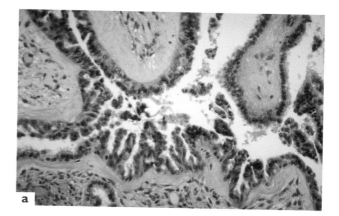
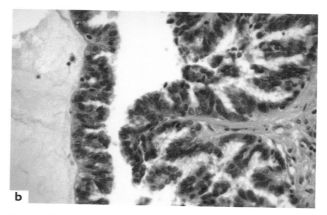

Figure 26.4 (a) and (b) Papillae covered with low-grade proliferative epithelium showing micropapillary tufting. Note the well-differentiated ciliated cells

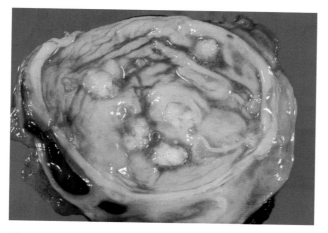

Figure 26.2 Several papillomatous foci can be seen inside a borderline cystic tumor of the ovary

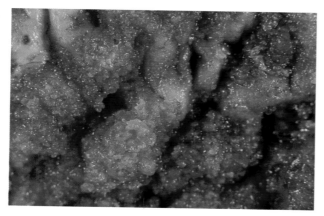

Figure 26.3 A close-up shows the papillary pattern of borderline foci in another serous borderline tumor of the ovary

management should be viewed with caution because of the higher recurrence rate.

Mucinous BOT

The mucinous form accounts for approximately 40% of all borderline tumors. Its spread tends to be limited to one ovary at the time of diagnosis (80–90% of stage I lesions, only 5% bilateral lesions).

Mucinous borderline neoplasms are typically large multilocular cysts (Figure 26.5), with a mean diameter of over 15 cm. Areas of necrosis and hemorrhage can be seen, as well as small papillae or nodules. The presence of surface vegetations is not uncommon, but ascites is rarely present. Histologically, the pseudostratified epithelium shows nuclear atypia (Figure 26.6).

The presence of stromal invasion (by atypical cells) excludes such tumors by definition from the borderline subgroup, but, in some cases, mucin can be found dissecting the stroma (pseudomyxoma ovarii).

Mucinous tumors of low malignant potential can be divided into two different subgroups with different histological characteristics: the Müllerian, endocervical type and the gastrointestinal type.

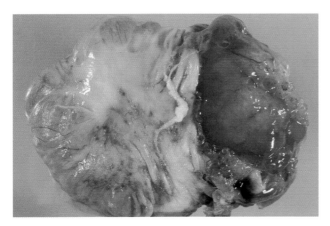

Figure 26.5 A large borderline tumor of the ovary with its mucinous content extruding through the right opening

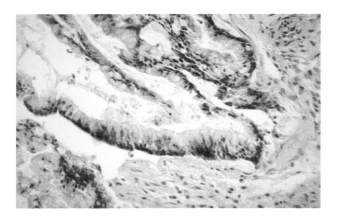

Figure 26.6 Pseudostratified epithelial lining of the cyst showing hyperchromatic nuclei and several goblet cells

Most tumors are of the intestinal variant, and the majority are encountered when still at stage I, with excellent survival rates. The endocervical variant is less frequent. As the micropapillary variant of the serous type, this subgroup more often involves both ovaries, but its prognosis is almost as good as for typical mucinous BOT[27].

A particular form is the pseudomyxoma peritoneii. It may occur as a complication in all mucinous neoplasms and is characterized by a more or less chronic form of mucinous ascites with peritoneal implants, producing a gelatinous substance. It is generally associated with a defect in the primary cyst wall, leading to spontaneous spillage.

This condition may lead to abdominal pain or discomfort, and even to bowel obstruction.

A concomitant intestinal lesion is found in almost every case, but, even after careful exploration of the intestines, some tumors still appear to be of ovarian origin.

Because of the high probability of an occult intestinal lesion, careful surgical exploration of the appendix and all the intestines is necessary. Furthermore, routine appendec-tomy should be performed in all cases of pseudomyxoma peritoneii.

Endometrioid tumors

These tumors are often associated with peritoneal or ovarian endometriosis (in 30–50% of cases). However, peritoneal implants can be distinguished from endometriosis by the lack of hemorrhage and endometriotic stroma. Two different subtypes are known. The first develops on an adenofibrous background. The second consists of back-to-back glands and shows no adenofibrous matrix. Both types tend to be cystic, and recurrence seems to be infrequent.

Brenner tumors

This very rare variant seems generally to behave as a benign tumor, and stromal invasion is exceptionally infrequent. This BOT is usually cystic and bordered by epithelium formed of several cell layers, resembling a non-invasive papillary urothelial cell carcinoma.

Clear cell tumors

Clear cell tumors are another rare subspecies of borderline tumors, consisting of mostly fibrous tissue with glandular and tubal elements in a one-cell-layer epithelium.

Peritoneal implants

If stromal invasion is observed in the primary ovarian lesion, it should be classified and treated as malignant cancer. On the other hand, the presence of microinvasive lesions on the peritoneal surface is often encountered in higher-stage disease[32]. These are not considered as metastases but referred to as implants (Figure 26.7). The impact on long-term survival is still uncertain with this type of implant, but they seem to constitute one of the most unfavorable elements in disseminated disease[4,11].

Some authors consider these peritoneal lesions not as local dissemination, but as independent primary lesions. This theory of multifocal disease[33] is supported by the polyclonal origin of these lesions. Some cases of BOT could therefore be considered as peritoneal disease, not necessarily of ovarian origin alone.

MOLECULAR BIOLOGY

Genetic alterations are common in most malignant tumors. The semimalignant BOT is no exception. At least 50% of all borderline lesions present with at least one karyotypic anomaly. To date, cases of monosomy or trisomy of 19 different chromosomes have been reported[34,35]. Several of these anomalies are more specific to one or the other tumor type.

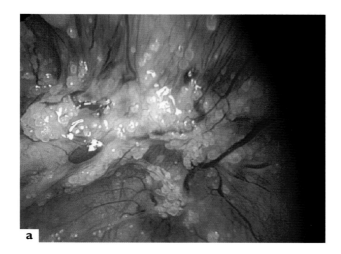

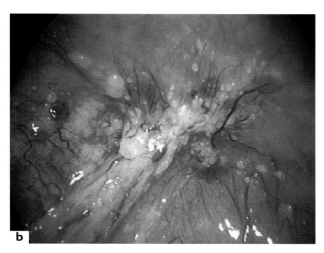

Figure 26.7 (a) and (b) Peritoneal implants of a stage III serous borderline tumor of the ovary (BOT). Even if these lesions with their extensive neovascularization have the appearance of invasive implants, the non-infiltrative nature was confirmed by histological examination

Gain of chromosome 12 is more frequent in serous BOT (23% vs. 8% in mucinous BOT). Gain of chromosome X is observed in 42% of mucinous BOT and 30% of the serous variant, while gain of chromosome 8 has not been noted in typical mucinous BOT. It is, on the other hand, more commonly encountered in serous and endocervical-mucinous borderline lesions or invasive ovarian carcinomas. Loss of chromosome X is much more common in invasive carcinomas.

These data[36,37] are somewhat at odds with the multistep progression model for the progression of BOT to invasive carcinoma. Future studies might be able to identify some genetic pattern in BOT subgroups predisposing them to malignant transformation.

Several proteins are currently under investigation. One candidate is the HER-2 gene encoding epidermal growth factor. Some series show that this oncoprotein is amplified

in 25–66% of ovarian carcinomas and that its overexpression is less common in BOT[38]. A possible link between tumor progression and this gene still needs to be confirmed. Other possible genetic markers of poor prognosis and progression towards invasive disease might be the OVCA-1, OVCA-2, BRCA or p53 genes.

The importance of a genetic prognostic tool for borderline disease is understood by most gynecological oncologists, but all studies published so far involve very small series, and much more epidemic data are needed. The low incidence of the different BOT types and the even lower probability of malignant transformation of borderline disease make it very difficult to gather enough material to perform such studies on a larger scale. Multicentric efforts will therefore be needed in the future to enable further progress to be made in this area.

DIAGNOSIS

Symptoms

Borderline tumors of the ovary show the same clinical symptoms as those for invasive epithelial cancers[4,21,39]:

- Abdominal discomfort or pain
- Abdominal enlargement
- Sensation of an abdominal mass
- Menometrorrhagia

Many patients have no symptoms, and the ovarian mass is detected during a routine check-up, or investigation for an infertility problem. Any newly discovered ovarian mass (mostly cysts) should be carefully evaluated.

Ultrasound scans

The first examination should be a transvaginal ultrasound scan[40]. The proximity of the probe to the ovary allows relatively precise resolution. This examination has high sensitivity (87–95%) if performed by an experienced operator using the latest technology.

Criteria used to evaluate the benign nature of a cyst by ultrasound are the following[39]:

(1) The cyst diameter: size below 5 cm suggests a benign cyst. A diameter above 10 cm, on the other hand, suggests either a malignant cyst or a benign mucinous cyst.

(2) The homogeneity of the cyst content: homogeneous content of low echogenicity in a unilocular cyst is in favor of a non-malignant lesion. On the other hand, the presence of hyperechogenic areas and septa is suspect (Figure 26.8).

(3) The absence of intracystic vegetations: the presence of such vegetations is certainly not proof of malignancy but is at least suspect (Figure 26.9).

Laparoscopic reimplantation of cryopreserved ovarian tissue

J Donnez, M M Dolmans, D Demylle, P Jadoul, C Pirard, J Squifflet,
B Martinez-Madrid, A Van Langendonckt

INTRODUCTION

The treatment of childhood malignant disease is becoming increasingly effective. Aggressive chemotherapy and radiotherapy, and bone-marrow transplantation, can cure more than 90% of girls and young women affected by such disorders. However, the ovaries are very sensitive to cytotoxic treatment, especially to alkylating agents and ionizing radiation, generally resulting in loss of both endocrine and reproductive function[1]. Moreover, uterine irradiation at a young age reduces adult uterine volume[2].

By 2010, about one in 250 people in the adult population will be childhood-cancer survivors[3]. Several potential options are available to preserve fertility in patients facing premature ovarian failure, including immature and mature oocyte cryopreservation, and embryo cryopreservation[4,5]. For patients who need immediate chemotherapy, the cryopreservation of ovarian tissue is a possible alternative[4,6,7]. The aim of this strategy is to reimplant ovarian tissue into the pelvic cavity (orthotopic site) or a heterotopic site such as the forearm once treatment is completed and the patient is disease-free[4,8–10].

Oktay et al. reported laparoscopic transplantation of frozen–thawed ovarian tissue to the pelvic side wall[8], forearm[9], and beneath the skin of the abdomen. A four-cell embryo was obtained from 20 oocytes retrieved from tissue transplanted to the abdomen, but no pregnancy occurred after transfer[11]. Radford et al.[10] reported a patient with a history of Hodgkin's disease treated by chemotherapy, in whom ovarian tissue had been biopsied and

cryopreserved 4 years after chemotherapy and later reimplanted. In this case, histological section of ovarian cortical tissue revealed only a few primordial follicles because of the previous chemotherapy. After reimplantation, the patient had only one menstrual period.

In 1995, the Catholic University of Louvain ethics committee approved a protocol to assess the safety and efficacy of the cryopreservation of ovarian tissue in women treated with high doses of chemotherapy, which could induce ovarian failure.

Here, we describe the outcome of orthotopic autotransplantation of cryopreserved ovarian tissue in three patients.

METHODS

Patient 1

In 1997, a 25-year-old woman presented with clinical stage IV Hodgkin's lymphoma. Ovarian tissue cryopreservation was undertaken before chemotherapy. We obtained written informed consent. By laparoscopy, we took five biopsy samples – about 12–15 mm long and 5 mm wide – from the left ovary (Figure 27.1). Freezing of ovarian tissue was carried out according to the protocol described by Gosden et al.[6]. We immediately transferred biopsy samples to the laboratory in Leibovitz L-15 medium supplemented with GlutaMAX™ (Invitrogen, Paisley, UK), where the remaining stromal tissue was gently removed. We cut four biopsy samples of cortex into 70 small cubes of 2×2 mm, and one strip of 12×4 mm was left whole. These fragments of ovarian tissue were suspended in the cryoprotective medium. We placed all the fragments into precooled 2-ml cryogenic vials (Simport, Quebec, Canada) filled with Leibovitz medium, supplemented with 4 mg/ml of human serum albumin (Red Cross, Brussels, Belgium) and 1.5 mmol/l DMSO (dimethylsulfoxide) (Sigma, St Louis, MO, USA). The cryotubes were cooled in a programmable freezer (Kryo 10, Series III; Planer, Sunbury-on-Thames, UK) using the following program: (1) cooled from 0 to $-8°C$ at $-2°C/min$; (2) seeded manually by touching the cryotubes with forceps prechilled in liquid nitrogen; (3) cooled to $-40°C$ at $-0.3°C/min$; (4) cooled to $-150°C$ at $-30°C/min$; and (5) transferred to liquid nitrogen ($-196°C$) immediately for storage.

Removal of the whole ovary was not an option, because one can never exclude recovery of ovarian function after

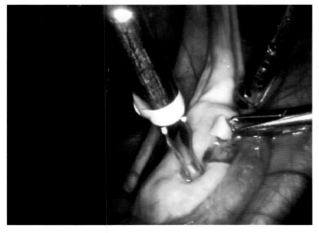

Figure 27.1 Biopsy of the cortex. Only cortical pieces 12–15 mm long and 5 mm wide must be biopsied

chemotherapy. Indeed, premature ovarian failure after chemotherapy is dependent on age, drug used and dose given, and does not happen in all cases. After laparoscopy, the patient received MOPP/ABV hybrid chemotherapy (mechlorethamine, vincristine, procarbazine, prednisone, doxorubicin, bleomycin, vinblastine) from August 1997 to February 1998, followed by radiotherapy (38 Gy).

The patient became amenorrheic shortly after the initiation of chemotherapy. After chemotherapy and radiotherapy, concentrations of follicle stimulating hormone (FSH) were 91.1 mIU/ml, luteinizing hormone (LH) 85 mIU/ml and estradiol 17 pg/ml, confirming castration. This ovarian failure profile was confirmed 3 months later. Hormone replacement therapy (HRT) was started in June 1998 and then stopped in January 2001 because the patient wanted to become pregnant. A thorough evaluation by oncologists showed that she was disease-free.

After the cessation of HRT, concentrations of FSH, LH and 17β-estradiol returned to levels consistent with ovarian failure. From January 2001 to December 2002 the patient had only one ovulatory cycle.

Reimplantation

We performed the first laparoscopy 7 days before reimplantation to create a peritoneal window by means of a large incision just beneath the right ovarian hilus, followed by coagulation of the edges of the window (Figure 27.2a). The goal was to induce angiogenesis and neovascularization in this area.

We performed a second laparoscopy 7 days after creation of the peritoneal window. A biopsy sample of 4–5 mm in size was taken from each of the atrophic ovaries to check for the presence or absence of primordial follicles.

We thawed the cryogenic vials at room temperature (between 21 and 23°C) for 2 min and immersed them in a water bath at 37°C for another 2 min. We immediately transferred ovarian tissue from the vials to tissue culture dishes (Becton Dickinson, NY, USA) in Leibovitz medium and subsequently washed the tissue three times with fresh medium to remove cryoprotectant before further processing.

Thawed ovarian cortical tissue was placed in sterile medium and immediately transferred to the operating theater. We pushed the large strip and 35 small cubes of frozen–thawed ovarian tissue into the furrow created by the peritoneal window, very close to the ovarian vessels and fimbria on the right side (Figure 27.3). No suture was used. An extensive neovascular network was clearly visible in this space (Figure 27.2b). We used vital fluorescent staining (Molecular Probes, Leiden, The Netherlands) to confirm the survival of primordial follicles after freeze–thawing[12].

After long discussions with the oncologists and the patient, a third laparoscopy was proposed. At least three reasons were given to justify the procedure: (1) to check the viability of the orthotopic grafts, 4 months after

transplantation, by laparoscopic visualization and histological analysis; (2) to check for the absence of any cellular growth anomalies (peritoneal fluid, histology), the cortical strip and cubes having been biopsied before chemotherapy; and (3) to reimplant the remaining ovarian cortical cubes, by request of the patient, who was now aged 32 years. Indeed, if pregnancy had not ensued from the reimplanted tissue, she would have considered oocyte donation. A validated technique will probably not need so many surgical procedures in the future.

Results

FSH and LH concentrations were at castrated levels, and vaginal echography failed to show any ovarian activity, until 5 months after reimplantation. The day before the third laparoscopy, ultrasonography clearly showed the presence of a follicle outside the ovaries, both of which appeared atrophic. The atrophic ovaries were visualized as

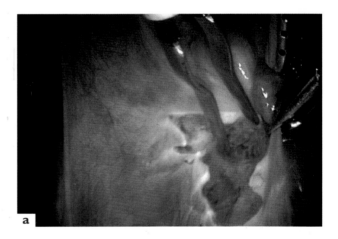

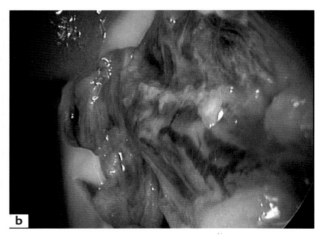

Figure 27.2 Site of transplantation. (a) During the first laparoscopy (7 days before transplantation), a peritoneal window was created and the edges of the window were coagulated. (b) Seven days later (day of reimplantation), an extensive vascular network was clearly visible in this space

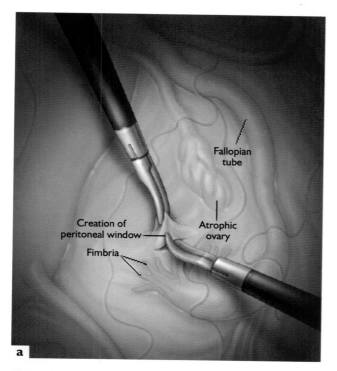
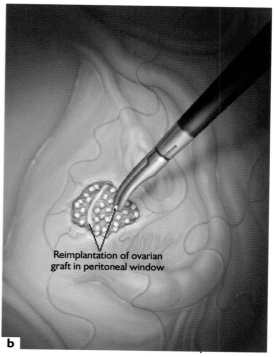

Figure 27.3 Laparoscopic creation of a peritoneal window and subsequent development of a vascular network. During the first laparoscopy (7 days before transplantation), a peritoneal window was created, and the edges of the window were coagulated (a). The large strip and small cubes were then placed in the peritoneal window (b)

dense echogenic structures measuring about 2 cm long and 0.75–1 cm wide. The follicular structure could be seen clearly separated (0.5–1 cm) from the right ovary. At this laparoscopy, the ovaries were still atrophic, without any signs of ovarian activity. At the site of reimplantation, the follicular structure seen at vaginal echography was visible, and was subsequently biopsied (Figure 27.4a). The biopsy sample showed that granulosa cells were present, as proved by the presence of cells immunohistochemically expressing inhibin A (Figure 27.4b)[13]. The grafted cubes could also be seen, and one of them was biopsied for the assessment of primordial follicle survival (Figure 27.5). Follicular viability was proved by the presence of two primordial follicles, which were colored by vital fluorescent staining (Figure 27.5). The remaining 32 cubes were then reimplanted at the site of the ovarian graft biopsy on the right side. At that time, a slight reduction in LH and FSH was noted, concomitantly with follicular development in the grafted area.

From 5 to 9 months after reimplantation, ultrasonography revealed the development of a follicle, followed by corpus luteum formation with every menstrual cycle at the site of reimplantation; this corresponded with an estradiol concentration of more than 100 pg/ml and a progesterone level of 12–37 ng/ml. Amounts of LH and FSH were lower than those observed before reimplantation. This change led to the restoration of consecutive menstrual bleeding every month. At 9.5

months, FSH concentrations rose to 78.7 mIU/ml, and returned to normal values 7 days later. Three weeks later, a follicle of 2.6 cm in size had developed on the right side, clearly outside the right ovary (Figure 27.6a). Both native ovaries were well visualized and obviously atrophic. Eighteen days after ovulation, calculated by basal body temperature, the concentration of human chorionic gonadotropin was 2853 mIU/ml. We should stress that conception arose spontaneously, since neither ovarian stimulation nor *in vitro* fertilization (IVF) had been carried out. Because we do not yet know whether transplanted tissue can sustain ovarian steroid hormone support during pregnancy, we initiated progesterone treatment (administered vaginally at a dose of 600 mg per day). Vaginal ultrasonography at 8 weeks confirmed a viable intrauterine pregnancy (Figure 27.6b). Triple test evaluation and ultrasonography did not reveal any anomalies. The pregnancy resulted in the live birth of a healthy girl, weighing 3.72 kg, with an Apgar score of 9 at 1 min, 9 at 5 min and 9 at 10 min.

Patient 2

In 1999, a 21-year-old woman presented with complications (spleen abscess and cerebral thrombosis) due to homozygous sickle cell anemia. Bone marrow transplantation (BMT) was proposed to the patient, her sister being human leukocyte antigen (HLA)-compatible.

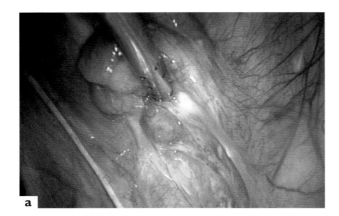

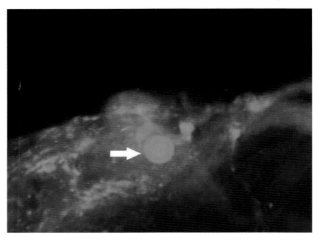

Figure 27.5 Biopsy sample of a frozen–thawed cube, 5 months after reimplantation. Vital fluorescent staining by calcein-AM and ethidium homodimer 1 indicated viable primordial follicles, colored in green (arrow). Original magnification ×20

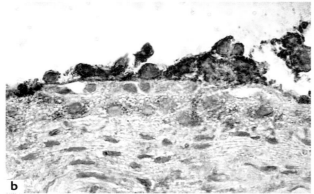

Figure 27.4 Follicle from the grafted tissue. (a) Laparoscopic view of the follicular structure at the site of the large strip implantation. (b) Histology of the follicular wall showing the presence of cells expressing inhibin A (brown). Original magnification ×100

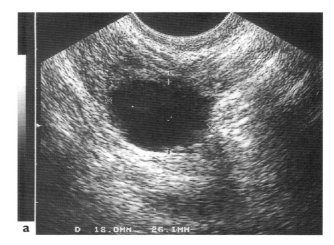

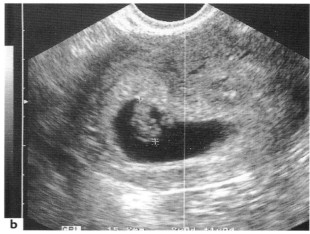

Figure 27.6 Vaginal ultrasonography. (a) Vaginal echography showing a follicle of 18×26 mm in size at the site of ovarian cortex transplantation. (b) Ongoing intrauterine pregnancy (8 weeks). Crown–rump length 15 mm, cardiac activity +

Ovarian tissue cryopreservation was undertaken before chemotherapy.

Using laparoscopy, we performed a right oophorectomy. Removal of the whole ovary was decided upon in the present case, because ovarian failure is almost always induced after chemotherapy given prior to BMT[14,15].

After laparoscopy, the patient received two alkylating agents (busulfan 16 mg/kg; cyclophosphamide 120 mg/kg). In July of that year, bone marrow transplantation was carried out.

The patient became amenorrheic immediately after the initiation of chemotherapy. Concentrations of follicle stimulating hormone (FSH) were 48.2 mIU/ml, luteinizing hormone (LH) 18.5 mIU/ml and estradiol < 10 pg/ml, confirming castration. This ovarian failure profile was confirmed 3 and 5 months later, and HRT was started in December 1999 and stopped in December 2002.

After the cessation of HRT, bimonthly measurements of FSH, LH and 17β-estradiol concentrations proved the absence of ovulatory cycles from December 2002 to August 2004. The measurement of ovarian volume by ultrasound revealed a volume of 14.1×1×1 cm. No remaining follicles where visible by ultrasound during this

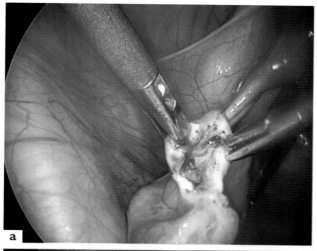

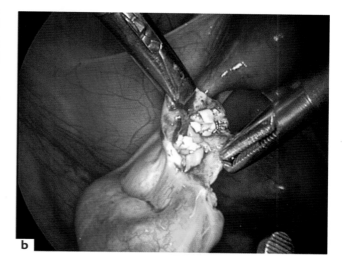

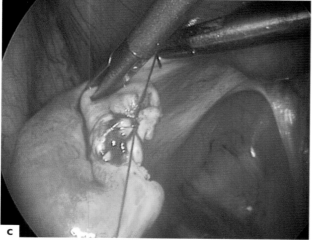

Figure 27.7 (a) Seven days after the ovarian incision, an intraovarian vascular network was clearly visible. (b) Twenty-five cubes were placed in the ovary. (c) Only one suture (Vicryl® 5-0) was used to reapproximate the edges of the incised cortex

20-month period. The decision to reimplant the cryopreserved tissue was therefore taken.

Reimplantation

A first laparoscopy was performed 7 days before reimplantation, not only to create a peritoneal window just beneath the left ovarian hilus, as previously described, but also to perform an ovarian incision along the longitudinal ovarian axis. The edges of the window and the ovarian incision were coagulated in order to induce neovascularization in this area.

Knowing from experimental data that the ovary itself, even if atrophic, may be an ideal site for reimplantation, we decided to prepare simultaneously two sites for reimplantation[16,17] (and Dolmans *et al.*, personal communication).

A biopsy measuring 0.5 cm in size was taken from the left atrophic ovary (1.5×1 cm in size). A second laparoscopy was carried out 8 days later. It was decided to thaw only part of the cryopreserved tissue. Forty cubes were thawed according to the previously described technique, and immediately transferred to the operating theater. We placed 15 cubes in the peritoneal window and 24 cubes in the intraovarian area (Figure 27.7).

Results

On the day of reimplantation, the left ovary was atrophic, but the intraovarian area, which had been incised and slightly coagulated, demonstrated an extensive vascular network. Angiogenesis was less pronounced in the area of the peritoneal window.

No primordial follicles were found in serial sections of the biopsy of 0.5 cm in size taken from the left atrophic ovary. This biopsy from an atrophic ovary (measuring 1×1.5 cm) must be considered representative, since it corresponds to about 10% of the residual value.

From the day of reimplantation to 4 months later, FSH, LH and 17β-estradiol levels ranged from 32 to 45 mIU/ml (FSH), 15 to 22 mIU/ml (LH) and 10 to 14 pg/ml (17β-estradiol) (Figure 27.8). At 4.5 months, FSH and LH concentrations decreased to 20.8 and 10.2 mIU/ml, respectively, while the 17β-estradiol level rose to 58 pg/ml. Ultrasonography demonstrated the presence of an intraovarian follicle of 9.2 mm, which grew to 14 mm (Figure

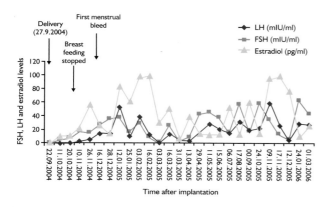

Figure 27.8 Follicle stimulating hormone (FSH), luteinizing hormone (LH) and 17β-estradiol levels of patient 2

27.9a). Three days later, sequential serum concentrations of LH demonstrated a peak, leading to the development of a corpus luteum of 21.2 mm in size (Figure 27.9b). The luteal phase was confirmed by a progesterone level of 6.5 ng/ml. During the luteal phase, FSH and LH concentrations decreased to 15 and 10 mIU/ml, respectively. The patient menstruated 14 days after the LH peak.

After this first cycle, FSH levels rose to 34 mIU/ml for 6 weeks, concomitant with 17β-estradiol levels of ≤ 15 pg/ml. Thereafter, 17β-estradiol concentrations rose from 15 to 42 pg/ml, concomitant with a decrease in FSH, which nevertheless remained at around 20 mIU/ml. Ultrasonography revealed the presence of two small intraovarian follicles, which achieved a maximum size of 11 mm. The patient experienced menstrual bleeding.

Following this cycle, FSH and 17β-estradiol values returned to castrated levels, 35.2 mIU/ml and 11 pg/ml, respectively, for another 4–5 weeks, before hormone measurements and ultrasound proved the presence of follicular maturation. Indeed, the 17β-estradiol level increased to 53 pg/ml and the FSH concentration decreased to 18.2 mIU/ml. Ultrasound revealed a follicle of 16 mm in size emerging from the tissue grafted into the peritoneal window, close to the ovary, but clearly separated from it. After these three cycles, FSH and LH values returned to castrated levels. No ovarian activity was detected, and a second transplantation was recently carried out.

Patient 3

A third transplantation of cryopreserved tissue was carried out in June 2005.

A patient of 25 years of age presented with a clinical diagnosis of stage IIIa Hodgkin's disease. She received ABVD (doxorubicin, bleomycin, vinblastine, dacarbazine) chemotherapy in November 1997. In April 1998, a relapse was diagnosed, and ovarian tissue cryopreservation was carried out by means of a left oophorectomy. In May 1998,

she received MOPP chemotherapy and total body irradiation before peripheral stem cell transplantation.

As complications, the patient presented with vascular necrosis of the left knee and both hips, alveolitis and premature ovarian failure (FSH 72 mIU/ml).

With the agreement of both the oncology department and the ethics committee, the reimplantation of five pieces (~ 1 × 0.5 cm) of frozen–thawed ovarian tissue was carried out on the medulla of the remaining ovary (Figure 27.10). At the time of reimplantation, Ovidol® and gonadotropin-releasing hormone (GnRH) antagonists were given.

Five months after reimplantation, LH and FSH were still at castrated levels. Six months after reimplantation, we observed the first follicular maturation (to a size of 20 mm) and an increase of estradiol level to 194 pg/ml.

DISCUSSION

Unfortunately, in most female cancer patients, aggressive chemotherapy and radiotherapy lead to ovarian failure. The restoration of ovarian function after such treatment has two main goals: to improve quality of life and restore reproductive function. For patients who need immediate chemotherapy, ovarian tissue cryopreservation, undertaken before cancer treatment starts, could be a means of preserving fertility without delaying the initiation of chemotherapy. However, one major concern surrounding the use of ovarian cortical strips for orthotopic auto-transplantation is the potential risk that the frozen–thawed ovarian cortex might harbor malignant cells, which could induce recurrence of disease after reimplantation. Shaw et al.[18] reported that ovarian grafts from AKR mice (a strain with high incidence of spontaneous T cell lymphomas) could transfer lymphoma to recipient animals. Nevertheless, findings of other studies have suggested that ovarian tissue transplantation in Hodgkin's disease is safe[19–21].

In our study, the histological assessment of ovarian cortex before and after reimplantation found no evidence of disease. However, confirmation of the absence of malignant cells by light microscopy might not be sufficient, especially in other types of cancer (e.g. hematogenous or systemic neoplasms)[22]. Screening methods to detect minimal residual disease must be developed to eliminate the risk of cancer cell transmission with reimplantation[5].

To date, ovarian tissue has been successfully cryopreserved and transplanted in rodents, sheep and marmoset monkeys[11,23,24]. Successful fertilization and pregnancy has been described[25] after egg collection from fresh transplanted ovarian tissue in a primate: the grafted tissue functioned without any surgical connection to major blood vessels. Experimental studies have indicated that the fall in number of primordial follicles in grafted tissue is due to hypoxia, and the delay before reimplanted cortical tissue becomes revascularized. The loss of primordial

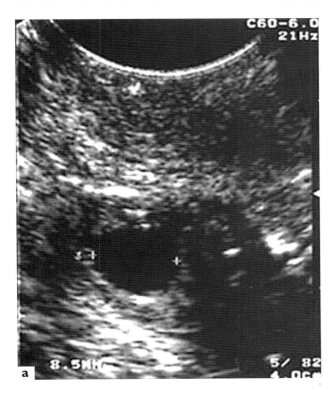

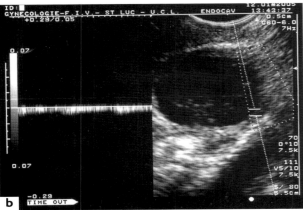

Figure 27.9 (a) Four and a half months after reimplantation, ultrasonography demonstrated the presence of a follicle of 9.2 mm in size, which reached 14 mm 3 days before the luteinizing hormone peak. (b) One week later, a corpus luteum of 21.2 mm was clearly visible, concomitant with the presence of a serum progesterone level of 6.5 ng/ml

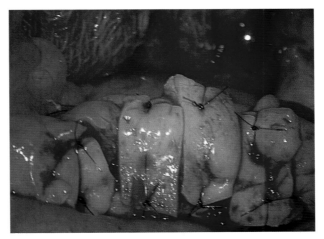

Figure 27.10 Five pieces of cryopreserved ovarian tissue were sutured to the medulla of the remaining ovary

of the abdomen. Temperature and pressure changes in the subcutaneous space could damage oocytes.

We have previously shown that peritoneal tissue is superior to subcutaneous tissue as a site of transplantation, with the loss of fewer follicles in peritoneal tissue[10]. Our model also showed effective revascularization in the peritoneal layer, and led us to propose orthotopic transplantation. In the first three cases we describe, vaginal echography and laparoscopy revealed a follicular structure 5 months after frozen–thawed ovarian tissue transplantation. The grafted tissue was biopsied, and histological analysis and fluorescent probe staining revealed the presence of viable primordial follicles and a follicular structure with inhibin A-marked cells. Follicles at an early growth stage need more than 85 days to reach the antral stage[29]. Primordial follicles obviously need even more. The appearance of the first follicle in the grafted tissue 5 months after reimplantation in patients 1, 2 and 3 is totally consistent with the expected time course. This time interval observed in our study between the implantation of cortical tissue and the first estradiol peak (5 months) is also consistent with data obtained from sheep and human-beings[10,27].

The relatively high level of FSH (> 20 mIU/ml) must be associated with a decline in inhibin secretion, as suggested by the sheep model[30,31], or with slower follicular growth from a poor follicular reserve in the graft. Indeed, because of the loss of primordial follicles in the transplants, the follicular density was low, but in any case, the total amount of cortical tissue transplanted is fairly unimportant. After transplantation, the patients would have been regarded as poor responders, because, of the 500–1000 primordial follicles that would have been transplanted, more than 50% would have been lost due to hypoxia[26].

Cryopreservation should not be reserved solely for women with malignant disease. Indeed, bone marrow transplantation (BMT) has been increasingly used for non-cancerous diseases in recent decades, but the high doses of

follicles in cryopreserved ovarian tissue after transplantation is estimated to be 50–65% in some studies[7,26,27]. In one trial, in which ovarian cortex was grafted onto the uterine horn and under the skin, the loss was more than 90%[28].

Oktay et al.[11] suggested that oocyte quality might be compromised by transplantation to a heterotopic site. Indeed, they only obtained a four-cell embryo from 20 oocytes retrieved from tissue transplanted under the skin

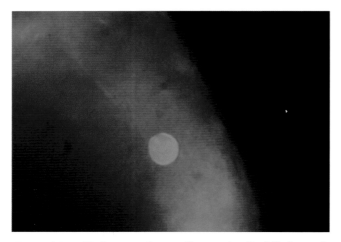 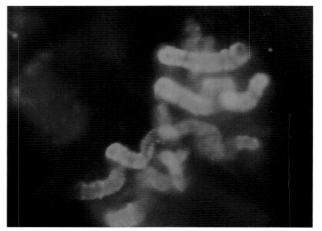

Figure 28.5 High survival rate of stromal cells, follicles and vessels in a cryopreserved whole ovary (viable cells are stained green with calcein-AM and dead cells are stained red with ethidium homodimer 1)

vascularization and minimize post-transplantation ischemia responsible for the reduction in follicular density.

CONCLUSION

The cryopreservation of ovarian tissue should be seriously considered for any patient undergoing treatment likely to impair future fertility, the indications being pelvic, extrapelvic and/or systemic diseases. The age of the patient should be taken into consideration, because the contents of the ovary are not the same in prepubertal and postpubertal women. Because a decline in fertility is now well documented after the age of 38 years, the procedure should probably be restricted to patients below this limit. In any case, irradiation and chemotherapy appear to be less harmful to the gonads of prepubertal than those of postpubertal women[88–90].

There may be many potential indications for ovarian tissue cryopreservation. Indeed, careful evaluation of all the parameters, such as the type of disease, survival prognosis, age and the dose and type of treatment, should be carried out before candidate selection for such procedures. On the other hand, respecting the code of good practice, all patients who may become infertile have the right to receive proper consideration of their interests for future possibilities in the field of ovarian function preservation. The selection of cases should be carried out on the basis of a multidisciplinary staff discussion including oncologists, gynecologists, biologists, psychologists and pediatricians. Counseling should be given, and informed consent obtained from the patient.

We believe that it is preferable to remove only one ovary if possible, to avoid the psychological stress of surgical castration in a young patient, because cases of spontaneous pregnancy have been described after total body irradiation[91–93] and because, in many cases, the remaining ovary will be able to resume all endocrine functions after some years. Moreover, the thousands of primary follicles that are contained in a single ovary of a young patient are more than sufficient to ensure fertility after cryopreservation.

After unilateral ovariectomy and/or cryopreservation of multiple cortical slices, different options are now available:

- Isolation of immature oocytes or preantral follicles and *in vitro* maturation to metaphase II oocytes

- Autotransplantation, either orthotopic with restoration of natural fertility[6], or heterotopic, requiring ovarian stimulation and IVF[94]

- Heterotransplantation in patients suffering from premature ovarian failure[95]

It has been demonstrated that cryopreserved primordial follicles can survive after thawing, and that growth and maturation are possible under certain conditions. Research must now focus on the best way to use thawed tissue. It is probable that the answer lies in the use of culture environments adapted to each stage of follicular development. If autografting is the aim of cryopreservation of ovarian tissue, testing for malignant cells in the tissue must be carried out using adequate techniques. This is especially true for hematological malignancies. The idea of 'oocyte banking' is attractive, but it requires sustained efforts to achieve better results with ovarian tissue cryopreservation techniques and *in vitro* oocyte maturation procedures.

Live births obtained after transplantation of frozen–thawed ovarian tissue give hope to young cancer patients, but great efforts are still required in research programs in order to determine whether active angiogenesis can be induced to accelerate the process of neovascularization in grafted tissue, whether isolated human follicles can be grafted or indeed whether grafting an entire ovary with its vascular pedicle is a valuable option.

REFERENCES

1. Blatt J. Pregnancy outcome in long-term survivors of childhood cancer. Med Pediatr Oncol 1999; 33: 29–33

2. Torrents E, Boiso I, Barri PN, et al. Applications of ovarian tissue transplantation in experimental biology and medicine. Hum Reprod Update 2003; 9: 471–81

3. Donnez J, Dolmans MM, Martinez-Madrid B, et al. The role of cryopreservation for women prior to treatment of malignancy. Curr Opin Obstet Gynecol 2005; 17: 333–8

4. The Ethics Committee of the American Society for Reproductive Medicine. Fertility preservation and reproduction in cancer patients. Fertil Steril 2005; 83: 1622–8

5. Stachecki JJ, Cohen J. An overview of oocyte cryopreservation. Reprod Biomed Online 2004; 9: 152–63

6. Donnez J, Dolmans MM, Demylle D, et al. Livebirth after orthotopic transplantation of cryopreserved ovarian tissue. Lancet 2004; 364: 1405–10

7. Meirow D, Levron J, Eldar-Geva T, et al. Pregnancy after transplantation of cryopreserved ovarian tissue in a patient with ovarian failure after chemotherapy. N Engl J Med 2005; 353: 318–21

8. Sonmezer M, Oktay K. Fertility preservation in female patients. Hum Reprod Update 2004; 10: 251–66

9. Seli E, Tangir J. Fertility preservation options for female patients with malignancies. Curr Opin Obstet Gynecol 2005; 17: 299–308

10. Winkel CA, Fossum GT. Current reproductive technology: considerations for the oncologist. Oncology (Huntingt) 1993; 7: 40–51

11. Brown JR, Modell E, Obasaju M, et al. Natural cycle in-vitro fertilisation with embryo cryopreservation prior to chemotherapy for carcinoma of the breast. Hum Reprod 1996; 11: 197–9

12. Oktay K, Buyuk E, Davis O, et al. Fertility preservation in breast cancer patients: IVF and embryo cryopreservation after ovarian stimulation with tamoxifen. Hum Reprod 2003; 18: 90–5

13. Oktay K, Buyuk E, Libertalla N, et al. Fertility preservation in breast cancer patients: a prospective controlled comparison of ovarian stimulation with tamoxifen and letrozole for embryo cryopreservation. J Clin Oncol 2005; 23: 4347–53

14. Porcu E. Cryopreservation of oocytes: indications, risks and outcome. Abstracts of the 21st Annual Meeting of the European Society of Human Reproduction and Embryology. Hum Reprod 2005; 20 (Suppl 1): i50, O–137

15. Chen C. Pregnancy after human oocyte cryopreservation. Lancet 1986; 1: 884–6

16. Lutchman Singh K, Davies M, Chatterjee R. Fertility in female cancer survivors: pathophysiology, preservation and the role of ovarian reserve testing. Hum Reprod Update 2005; 11: 69–89

17. Porcu E, Fabbri R, Seracchioli R, et al. Birth of a healthy female after intracytoplasmic sperm injection of cryopreserved human oocytes. Fertil Steril 1997; 68: 724–6

18. Fabbri R, Porcu E, Marsella T, et al. Human oocyte cryopreservation: new perspectives regarding oocyte survival. Hum Reprod 2001; 16: 411–16

19. Nagy ZP, Cecile J, Liu J, et al. Pregnancy and birth after intracytoplasmic sperm injection of in-vitro matured germinal vesicle stage oocytes: case report. Fertil Steril 1996; 65: 1047–50

20. Gook DA, Schiewe MC, Osborn SM, et al. Intracytoplasmic sperm injection and embryo development of human oocytes cryopreserved using 1,2-propanediol. Hum Reprod 1995; 10: 2637–41

21. Pickering SJ, Braude PR, Johnson MH, et al. Transient cooling to room temperature can cause irreversible disruption of the meiotic spindle in the human oocyte. Fertil Steril 1990; 54: 102–8

22. Gook DA, Osborn SM, Johnston WI. Cryopreservation of mouse and human oocytes using 1,2-propanediol and the configuration of the meiotic spindle. Hum Reprod 1993; 8: 1101–9

23. Gook DA, Osborn SM, Bourne H, et al. Fertilization of human oocytes following cryopreservation: normal karyotypes and absence of stray chromosomes. Hum Reprod 1994; 9: 684–91

24. Vincent C, Johnson MH. Cooling, cryoprotectants, and the cytoskeleton of the mammalian oocyte. Oxf Rev Reprod Biol 1992; 14: 73–100

25. Gosden RG. Prospects for oocyte banking and in vitro maturation. J Natl Cancer Inst Monogr 2005; 34: 60–3

26. Yoon TK, Chung HM, Lim JM, et al. Pregnancy and delivery of healthy infants developed from vitrified oocytes in a stimulated in vitro fertilization–embryo transfer program. Fertil Steril 2000; 74: 180–1

28. Katayama KP, Stehlik J, Kuwayama M, et al. High survival rate of vitrified human oocytes results in clinical pregnancy. Fertil Steril 2003; 80: 223–4

28. The Practice Committee of the American Society for Reproductive Medicine. Ovarian tissue and oocyte cryopreservation. Fertil Steril 2004; 82: 993–8

29. Falcone T, Attaran M, Bedaiwy M, et al. Ovarian function preservation in the cancer patient. Fertil Steril 2004; 81: 243–57

30. Boiso I, Marti M, Santalo J, et al. A confocal microscopy analysis of the spindle and chromosome configurations of human oocytes cryopreserved at the germinal vesicle and metaphase II stage. Hum Reprod 2002; 17: 1885–91

31. Cha KY, Koo JJ, Ko JJ, et al. Pregnancy after in vitro fertilization of human follicular oocytes collected from nonstimulated cycles, their culture in vitro and their transfer in a donor oocyte program. Fertil Steril 1991; 55: 109–13

32. Trounson A, Wood C, Kausche A. in vitro maturation and the fertilization and developmental competence of oocytes recovered from untreated polycystic ovarian patients. Fertil Steril 1994; 62: 353–62

33. Tucker MJ, Wright GH, Morton PC, et al. Birth after cryopreservation of immature oocytes with subsequent in vitro maturation. Fertil Steril 1998; 70: 578–9

frozen–thawed human ovarian xenografts in nude mice. Fertil Steril 2000; 74: 122–9

12. Baird DT, Webb R, Campbell BK, et al. Long-term ovarian function in sheep after ovariectomy and transplantation of autografts stored at –196°C. Endocrinology 1999; 140: 462–71

13. Demirci B, Salle B, Frappart L, et al. Morphological alterations and DNA fragmentation in oocytes from primordial and primary follicles after freezing–thawing of ovarian cortex in sheep. Fertil Steril 2002; 77: 595–600

14. Wang X, Chen H, Yin H, et al. Fertility after intact ovary transplantation. Nature 2002; 415: 385

15. Yin H, Wang X, Kim SS, et al. Transplantation of intact rat gonads using vascular anastomosis: effects of cryopreservation, ischemia and genotype. Hum Reprod 2003; 18: 1165–72

16. Jeremias E, Bedaiwy MA, Gurunluoglu R, et al. Heterotopic autotransplantation of the ovary with microvascular anastomosis: a novel surgical technique. Fertil Steril 2002; 77: 1278–82

17. Scott JR, Keye WR, Poulson AM, Reynolds WA. Microsurgical ovarian transplantation in the primate. Fertil Steril 1981; 36: 512–15

18. Mhatre P, Mhatre J, Magotra R. Ovarian transplant: a new frontier. Transplant Proc 2005; 37: 1396–8

19. Bedaiwy A, Jeremias E, Gurunluoglu R, et al. Restoration of ovarian function after autotransplantation of intact frozen–thawed sheep ovaries with microvascular anastomosis. Fertil Steril 2003; 79: 594–602

20. Arav A. Animal models for whole ovary cryopreservation and transplantation. Invited presentation. In Program and Symposium Syllabus of the Workshop on Mammalian Oogenesis and Folliculogenesis: in vivo and in vitro approaches. European Society of Human Reproduction and Embryology, Frascati, Italy, 2003: 46

21. Martinez-Madrid B, Dolmans MM, Van Langendonckt A, et al. Freezing entire human ovaries with a passive cooling device. Fertil Steril 2004: 82: 1390–4

22. Eppig JJ. Further reflections on culture systems for the growth of oocytes in vitro. Hum Reprod 1994; 9: 974–6

23. Hovatta O, Wright C, Krausz T, et al. Human primordial, primary and secondary ovarian follicles in long-term culture: effect of partial isolation. Hum Reprod 1999; 14: 2519–24

24. Dolmans MM, Michaux N, Camboni A, et al. Evaluation of Liberase, a purified enzyme blend, for the isolation of human primordial and primary ovarian follicles. Hum Reprod 2006; 21: 413–20

Laparoscopic ovarian transposition before radiotherapy

30

P Jadoul, J Squifflet, J Donnez

INTRODUCTION

Pelvic radiotherapy is frequently used to treat pelvic tumors in premenopausal women. It has already been stated that a dose of 5–20 Gy administered to the ovary is sufficient to impair gonadal function completely[1–3], whatever the age of the patient.

Ovarian transposition should be indicated in all women requiring radiotherapy for gynecological or non-gynecological malignancy.

All the indications for laparoscopic ovarian transposition should also be indications for ovarian tissue cryopreservation, and ovarian tissue-banking facilities should be available. Indeed, even if chemotherapy is not initially proposed to the patient, it must always be considered as a possibility after surgery which could impair gonadal function, even in a transposed ovary.

EFFECTS OF RADIOTHERAPY ON OVARIAN FUNCTION

Several procedures have been proposed[1,4–6] to preserve ovarian function when radiotherapy is needed in the pelvis. In 1993, Haie-Meder et al.[3] reported the outcome of ovarian preservation after lateral transposition in young women requiring radiotherapy with or without chemotherapy. In their study, the predictive factors of ovarian function preservation after radiotherapy were age, irradiation field and dose, and the association of chemotherapy.

Age and hormonal status at diagnosis

Age in itself is a predictive factor of ovarian function. The physiological decrease in the number of primordial follicles with age makes the ovaries more sensitive to any aggressive treatment, such as chemotherapy and/or radiotherapy. In patients treated for Hodgkin's disease, Schilsky et al.[7] reported a significantly shorter time from diagnosis to amenorrhea in patients > 25 years of age. Gradishar and Schilsky[8] suggested that patients < 25 years of age would not experience any significant therapy-related dysfunction for 5–10 years following the completion of chemotherapy.

From the literature published to date, it is impossible to determine whether the prepubertal ovary is less susceptible to the effects of irradiation than is the adult ovary. An alternative explanation for an apparently increased resistance to damage of a young girl's ovary may simply be a reflection of the earlier age and larger number of oocytes within the ovary, rather than any effect of puberty. Furthermore, in addition to direct gonadal damage, irradiation may also affect the uterus, thus decreasing the chance of successfully carrying a pregnancy to full term.

Irradiation field and dose

Ovarian preservation according to the type of irradiation is determined by measurements on a phantom[3]. There is a significant difference in ovarian preservation according to the irradiation field. Pelvic irradiation and inverted irradiation carry the highest probability of ovarian failure (Table 30.1).

In cases of supradiaphragmatic irradiation, the risk of impairment of gonadal function is ~ 10%, while with infradiaphragmatic irradiation, this risk increases to 35%[3]. These percentages are dependent on the total dose and distribution of the dose administered. The risk of ovarian failure according to the dose of radiotherapy is summarized in Table 30.2.

Women who received a dose of ≤ 5 Gy of ovarian irradiation had a higher probability of ovarian function preservation than patients who received > 5 Gy[3]. In addition to dose, age also has an impact on ovarian function preservation.

Lushbaugh and Casaren[1] suggested that the total dose inducing menopause was 6 Gy in women ≥ 40 years of age, while it could be as high as 20 Gy in girls. In the study by Haie-Meder et al.[3], all the prepubescent girls became pubescent, while the same range of doses caused menopause in 32% of patients > 25 years of age. The dose to the ovaries, however, was the most important predictive factor of ovarian function preservation (≤ 5 Gy vs. > 5 Gy).

Table 30.1 Toxicity of radiotherapy according to irradiation field

Site of radiotherapy	Risk of premature ovarian failure (%)
Supradiaphragmatic	10
Infradiaphragmatic	35
Total body irradiation	> 50

Laparoscopic preservation of female fertility

31

H Baakdah, T Tulandi

It is estimated that about 650 000 new cases of cancer in females are diagnosed annually[1], and 8% occur in women under the age of 40 years[2]. Fortunately, advances in cancer therapy have improved the long-term survival of young patients suffering from malignancies. In fact, many childhood lymphomas and leukemias can now be cured. However, cancer treatment sometimes carries adverse side-effects, including loss of gonadal function and sterility in both sexes.

The preservation of fertility in males by sperm freezing is already well established, although it is still an imperfect technology. There have been few options for young women undergoing cancer treatment, but the advent of new methods for preserving gonadal function and fertility is promising. Today, we can cryopreserve embryos, oocytes and ovarian tissue, and in those undergoing pelvic irradiation, laparoscopic ovarian suspension can be considered[3]. In this review, we discuss the use of laparoscopy in the preservation of fertility in females.

LAPAROSCOPIC OVARIAN SUSPENSION

In women undergoing pelvic irradiation, the ovaries can be moved out of the radiation field to avoid the direct effects of ionizing radiation; this procedure is called ovarian suspension, ovarian transposition or oophoropexy. The procedure has been performed for more than three decades in women with Hodgkin's disease receiving pelvic or para-aortic lymph-node irradiation at staging laparotomy[4–7].

There are two types, lateral or medial ovarian transposition. In medial ovarian transposition, the ovaries are transposed behind the uterus and protected with a lead block during irradiation. However, considerable amounts of radiation are still received. Lateral ovarian transposition, repositioning the ovaries out of the radiation field, is more effective. It can be done during the initial staging laparotomy or during laparotomy for debulking the tumor. In patients who do not need a laparotomy, ovarian transposition can be performed by laparoscopy. The laparoscopic approach is certainly less invasive and yet effective.

Ovaries have been transposed to a variety of sites and levels, from the base of the round ligament to the level of the lower kidney pole[8–22]. It seems that the ovaries should be transposed at least to a level above the pelvic brim. Transposition to this level can be achieved without separating the Fallopian tubes from their uterine origin. This

allows the possibility of spontaneous conception[23]. However, transient ovarian failure following this procedure has been reported[24].

Concerns with ovarian transposition include the uncommon development of radiation-induced cancer in the transposed ovaries[23]. Anderson et al.[25] studied 82 premenopausal women with early-stage carcinoma of the cervix who underwent ovarian transposition. Only one patient was found to have metastatic disease to the ovary 17 months later. Similar to normally located ovaries, ovarian cysts can be found in the transposed ovaries.

Technique of laparoscopic lateral ovarian transposition

To facilitate relocation of the ovaries above the pelvic brim, we use three trocars: the primary trocar is inserted 2 cm above the umbilicus and two secondary trocars are inserted at the same level. Peritoneal lavage for cytological examination is first done. A thorough examination of the abdominal cavity, including the liver and diaphragm, should be carried out. The course of the ureter is first followed, and then the ovarian ligament is electro-coagulated and transected. Dissection is continued on the mesovarium as far as the infundibulopelvic ligament, but the vascular pedicle inside the ligament is left intact[13].

The ovary is then mobilized superiorly and laterally to the site above the pelvic brim. If mobilization is inadequate, a relaxing incision on the peritoneum inferior to the ovary is performed. In our experience, the tubes do not have to be transected. This helps future spontaneous conception[13,23]. To prevent the return of the ovaries to the pelvic cavity, the transposed ovaries should be securely anchored to the peritoneum. We use two sutures of 4-0 polydioxanone. In a case where the ovaries were anchored with hemoclips only[26], the ovaries slipped back into the pelvic cavity and the patient became menopausal after irradiation. At the end of the procedure, the ovary is marked with a metal clip bilaterally. This is to facilitate future location of the ovaries by ultrasound or other imaging techniques.

OVARIAN CRYOPRESERVATION

The treatment of childhood malignant disease is becoming increasingly effective. More than 90% of girls and young women affected by malignant diseases can be treated by aggressive chemotherapy and radiotherapy, and bone

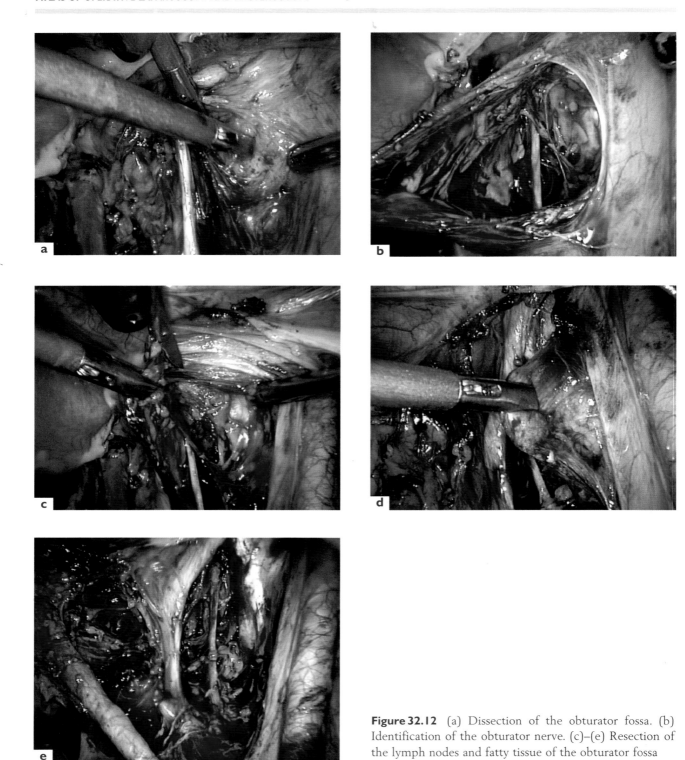

Figure 32.12 (a) Dissection of the obturator fossa. (b) Identification of the obturator nerve. (c)–(e) Resection of the lymph nodes and fatty tissue of the obturator fossa

infection associated with vaginal hysterectomy, thus decreasing the postoperative hospitalization and recovery time.

The results of radical laparoscopic hysterectomy ('Wertheim's' procedure) performed with lymphadenectomy are clearly less favorable. In spite of the less painful postoperative convalescence, significantly faster recovery

of bowel movement, less pronounced drop in the hemoglobin rate and reduced hospitalization costs[27], the procedure has several disadvantages. The relatively long operating time (6–8 h) and the rather difficult technical approach of this procedure[12,27] lead us to conclude that this technique (of which only a few cases have been published) still requires further research and evaluation,

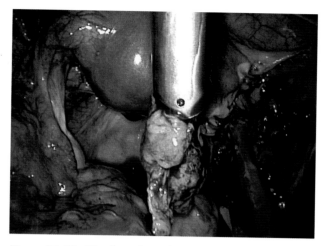

Figure 32.13 The lymph nodes are removed through a 10-mm trocar

especially in oncological surgery. Continued studies involving greater numbers of women should thus demonstrate the potential advantages of laparoscopic surgery compared with laparotomy, but also its harmful effects, such as tumor dissemination due to internal trauma during uterine mobilization or lymph node removal.

All surgical maneuvers are more or less feasible by laparoscopy; the important thing to consider with regard to this new approach to radical uterine surgery is not its feasibility, but rather whether it is justifiable and safe[27]. As already stated in this chapter, lymphangiography is unable to visualize internal iliac and other medical node groups. Computed tomography scanning and magnetic resonance imaging are not sufficiently sensitive if the nodes are not macroscopically enlarged. PET appears to be an interesting tool, and is being evaluated in different malignancies. It is probably a very sensitive method, but not specific enough[28]. As a consequence, lymph node biopsy remains the only reliable method for appraising the status of pelvic nymph nodes.

Pelvic lymph node sampling by a retroperitoneal endoscopic approach has been described[18]. Progress in laparoscopic surgery allows a surgically satisfactory pelvic lymphadenectomy to be performed, removing the obturator, external iliac and hypogastric lymph nodes. Dargent and Salvat[18] have described a panoramic retroperitoneal approach, while Querleu and Leblanc have reported the technique of pelvic lymphadenectomy[6,20] and para-aortic lymphadenectomy by laparoscopy[20].

The principal indication for laparoscopic lymphadenectomy in gynecological oncology is the staging of carcinoma of the cervix[6]. The risk of involvement of para-aortic nodes is very low (<1%) if the pelvic nodes are negative histologically. Stage Ib–IIa–IIb cancer with negative pathological staging may be cured by radical vaginal or abdominal surgery. However, radical hysterec-

tomy is not justified when metastatic nodes are present. Pretreatment laparoscopic staging of stage I endometrial carcinoma is not very useful, since the prevalence of lymph node metastasis is very low in this condition. Laparoscopic lymphadenectomy may be included in the surgical step of treatment, in association with vaginal surgery[3].

REFERENCES

1. Schauta R. Techniques chirurgicales. In Encyclopedie Médico Chirurgicale. Paris: Elsevier Science, 1961: 41–735
2. Mage G, Wattiez A, Chapron C, et al. Hystérectomie per-coelioscopique: résultats d'une série de 44 cas. J Gynecol Obstet Biol Reprod 1992; 21: 436–44
3. Donnez J, Nisolle M, Anaf V. Place de l'endoscopie dans le cancer de l'endomètre. In Dubuisson JB, Chapron C, Bouquet de Joliniere J, eds. Coelioscopie et Cancerologie en Gynecologie. Paris: Arnette, 1993: 77–82
4. Photopulos GJ, Stovall TG, Summitt RL Jr. LAVH, bilateral salpingoophorectomy, and pelvic lymph node sampling for endometrial cancer. J Gynecol Surg 1992; 8: 91–4
5. Plentl AA, Friedman EA. Lymphatic System of the Female Genitalia: The Morphologic Basis of Oncologic Diagnosis and Therapy. Philadelphia: WB Saunders, 1971: 57–74
6. Querleu D, Leblanc E, Castelain G. Laparoscopic pelvic lymphadenectomy in the staging of early carcinoma of the cervix. Am J Obstet Gynecol 1991; 164: 579–81
7. Perez CA, Korba A, Sharma S. Dosimetric considerations in irradiation of carcinoma of the vagina. Int J Radiol Oncol Biol Phys 1977; 2: 639–45
8. Querleu D, Leblanc E, Castelain B. Lymphadénectomie pelvienne sous contrôle coelioscopique. J Gynecol Biol Reprod 1990; 19: 576–8
9. Dargent D. A new future for Schauta's operation through presurgical retroperitoneal pelviscopy. Eur J Gynecol Oncol 1987; 8: 292–6
10. Svardi J, Vidaurreta J, Bermudez A, et al. Laparoscopically assisted Schauta operation: learning experience at the gynecologic oncology unit, Buenos Aires, University Hospital. Gynecol Oncol 1999; 75: 361–5
11. Nezhat GR, Burrel MO, Nezhat FR, et al. Laparoscopic radical hysterectomy with para-aortic and pelvic node dissection. Am J Obstet Gynecol 1992; 166: 864–5
12. Canis M, Mage G, Wattiez A, et al. La chirurgie endoscopique at-elle une place dans la chirurgie radicale du cancer du col utérin? J Gynecol Obstet Biol Reprod 1990; 19: 921–6
13. Dargent D, Martin X, Mathevel P. Laparoscopic assessment of the sentinel lymph node in early stage cervical cancer. Gynecol Oncol 2000; 79: 411–15
14. Vercamer R, Janssens J, De P Usewils RI, et al. Computerised tomography and lymphography in the

presurgical staging of early carcinoma of the uterine cervix. Cancer 1987; 60: 1745–50

15. King LA, Talledo OE, Gallup DG, et al. Computed tomography in evaluation of gynecological malignancies: a prospective analysis? Am J Obstet Gynecol 1986; 60: 1055–61

16. Walsh JM, Goplerud DR. Prospective comparison between clinical and CT staging in primary cervical carcinoma. Am J Roentgenol 1981; 137: 997–1003

17. Wurtz A, Mazman E, Gosselin B, et al. Bilan anatomique des adénopathies rétropéritonéales par endoscopie chirurgicale. Ann Chir 1987; 41: 258–63

18. Dargent D, Salvat J. L'Envahissement Ganglionnaire Pelvien. Paris: Midsi/McGraw-Hill, 1989

19. Reich H. New techniques in advanced laparoscopic surgery. Clin Obstet Gynecol 1989; 3: 655–81

20. Querleu D, Leblanc E. Laparoscopic pelvic lymphadenectomy. In Sutton C, Diamond M, eds. Endoscopic Surgery for Gynecologists. London: WB Saunders, 1993: 172–8

21. Vergote I, De Wever I, Tjalma W, et al. Neoadjuvant chemotherapy or primary debulking surgery in advanced ovarian carcinoma: a retrospective analysis of 285 patients. Gynecol Oncol 1998; 71: 431–6

22. Clough KB, Ladonne JM, Nos C, et al. Second look for ovarian cancer: laparoscopy or laparotomy? A prospective comparative study. Gynecol Oncol 1999; 72: 411–17

23. Reich H, McGlynn F, Wickie W. Laparoscopic management of stage 1 ovarian cancer: a case report. J Reprod Med 1990; 35: 601

24. Dexus S, Cusido MT, Suris JC, et al. Lymphadenectomy in ovarian cancer. Eur J Gynaecol Oncol 2000; 21: 215–22

25. Leblanc E, Querleu D, Narducci F, et al. Surgical staging of early invasive epithelial ovarian tumors. Semin Surg Oncol 2000; 19: 36–41

26. Morice P, Pautier P, Mercier S, et al. Laparoscopic prophylactic oophorectomy in women with inherited risk of ovarian cancer. Eur J Gynaecol Oncol 1999; 20: 202–4

27. Canis M, Mage G, Wattiez A, et al. Vaginally assisted laparoscopic radical hysterectomy. J Gynecol Surg 1992; 8: 103–5

28. Anderson H, Price P. What does positron emission tomography offer oncology? Eur J Cancer 2000; 36: 2028–35

Indications for lymphadenectomy in stage I/IIa endometrial cancer

33

J Squifflet, J Donnez

Endometrial carcinoma is the most common pelvic malignancy in the Western world. Because most patients present with early-stage disease, the prognosis of endometrial carcinoma is generally good, with a survival rate between 90 and 95%. Due to this favorable outcome in most cases, the goal is to select patients at increased risk of relapse who might benefit from more extensive surgical procedures and adjuvant therapies, and to avoid over-treatment of low-risk cases that would be exposed to the risk of excess morbidity.

The decision to perform lymphadenectomy is dependent upon preoperative assessment and the risk of nodal metastases.

The number of early-stage versus advanced-stage cases observed in clinics depends on different factors. First, we know that the longer a patient experiences post-menopausal bleeding, the more advanced the stage of disease may be. If patients were more aware of the need to present for treatment as soon as possible in the case of postmenopausal bleeding, we would diagnose the disease at an earlier stage. In populations of lower socioeconomic status and education potential, with no medical follow-up or screening, the time between the onset of symptoms and diagnosis could be even longer, and the stage of disease more advanced.

MEDICAL ADVICE

In our department, all patients presenting with post-menopausal bleeding undergo a classic clinical evaluation (Papanicolaou (PAP) smear with evaluation of the size and mobility of the uterus). A normal PAP smear is not sufficient to exclude endometrial cancer in symptomatic women, but an abnormal result is more frequently associated with more advanced disease. The presence of atypical glandular cells (AGUS) or normal endometrial cells increases the risk of extrauterine disease[1-3].

The normal thickness of the endometrium during transvaginal sonography is less than 4–5 mm. It appears as a thin symmetrical and regular line. In these conditions, the risk of endometrial cancer is very low. Above this threshold, or in the case of an irregular or asymmetrical appearance of the endometrium, an office hysterectomy (Storz optic 2.7 mm) or endometrial biopsy is proposed.

A recent comparison of saline infusion sonography and office hysteroscopy revealed similar patient ratings of pelvic pain during the procedures. Sensitivity and specificity coefficients, as well as negative and positive predictive values, were higher with office hysteroscopy[4]. Office hysteroscopy can evaluate the range of the disease, and even its extension through the cervix. Endometrial biopsy is performed after hysteroscopy to determine the histological grade and differentiation, and the histological type of the lesions.

An elevated CA125 level could be a marker of extrauterine disease in a case of endometrial cancer. In a non-multivariable evaluation, it is difficult to identify a cut-off value below which lymphadenectomy can be avoided, and above which lymphadenectomy should be proposed. Dotters showed that a CA125 level > 20 U/ml, with a grade 3 tumor, correctly predicted 87% of patients requiring complete surgical staging. In stage I disease with a histological grade of 1 or 2 and a CA125 level below 20 U/ml, the risk of nodal metastases is low[5,6].

Magnetic resonance imaging (MRI) could be proposed for the evaluation of myometrial invasion and retro-peritoneal node involvement (pelvic and lumboaortic area). In the case of more advanced disease, a computed tomography (CT) scan of the abdomen and the chest should be proposed (Table 33.1).

Table 33.1 Clinicopathological prognostic factors in endometrial cancer

FIGO stage (1998)	Corpus–cervix and peritoneal cytology
Histological subtype	Endometrioid or non-endometrioid (serous–papillary
Myometrial invasion	and clear cell)
Lymphovascular space invasion	
Tumor size	
Age	

FIGO, International Federation of Gynecologists and Obstetricians

Table 33.2 Risks of pelvic lymph node metastases in stage I disease[7]

Depth	Grade 1 (%)	Grade 2 (%)	Grade 3 (%)
Endometrium	0	3	0
Inner third	3	5	9
Middle third	0	9	4
Outer third	11	19	34

In stage I disease, the risk of nodal involvement depends on the grade of the lesion and the myometrial invasion. We have identified three different types of disease in terms of nodal involvement (Table 33.2):

- Low risk of nodal involvement with a 5-year survival rate >90% (grade 1, stage Ia or Ib; grade 2, stage Ia and Ib)

- Intermediate risk of nodal involvement with a 5-year survival rate between 80 and 90% (grade 1, stage Ic; grade 2, stage Ic; grade 3, stage Ia and Ib)

- High risk of nodal involvement with a 5-year survival rate below 70% (grade 3, stage Ic)

RATIONALE FOR LYMPHADENECTOMY

Since 1988, pelvic node involvement has represented stage IIIc disease in the International Federation of Gynecologists and Obstetricians (FIGO) classification of endometrial cancer, and hence avoiding lymphadenectomy could result in incomplete staging of the neoplasia.

The rate of positive nodes found in stage I disease ranges from 4.7 to 11%. The size of pelvic lymph nodes does not predict metastatic involvement in patients with endometrial cancer. Fewer than 30% of positive nodes are palpable[8]. In 1996, Reich et al.[9] showed that 54% of positive nodes measured less than 10 mm, while at least 29% of negative nodes were larger than 10 mm.

Palpation during intraoperative evaluation is not reliable to detect node metastases[10]. Furthermore, nodes may be positive even in low-risk patients[11,12].

In a meta-analysis, Nijman et al.[13] found an average of 11 nodes (range 0–42) removed during lymphadenectomy for endometrial cancer, with seven at the 10th centile. For Kilgore et al.[14] and Cragun et al.[15], the extent of lymphadenectomy (more than 11 nodes removed) in high-risk patients (poorly differentiated tumors, stage Ic, grade 3) correlates with better survival. For these reasons, simple node sampling is unreliable for diagnosis

Furthermore, lymphadenectomy in intermediate- and high-risk patients may identify subgroups of patients at very low risk of recurrence, who could avoid total pelvic radiotherapy.

When brachytherapy is performed after complete staging surgery in endometriotic carcinoma, we observe a mean recurrence of 6%, with all recurrences located outside the pelvis[16–19]. Thus, external pelvic radiotherapy may be avoided in a case of negative nodes, and brachytherapy should be proposed in the case of a high-risk patient (Gynecologic Oncology Group (GOG) study, reference 24).

WHICH NODES SHOULD BE REMOVED?

Lymphatic spread is more common in external iliac nodes. For Mariani et al.[20], external iliac and obturator nodes are more frequently the first site of metastases in cases of involvement of the uterine corpus.

In stage II disease (cervical involvement), the first sites of metastases are the common iliac nodes. In a review of the use of sentinel lymph node identification in endometrial cancer, the sentinel lymph node was found between the common iliac vessels and the ilio-obturator vessels in 60–92% of cases[21].

EFFECTIVENESS OF RADIOTHERAPY

Three large randomized controlled trials are presented. In 1980, Aalders et al.[22] (Norwegian Radium Hospital Study) published a study of 540 stage I patients. Total abdominal hysterectomy with bilateral salpingo-oophorectomy was systematically performed, with a follow-up of 10 years. The patients were randomized between brachytherapy and brachytherapy with pelvic irradiation. Overall survival was not statistically significantly different (90% vs. 87%), but locoregional recurrence rates were lower in the pelvic irradiation group (1.9% vs. 6.9%; $p < 0.01$).

A subgroup of cases (grade 3, stage Ic) benefited more from pelvic irradiation, showing a decrease in local recurrence and death from the disease. Significantly more deaths and recurrences were encountered among patients with tumor cells in endothelial spaces than among those without vessel invasion (26.7% vs. 9.1%; $p < 0.01$).

In 2000, Creutzberg *et al.* published a randomized controlled trial of 715 cases (Post Operative Radiation Therapy in Endometrial Cancer (PORTEC) I study)[23]. Patients presenting with stage I disease underwent total abdominal hysterectomy with bilateral salpingo-oophorectomy, without lymphadenectomy.

Stage Ic, grade 3 and all Ia stages were excluded. The median follow-up was 52 months. After surgery, patients received either external radiation (46 Gy) or no further treatment. The 5-year locoregional recurrence rate was 4% in the radiation group vs. 14% in the control group ($p < 0.001$). There was no difference in distant metastases between the two groups (8% vs. 7% for the control group).

As vaginal recurrence could be controlled by surgery and/or radiotherapy if none was previously given, the 3-year survival rate after recurrence was 69%. In the case of vaginal recurrence after pelvic radiotherapy, overall survival at 3 years was less than 25%. However, in the case of pelvic or distant relapse, the prognosis was very poor; the 3-year survival rate was just 13%.

Overall survival was 85% in the control group and 81% in the radiotherapy group. Most of the deaths that occurred were not related to the endometrial disease (Tables 33.3 and 33.4).

In 2004, Keys *et al.* (GOG study) presented a study of 392 patients who underwent total abdominal hysterectomy with bilateral salpingo-oophorectomy, and with lymphadenectomy[24]. In the case of negative nodes,

patients were further randomized to receive pelvic radiotherapy (50 Gy) or not. The disease-free survival rate after 4 years was 86% in the no-treatment group versus 92% in the radiotherapy group, but there was no difference in overall survival. A decreased pelvic recurrence rate was observed in the radiotherapy group compared with the control group: 1.7% vs. 12%.

In this study, a high-intermediate-risk subgroup was identified: grade 3, presence of lymphovascular space involvement, deep myometrial invasion and age (above 70 years). A high intermediate risk is defined as: above 70 years of age with one of the risk factors; or above 50 years of age with two of the risk factors; or three of the risk factors. This corroborates the findings of other studies that lymphadenectomy and radiotherapy may have an impact on survival in a subgroup of patients with poor prognosis.

INDICATIONS FOR LYMPHADENECTOMY

Lymphadenectomy may clearly be avoided in endometrioid adenocarcinoma of stage I, grade 1 or 2, when the disease is limited to the inner part of the myometrium and the size of the lesion is less or equal to 2 cm[25]. In these circumstances, the risk of nodal metastases is less than 5%, and may even be 0%. However, numerous studies suggest that at least 20% of stage I patients are understaged by surgery[26].

Table 33.3 Complications

Study	Treatment	Gastrointestinal grade 3 or 4 (%)
PORTEC[23]	Radiotherapy	3
GOG[24]	Lymphadenectomy + radiotherapy	8
	Brachytherapy	0–1

PORTEC, Post Operative Radiation Therapy in Endometrial Cancer; GOG, Gynecologic Oncology Group

Table 33.4 Recurrence rate

Study	No radiotherapy (%)	Radiotherapy (%)	p Value
PORTEC[23]	14	4	<0.05
Aalders *et al.*[22]	7 (brachytherapy)	2	<0.05
GOG[24]	12	3	<0.05
vaginal and pelvis site only after 24 months	7.4	1.6	<0.05
GOG[24] Hir	26	6	<0.05
GOG[24] Lir	6	2	Ns

PORTEC, Post Operative Radiation Therapy in Endometrial Cancer; GOG, Gynecologic Oncology Group; Hir, high intermediate risk; Lir, low intermediate risk

In stage I disease with pelvic lymphadenectomy and no brachytherapy, Orr et al.[27] observed survival rates of 100%, 97% and 93% in stage Ia, Ib and Ic disease, respectively. Good results may therefore be obtained in correctly staged patients even in the absence of radiotherapy.

The challenge is correctly evaluating all the low- and high-risk patients preoperatively. Of course, anatomo-pathological evaluation is the only available technique to evaluate lymphovascular space involvement.

The grade of the lesions may also be under- or overestimated between the preoperative evaluation and post-surgery[28]. Tumor grade was found to change, from the diagnostic dilatation and curettage (D&C) specimen to the definite surgical specimen, in 31% of all cases and in 50% of all grade 3 lesions. Sixteen per cent of grade 1 and 2 lesions were overgraded to grade 3, and up to 50% of grade 3 lesions may have been undergraded to grade 1 or 2.

Myometrial invasion may be assessed by ultrasonography, transvaginal ultrasonography or MRI, but, in clinical practice, these evaluations do not always correlate with anatomopathological findings.

Preliminary data from the UK Medical Research Council ASTEC study (Randomized Trial of Lymphadenectomy and of Adjuvant External Beam Radiotherapy in the Treatment of Endometrial Cancer) were recently presented at the 14th Congress of the European Society of Gynecological Oncology in Istanbul. This multicenter randomized trial evaluated the impact of pelvic lymphadenectomy on the treatment of endometrial cancer located in the uterus.

More than 1400 patients were recruited between 1998 and March 2005. All patients were fit to receive lymphadenectomy, and all centers able to offer lymphadenectomy. Less than 10% of surgery was done by laparoscopy. After a median duration of 3 years of follow-up, disease-free survival and overall survival were not statistically different in the two groups. The incidence of complications, however, was higher in the lymph-adenectomy group (8% vs. 3% in the control group).

More than 80% of the lesions were classified as stage I. In the lymphadenectomy group, 9% of removed nodes were positive, and the mean number of nodes removed was 14. These data are preliminary, and need to be completed by further studies.

After surgical treatment, depending on the anatomopathological findings, two groups were identified: a low-risk group and a high-risk group. The high-risk group was further randomized to receive either radiotherapy or not. These data have not yet been presented.

In the future, with a longer follow-up, different subgroups may be identified. Indeed, we know that some groups have shown statistically significant survival benefits in poorly differentiated neoplasia with more than 11 nodes removed. In the study by Cragun et al.[15], the rates of pelvic and aortic nodal metastases were 5% and 3%, respectively, due to the exclusion of patients with grossly involved nodes.

Survival analysis showed a significant survival benefit for patients with grade 3 disease who had 11 or more nodes removed (5-year survival rate of 82% vs. 64%; $p < 0.01$). Patients with grade 1 or 2 disease did not show any survival difference, based on the number of nodes removed. Aortic node removal did not significantly influence survival (hazard ratio 1.29). The exclusion of patients with pelvic or aortic nodal metastases from the analysis still resulted in a significant survival benefit among patients with grade 3 cancer who had more than 11 nodes removed. Patients with 11 or more nodes removed had a lower rate of pelvic recurrence (1% vs. 5%; $p < 0.02$) and a similar rate of vaginal recurrence (2% vs. 3%).

The analysis by Cragun et al. suggests that lymphadenectomy should be considered for patients with grade 3 cancer, but there is no benefit for grade 1 or 2 disease. Lymphadenectomy should yield more than 11 pelvic nodes from multiple sites. This cut-off of 11 nodes is arbitrary, however. It is simply supported by statistical analysis. While it reflects the completeness of lymphadenectomy, its effectiveness is nevertheless dependent on the pathologist's evaluation of the surgical specimens.

The number of sections obtained per node and the application of immunohistochemistry for the detection of metastases also influences the results and the conclusions in the literature. In the study by Cragun et al.[15], it is interesting to note the persistence of improved survival rates among patients with grade 3 cancer from whom more than 11 nodes were removed, even in those with positive nodes who were excluded from the analysis.

The authors hypothesize that the removal of occult (micro) metastatic disease, not seen during histological examination, may have a therapeutic effect.

In conclusion, pelvic lymphadenectomy may be omitted in stage I endometrial cancer in cases of grade 1 or 2 lesions with less than 50% myometrial invasion and lesions less than 2 cm in size.

In cases of grade 3 lesions, factors such as deep myometrial invasion, vascular space involvement and especially age above 70 years seem to be correlated with a poorer prognosis. Nevertheless, physical status, life expectancy and associated morbidity could influence the feasibility and indications for lymphadenectomy in these patients. Indeed, lymphadenectomy could determine the risk of recurrence after surgery (low risk or high risk) and identify the necessary adjuvant treatment: extension of radiotherapy (external beam, brachytherapy, extension field) and/or chemotherapy.

In grade 3 lesions with deep myometrial invasion or non-endometrioid histological cancer, pelvic lymphaden-ectomy may even have a therapeutic effect.

This proves that preoperative evaluation of the patient has to be as complete as possible in order to identify the risk factors of pelvic node involvement.

REFERENCES

1. Fukuda K, Mori M, Uchiyama M, et al. Preoperative cervical cytology in endometrial carcinoma and its clinicopathologic relevance. Gynecol Oncol 1999; 72: 273–7

2. Larson DM, Johnson KK, Reyes CN Jr, Broste SK. Prognostic significance of malignant cervical cytology in patients with endometrial cancer. Obstet Gynecol 1994; 84: 399–403

3. DuBeshter B, Deuel C, Gillis S, et al. Endometrial cancer: the potential role of cervical cytology in current surgical staging. Obstet Gynecol 2003; 101: 445–50

4. Garuti G, Cellani F, Grossi F, et al. Saline infusion sonography and office hysteroscopy to assess endometrial morbidity associated with tamoxifen intake. Gynecol Oncol 2002; 86: 323–9

5. Dotters DJ. Preoperative CA125 in endometrial cancer: is it useful? Am J Obstet Gynecol 2000; 182: 1328–34

6. Kurihara T, Mizunuma H, Obara M, et al. Determination of a normal level of serum CA125 in postmenopausal women as a tool for preoperative evaluation and postoperative surveillance of endometrial carcinoma. Gynecol Oncol 1998; 69: 192–6

7. Creasman WT, Morrow CP, Bundy BN, et al. Surgical pathologic spread patterns of endometrial cancer; a Gynecologic Oncology Group study. Cancer 1987; 60: 2035–41

8. Creasman WT, Bornow RC, Morrow CP, et al. Adenocarcinoma of the endometrium: its metastatic lymph node potential. A preliminary report. Gynecol Oncol 1976; 4: 239–43

9. Reich O, Winter R, Pickel H, et al. Does the size of pelvic lymph nodes predict metastatic involvement in patients with endometrial cancer? Int J Gynecol Cancer 1996; 6: 445–7

10. Arango HA, Hoffman MS, Roberts WS, et al. Accuracy of lymph node palpation to determine need for lymphadenectomy in gynecologic malignancies. Obstet Gynecol 2000; 95: 553–6

11. Takeshima N, Umezawa S, Shimizu Y, et al. Pelvic lymph node metastasis in endometrial cancer. Nippon Sanka Fujinka Gakkai Zasshi 1994; 46: 883–8

12. Watanabe M, Aoki Y, Kase H, et al. Low risk endometrial cancer: a study of pelvic lymph node metastasis. Int J Gynecol Cancer 2003; 13: 38–41

13. Nijman HW, Khalifa M, Covens A. What is the number of lymph nodes required for an 'adequate' pelvic lymphadenectomy? Eur J Gynaecol Oncol 2004; 25: 87–9

14. Kilgore LC, Partridge EE, Alvarez RD, et al. Adenocarcinoma of the endometrium: survival comparisons of patients with and without pelvic node sampling. Gynecol Oncol 1995; 56: 29–33

15. Cragun J, Havrilesky L, Calingaert B, et al. Retrospective analysis of selective lymphadenectomy in apparent early-stage endometrial cancer. J Clin Oncol 2005; 23: 3668–75

16. Fanning J, Nanavati PJ, Hilgers RD. Surgical staging and high dose rate brachytherapy for endometrial cancer: limiting external radiotherapy to node-positive tumors. Obstet Gynecol 1996; 87: 1041–4

17. Orr JW Jr. Surgical staging of endometrial cancer: does the patient benefit? Gynecol Oncol 1998; 71: 335–9

18. Larson DM, Broste SK, Krawisz BR. Surgery without radiotherapy for primary treatment of endometrial cancer. Obstet Gynecol 1998; 91: 355–9

19. Mohan DS, Samuels MA, Selim MA, et al. Long-term outcomes of therapeutic pelvic lymphadenectomy for stage I endometrial adenocarcinoma. Gynecol Oncol 1998; 70: 165–71

20. Mariani A, Webb MJ, Keeney GL, et al. Predictors of lymphatic failure in endometrial cancer. Gynecol Oncol 2002; 84: 437–42

21. Barranger E, Cortez A, Grahek D, et al. Laparoscopic sentinel node procedure using a combination of patent blue and radiocolloid in women with endometrial cancer. Ann Surg Oncol 2004; 11: 344–9

22. Aalders J, Abeler V, Kolstad P, et al. Postoperative external irradiation and prognostic parameters in stage I endometrial carcinoma: clinical and histopathologic study of 540 patients. Obstet Gynecol 1980; 56: 419–27

23. Creutzberg CL, van Putten WL, Koper PC, et al. Surgery and postoperative radiotherapy versus surgery alone for patients with stage-1 endometrial carcinoma: multicentre randomized trial – PORTEC Study Group. Post Operative Radiation Therapy in Endometrial Carcinoma. Lancet 2000; 355: 1404–11

24. Keys H, Roberts J, Brunetto V, et al. A phase III trial of surgery with or without adjunctive external pelvic radiation therapy in intermediate-risk endometrial adenocarcinoma: a Gynecologic Oncology Group study. Obstet Gynecol Surv 2004; 59: 516–18

25. Mariani A, Webb MJ, Keeney GL, et al. Low-risk corpus cancer: is lymphadenectomy or radiotherapy necessary? Am J Obstet Gynecol 2000; 182: 1506–19

26. Orre JW, Roland PY, Leichter D, Orr PF. Endometrial cancer: is surgical staging necessary? Curr Opin Oncol 2001; 13: 408–12

27. Orr JW, Holimion JL, Orr PF. Stage I corpus cancer: is teletherapy necessary? Am J Obstet Gynecol 1997; 176: 777–9

28. Sant Cassia LJ, Weppelmann B, Shingleton H, et al. Management of early endometrial carcinoma. Gynecol Oncol 1989; 35: 362–6

whose anatomical structures are covered with fatty tissue, it is recommended first to locate the Cooper's ligament (Figure 34.3). This can be identified by palpation with a blunt instrument driven on the posterior surface of the abdominal wall, lateral to the umbilical ligament – acting the same way as a blind man seeking the edge of the pavement with his white stick.

The dissection is started by grasping the tissues located caudally to the external vein and gently pulling on them, while at the same time a second instrument tears the connective fibers and lymphatic channels joining the node-bearing tissues to the surrounding structures. It is common to find an inferior obturator vein at this level which crosses the nodes that are required; blunt dissection is generally enough to circumvent this. Once the subvenous nodes are freed, revealing the obturator nerve, the external iliac vein is traced back to point where it meets the internal iliac

vein. The same is done for the tissues located between the external iliac artery and the external iliac vein. The ascending dissection leads to bifurcation of the common iliac artery.

The next step concerns the node-bearing tissues located between the external iliac artery and the psoas muscle. One starts ventrally, at the level of the origin of the circumflex artery, and continues dorsally to the level of the common iliac artery. At this time, it is often necessary to make a lateral peritoneal incision in order to reflect upwards the ileocecal junction on the right side and the sigmoid colon on the left side. The ureter is identified at the level it crosses the vessels. If the infundibulopelvic ligament has not been divided and the posterior sheet of the broad ligament is intact, the ureter remains attached to its natural support. Both are pushed medially. The pararectal space is then opened (Figure 34.4). The node-bearing

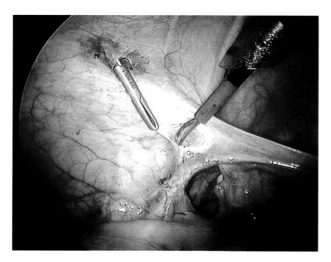

Figure 34.1 Incision of the peritoneum between the round ligament and the infundibulopelvic ligament (left side)

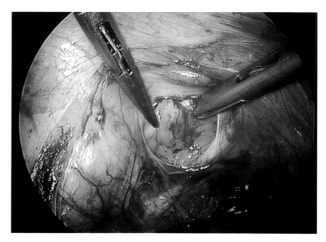

Figure 34.3 Identification of the Cooper's ligament which is crossed vertically by a collateral of the external iliac vein: the inferior obturatic vein

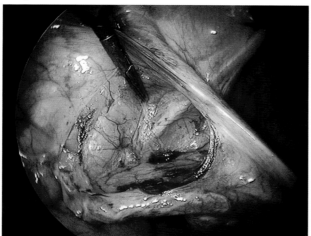

Figure 34.2 Identification of the superior vesical artery: traction medially onto the umbilical ligament

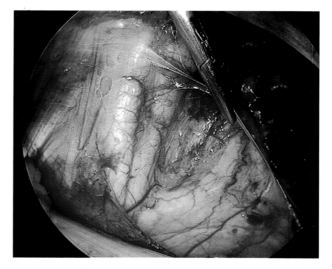

Figure 34.4 Opening the pararectal space

tissues alongside the inferior aspect of the common iliac artery and posterior aspect of the internal iliac artery are freed up.

The order in which the landmarks are identified and the different steps and techniques of dissection are performed varies from surgeon to surgeon. As for the technique of dissection, the simplest is the best, i.e. grasping the nodes with 'grasping forceps' (crocodile forceps) and tearing the surrounding structures with 'dissecting forceps' (cobra forceps). Such a technique (Figure 34.5) requires skill, but once this skill is acquired it is certainly less bloody: only the resistant structures, the blood vessels, have to be controlled before being divided, and they are few if the dissection is made in the appropriate way, not too far from and not too close to the nodes.

Two options are offered for removal of the nodes. The first is gathering them somewhere (in the uterovesical space, for example) and extracting them at the end of the procedure using an extracting bag. The second, and our preferred technique, is to use the Coelio-extractor®, which enables us to deliver the nodes one by one without contaminating the abdominal wall.

Querleu et al.[5] were the first to give data concerning the feasibility and safety of transumbilical transperitoneal laparoscopic pelvic dissection. For the 39 procedures they performed on patients affected by cancer of the cervix, stage Ib/IIb, the mean duration of the procedure was 80 min. No conversion to laparotomy was needed. The mean yield of nodes was 8.7. Positive nodes were found in five patients who were submitted to exclusive radiotherapy, as the 34 other patients were operated on and submitted either to abdominal radical hysterectomy (32 patients) or to vaginal radical hysterectomy (two patients). All the patients were reassessed after 5 years. The 5-year life-table survival rate was similar to the survival of a historical group matched for age, stage and therapy. Childers et al.[6]

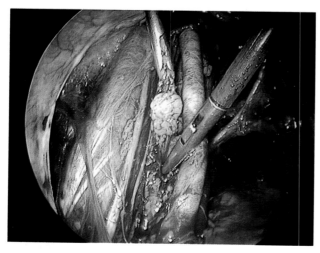

Figure 34.5 Dissection of the dorsal external iliac nodes: 'two forceps technique'

reported data collected from 18 procedures performed for cervical cancer, among which five were immediately submitted to abdominal radical hysterectomy and 13 were assessed before radiotherapy. No complications were observed. The duration of the staging procedure was 75–175 min for the patients assessed before radiotherapy. The lymph node yield was medially 31.4 (17–37) for the patients submitted to abdominal radical hysterectomy. One year later, data about 53 patients affected by endometrial cancer were presented[7]. All the patients were assessed with the laparoscope and 29 of them were submitted to pelvic lymphadenectomy plus aortic sampling. Three intra-operative complications occurred (one pneumothorax, one transection of the ureter and one bladder lesion) and three postoperative complications (two bowel obstructions and one left-side pulmonary collapse). The issue was addressed again 5 years later[8] for 125 patients. The rate of complications did not vary. However, the rate of conversion to laparotomy dropped from 8% (2/25) to 0% (0/100). At the same time, the operation time decreased from 196 min to 128 min ($p < 0.02$) and the hospital stay from 3.2 days to 1.8 days ($p < 0.0001$).

Since 1993, most of the published series[9–18] include data concerning the low aortic lymph node sampling, which was added to the pelvic dissection. Summarizing the data (Table 34.1), one can assume that the mean number of nodes retrieved with the scope was about 25 (plus five to ten aortic nodes). This number is close to the number of nodes retrieved in open surgery. Comparative studies confirmed that the numbers were about the same. Fowler et al.[9] pointed out that 25% of the pelvic nodes were still present at laparotomy after the patient had undergone a laparoscopic lymphadenectomy. However, no patient with negative nodes at laparoscopy had positive nodes at laparotomy. Moreover, Spirtos et al.[13], in a comparative study, obtained medially 20 pelvic nodes (plus eight para-aortic) in 13 patients operated on with a laparoscope versus 22 (plus seven para-aortic) in 16 patients operated on by laparotomy.

Concerning the safety of laparoscopic lymphadenectomy, the data collected in the Gynecologic Oncology Group (GOG) study[19] are the most informative. The mean number of retrieved nodes is 32.1 (16.6 on the left side and 15.5 on the right side). In spite of this record number, the results were judged incomplete in six of the 40 patients submitted to laparotomy after the laparoscopic lymphadenectomy. In fact, removing a high number of nodes is meaningless. The point is to remove the significant nodes. The extreme rarity of pelvic side-wall recurrences in laparoscopically pN_0 patients managed without laparotomic lymphadenectomy or radiotherapy indicates that laparoscopy enables us to remove the significant nodes, even if the total number of nodes is low (see later). If a criterion of safety had to be elected, photographic records taken at the end of the laparoscopic procedure would be the best. In the GOG study, the result was judged inadequate in three of the patients whose photographic records

21% in the patients assigned to the intraperitoneal approach and 15.3% in the patients assigned to the extraperitoneal approach. Using the extraperitoneal left-side laparoscopic approach, the rate of intra- and peroperative complications was low (see preceding section). As far as the actinic complications are concerned, their rate was also very low: two cases of radiation enteritis only (2.7%) in the 48 patients that we gathered with Denis Querleu[21]. So far, the extraperitoneal left-side laparoscopic aortic lymphadenectomy, which has the same informative value as the staging laparotomy while not carrying the same costs (hospital stay and surgical complications) or risks (actinic complications), deserves to be used widely in the pretherapeutic work-up of advanced-stage cervical cancer.

Laparoscopic aortic lymphadenectomy recognizes another helpful indication in the pre-exenteration work-up. If a recurrence occurs in a patient who has not been submitted to aortic dissection prior to the primary treatment, and if the indication is to perform a pelvic exenteration, one knows that this operation, which carries a high risk and exposes the patient to troublesome sequelae, is contraindicated in cases where the aortic nodes are involved because the chances for cure are very low. Rather than exposing this contraindication at the time the laparotomy has already been performed, one obtains a big advantage in exposing it by laparoscopic staging. In our experience[31], patients referred between April 1994 and June 1998 for recurrent cervical cancer confined to the pelvis according to the preoperative work-up (including normal CT scan) underwent a laparoscopic para-aortic assessment. All but one of the procedures were completely performed by laparoscopy. This patient was submitted to laparotomy for controlling a bleed from the right ovarian artery. Aortic nodes were not involved, but pelvic debulking was impossible. Among the seven other patients, aortic lymph node metastases were in evidence in two patients who were not submitted to pelvic exenteration. Among the five patients with no para-aortic lymph node involvement who were submitted to the exenteration, one developed a liver metastasis 4 months after surgery, one died with pelvic recurrence 16 months after surgery and three were still alive 2, 4 and 28 months after the surgery.

THE FUTURE: LAPAROSCOPIC ASSESSMENT OF THE SENTINEL NODE?

The concept of sentinel node assessment was born in 1992 at the time that the urologist Cabanas proposed the replacement of inguinofemoral dissection by the removal of the only node that was dyed after injection of blue dye close to the penile tumor that one had to manage. Such a policy enables avoidance of the heavy consequences that inguinofemoral dissection carries, while not increasing the chance for inguinofemoral recurrence. The same argument is put forward in the management of breast cancer and vulvar cancer. The conditions for such a lightening of the

management policy are, first, that the identification of the sentinel node is easy to perform and, second, that the negative predictive value of the assessment of this node is 100% or close to 100% as far as the status of the other regional nodes is concerned. Another and very important question concerns the therapeutic value of lymphadenectomy which is dismissed on the pretext that, as the sentinel node is not involved, the other regional nodes are also not involved.

Identification of the sentinel node in cervical cancer seems, according to the literature, to be difficult. O'Boyle et al.[32] tried to obtain it while injecting blue dye into the cervix before an abdominal radical hysterectomy was performed. Among the 40 assessed areas (20 patients), sentinel nodes were identified in 15 cases only. Verheijen et al.[33] injected technetium 99m colloidal albumin and blue dye around the tumor. In six out of ten eligible women who had a Wertheim–Meigs operation for cervical cancer stage Ib, one or more sentinel nodes could be detected by scintigraphy prior to the surgery. Intraoperative gamma-probe detection was successful in eight of the ten women, where visual detection found sentinel nodes in only four. Kamprath et al.[34] used colloidal technetium in 16 of 18 patients in whom sentinel nodes were detected. A median of 2.1 pelvic sentinel nodes was found in 16 patients and a median of 1.4 para-aortic sentinel nodes was found in five patients. No false negatives were registered by these authors; after systematic dissection, no metastatic nodes were found if the sentinel nodes were not involved. However, the practical interest of such a statement is low. As a matter of fact, the only drawback of systematic dissection is that it takes time; postoperative lymphedema is very rare, especially if no postoperative radiotherapy is given. Using laparotomy for identifying the sentinel node does not spare time. The same is true if laparoscopy is used, but the colloidal technetium technique leads in most cases to performance of an extended dissection.

The technique we propose differs from the others in that, first, we use the laparoscope, second, we do not use colloidal technetium but a blue dye and, third, we do not look directly for the blue-dyed nodes but for the blue-dyed lymphatic channels which are followed from inside to outside and lead to the sentinel node which, in most cases, is unique. Between October 1998 and September 2000, we operated on 52 patients using this technique. One or more lymphatic channels were identified in 87% of the cases which led to one blue-dyed node in 95% of the cases and to two separate nodes in 5% of the cases. While being more selective than the colloidal technetium technique, this technique has the same safety. Among the 95 sentinel nodes which were assessed, 13 were involved and 82 were not. Systematic dissection performed after sentinel node removal never showed in these 82 cases that other regional nodes were involved. Another advantage of the technique we propose is that it actually spares time in most cases. As a matter of fact, the sentinel node in 82 of the 95 cases (86%) was located at the contact of the external vein, either medial to it or caudal to it (between it and the obturator nerve (Figure 34.20)) or cephalic to it (between it and the external iliac artery). In all these cases, the place where the sentinel node was lying was ventral to the origin of the uterine artery. This means that we were able to identify and remove it less than 10 min after the start of the dissection.

Following the data given here, it seems that laparoscopic dissection undertaken after the injection of a blue dye into the cervix can, in most of the cases, be very much shortened. However, it is not certain that dismissing systematic dissection does not include a risk of enhancement of the rate of pelvic recurrences and, more precisely, of pelvic side-wall recurrences. In our 1986–1999 already-quoted personal experience, laparoscopically assisted vaginal radical hysterectomy, which was reserved for patients with no pelvic node involvement, was performed without appealing to the parametrial lymphadenectomy (see section 'Schauta–Stoeckel operation assisted by laparoscopy') in 168 cases and with parametrial lymphadenectomy in 73 cases. The rates of pelvic recurrence were 15.5% and 5.3%, respectively. No pelvic side-wall recurrences were observed in the second population. That means that, by increasing the radicality of the dissection, one lessens the chances for recurrence, even in patients apparently free of lymph node metastasis. Such a phenomenon could be explained by the data of molecular biology, which show that cancer can be present even if not morphologically evident. From the practical view, it seems not to be sensible to renounce systematic lymphadenectomy even if the sentinel node is not involved, with the exception of very early tumors (stage Ia and stage Ib less than 2 cm in size), in the management of which we have never observed recurrences whatever the technique of lymphadenectomy (176 cases).

CONCLUSION: WARNING!

Laparoscopic surgery does not improve the outcomes in the management of cancer. Worse than that, this surgery can be deleterious if the rules of safety are not respected. It is mandatory to avoid direct manipulation of the tumor. Therefore, the place of laparoscopic surgery has to be restricted to staging and to assisting radical surgery. A careful preoperative work-up is necessary to dismiss those cases at risk. On the other hand, one must not hesitate to convert to laparotomy if unexpected tumor bulk prevents the avoidance of direct manipulations. Actually, the advantage of laparoscopic surgery is only the lessening of surgical trauma while respecting better the forms and the functions. But that can lead, in the cases of early-stage cervical cancer in young patients, to surgery that makes possible the birth of normal babies. This result is worth the efforts of gynecological oncologists.

REFERENCES

1. Dargent D. A new future for Schauta's operation through pre-surgical retroperitoneal pelviscopy. Eur J Gynecol Oncol 1987; 8: 292–6
2. Whelan RL, Lee SW. Review of investigations regarding the etiology of port site tumor recurrence. J Laparoendosc Adv Surg Tech A 1999; 9: 1–16
3. Canis M, Botchorishvilli R, Wattiez A, et al. Cancer and laparoscopy, experimental studies: a review. Eur J Obstet Gynecol Reprod Biol 2000; 91: 1–9
4. Sonoda Y, Zerbe M, Barakat RR, et al. High incidence of positive peritoneal cytology in low-risk endometrial cancer treated by laparoscopically assisted vaginal hysterectomy (LAVH). Presented at the 31st Annual Meeting of the SGO, February 2000: Abstr 21
5. Querleu D, Leblanc E, Castelain B. Laparoscopic pelvic lymphadenectomy. Am J Obstet Gynecol 1991; 164: 579–81
6. Childers JM, Hatch K, Surwit EA. The role of laparoscopic lymphadenectomy in the management of cervical carcinoma. Gynecol Oncol 1992; 47: 38–43
7. Childers JM, Brzechffa PR, Hatch KD, et al. Laparoscopically assisted surgical staging (LASS) of endometrial cancer. Gynecol Oncol 1993; 51: 33–8
8. Melendez TD, Childers JM, Nour M, et al. Laparoscopic staging of endometrial cancer: the learning experience. J Soc Laparoendosc Surg 1997; 1: 45–9
9. Fowler JM, Carter JR, Carlson JW, et al. Lymph node yield from laparoscopic lymphadenectomy in cervical cancer: a comparative study. Gynecol Oncol 1993; 51: 187–92
10. Nezhat CR, Nezhat FR, Vurrel MO, et al. Laparoscopic radical hysterectomy and laparoscopi-

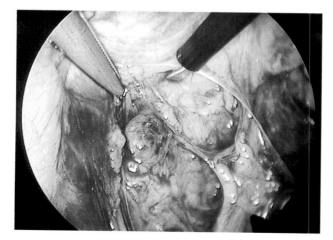

Figure 34.20 Main lymphatic channel and main lymphatic node (sentinel node) after injection of Patent Blue Violet in the cervix: the main lymphatic channel crosses the superior vesical artery and joins a node located alongside the podalic surface of the external vein

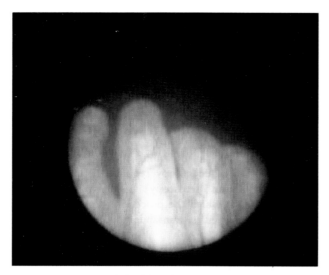

Figure 35.3 Normal fetal hand

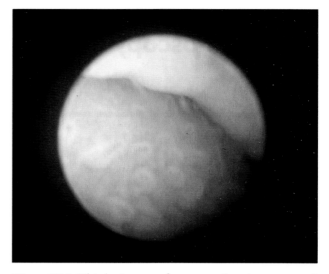

Figure 35.6 Third-trimester fetoscopy showing a normal fetal upper lip without cleft and, below, the tongue

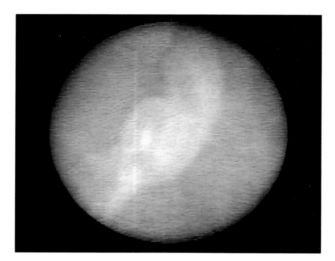

Figure 35.4 Umbilical cord and vessels

Ultrasound guidance is necessary for both routes in order to avoid the placenta and rule out any unknown multiple pregnancy or miscarriage. In the case of bleeding, saline or Ringer's lactate may be amnioinfused in order to improve the fetal view[6]. The use of CO_2 could induce acidosis, and should be avoided[10]. Glycine, used safely in animal models, may be a potential alternative[11]. The procedure can be performed on an outpatient basis under local or locoregional anesthesia. For both fetal immobilization and maternal sedation, remifentanyl has been shown to give similar results to those with diazepam, with better control of the maternal respiratory pattern[12]. Anti-D prophylaxis should be administered to rhesus-negative patients. Antibiotics should be given routinely in the case of transcervical procedures[7].

However, with improvements in ultrasound (endovaginal first-trimester scan), diagnostic interest in embryoscopy and fetoscopy has decreased, while their role as a fetal surgery tool has emerged during the past decade.

INDICATIONS

Diagnostic endoscopy

Prenatal diagnosis by fetal endoscopy should be offered in three distinct clinical conditions.

Suspicion of a first-trimester abnormality

As early endovaginal ultrasound is now able to diagnose major congenital anomalies[13], and as amniocentesis is indicated for aneuploidy diagnosis, fetoscopy may be done to confirm rapidly the final diagnosis. Fetoscopy may also be performed prior to dilatation and curettage for fetal

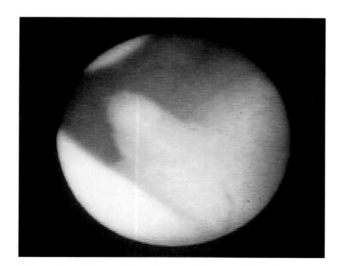

Figure 35.5 Normal female genitalia at 11th week

anomaly in order to exclude an unsuspected polymalformative syndrome. We previously reported two cases of conjoined twins in which combined ultrasound and endoscopy enabled us to confirm the diagnosis and allow early termination of the pregnancy[14] (Figure 35.7). Several cases of first-trimester anomalies confirmed by fetoscopy have been reported, such as multiple amniotic-band syndrome[15] and omphalocele[16]. A suspicion of neural tube defects in the presence of increased α-fetoprotein and a non-contributive ultrasound was also excluded by fetoscopy[8].

Polymalformative syndromes

Patients at risk of polymalformative syndromes affecting at least the face and/or the limb extremities are listed in Table 35.1. In patients with genetic syndromes transmitted with either recessive or dominant inheritance, fetoscopic diagnosis of a small defect may be performed at an earlier gestational age than can ultrasound. Among hand anomalies, mono-, a-, syn-, brachy-, campo-, clino- and polydactylism (Figure 35.8) may be diagnosed. A week-10 prenatal diagnosis of polydactylism associated with

recurrent Meckel–Gruber syndrome has been reported[17]. Ellis–van Creveld syndrome[6] was diagnosed at the 11th week in the presence of polydactylism. Gross facial anomalies such as cleft lip, anophthalmia and ear aplasia may be confirmed by fetoscopy as early as at the 10th week, as reported in the prenatal diagnosis of Smith–Lemli–Opitz and Fraser's cryptophthalmos syndromes[18,19]. Roberts' syndrome was excluded at 12 weeks, as no gross facial and limb malformations were seen[20]. Albinism was also diagnosed by fetoscopic view of the fetal hair color[21]. Club foot may also be diagnosed by fetoscopy (Figure 35.9).

Early fetal tissue sampling

Evans et al. reported two cases of endoscopically assisted fetal muscle biopsy performed for the prenatal diagnosis of Duchenne's muscular dystrophy[22]. Endoscopic guidance allowed diagnosis at an earlier gestational age, with an accurate site of biopsy. First-trimester umbilical vessel sampling was reported using transabdominal fetoscopy at between 8 and 12 weeks[23]. Directed skin biopsies in order to diagnose rare genodermatoses such as junctional epidermolysis bullosa[24] or trichothiodystrophy[25] have recently been reported.

Therapeutic endoscopy

Endoscopic fetoplacental surgery is now recognized as an effective alternative therapy in severe twin-to-twin transfusion syndrome (TTTS) and umbilical cord ligation in an abnormal twin pregnancy. Other experimental applications, such as for obstructive uropathy and congenital diaphragmatic hernia, have also been reported. For these indications, a larger-diameter sheath (> 2 mm) and parallel ports should be employed in order to use graspers, scissors, knot pushers and laser fibers. Fetal

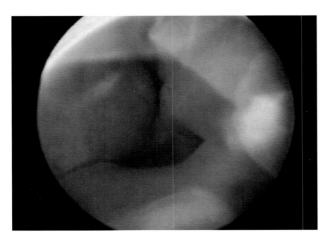

Figure 35.7 Thoraco-omphalopagus conjoined twins

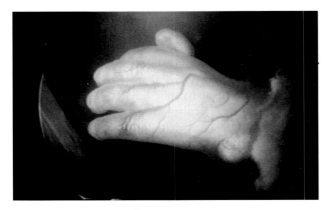

Figure 35.8 Hexadactylism

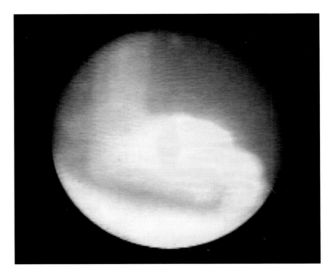

Figure 35.9 Club foot associated with neural tube defect

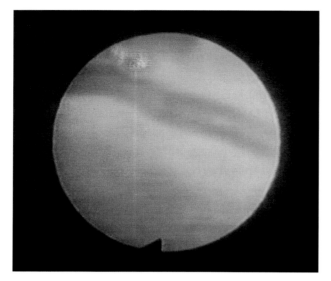

Figure 35.11 Endoscopic view of placental anastomoses in twin-to-twin transfusion syndrome (pre-laser coagulation)

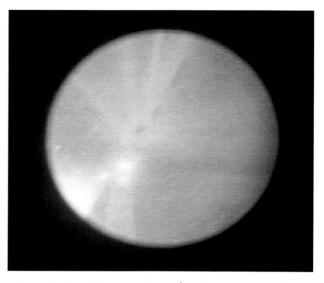

Figure 35.13 Fetoscopic view of an intertwin membrane with laser-operated septostomy

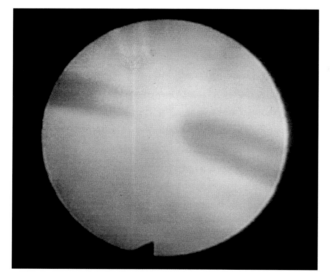

Figure 35.12 Endoscopic view of placental anastomoses in twin-to-twin transfusion syndrome (post-laser coagulation)

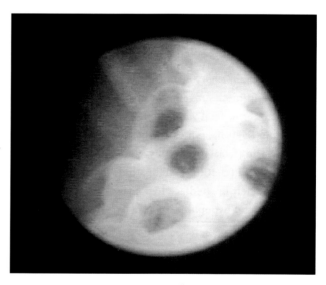

Figure 35.14 Fetoscopic view of an intertwin membrane with several laser shots

membranes (PROM) rate of 28%[43,44]. In the early cases, anterior placenta was associated with laparotomy, but in later studies laparotomy is not considered to be a contraindication to fetoscopy-guided laser coagulation[42,44].

Even if the study of Senat *et al.*[42] answered partly the question about efficacy of the technique in terms of fetal results, the associated maternal risk should still be borne in mind.

Septostomy This technique, involving intentional rupture of the intertwin septum, was reported by our team following one case of unintentional septostomy which led to an improvement in TTTS[45], and also by Saade *et al.*[46].

Other cases of septostomy have been reported, with differing outcomes[47,48], and a prospective randomized trial of amnioreduction versus septostomy before 24 weeks reported a similar survival rate (at least one infant, 78% vs. 80%)[49]. This study supports, however, the advantage of a single procedure in septostomy. A possible mechanism for the therapeutic effect of septostomy could be the equilibration of amniotic fluid between the two sacs, associated with correction of the unbalanced flow, mainly in the donor umbilical vessels and on the placental surface[50,53]. The involvement of amniotic fluid pressure changes has been suggested, but one article based on only two cases reports a similarly increased pressure in both

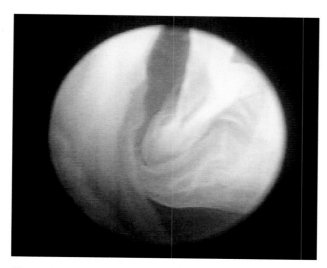

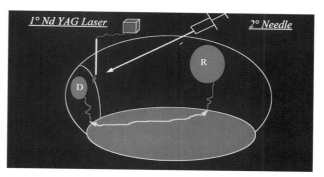

Figure 35.16 Septostomy techniques. Nd : YAG, neodymium : yttrium–aluminum-garnet; D, donor twin; R, recipient twin

Figure 35.15 Fetoscopic view of an intertwin membrane rupture following laser-operated coagulation

sacs[54]. In the donor twin, the filling of the amniotic sac may decrease cord compression, mainly when there is a velamentous insertion, a common finding in TTTS[55]. Another argument for the therapeutic effect of septostomy is the role of the intertwin septum in TTTS, as it is rare in monoamniotic twin pregnancy despite the presence of numerous placental anastomoses[55].

Technically, septostomy could be performed by fetoscopic Nd : YAG (neodymium : yttrium–aluminum–garnet) laser fulguration alone, or associated with placental anastomosis coagulation (Figures 35.13–35.15). However, in our latest cases, it was performed under ultrasound guidance by intentional needling of the intertwin membrane, as shown in Figure 35.16. Table 35.2 gives the combined results of the pioneer centers using this technique, with a mean survival rate of 65%[45,46,49]. The results of improved fetal hemodynamics (mainly umbilical artery Doppler)[46,50] are associated with increased donor urine production. This factor has been reported to be associated with a better survival rate[56].

The main specific risk associated with amniotomy is the iatrogenic creation of a pseudomonoamniotic twin pregnancy with cord entanglement[57]. However, this may be reduced by creating a small hole, as in twin pregnancy transeptal diagnostic amniocentesis[58]. Another potential

risk associated with septostomy is the presence of membrane flaps, which may induce amniotic band syndrome[59], and further compromising fetoscopic procedures such as cord ligation[60,61].

Cord occlusion in abnormal twin pregnancy

In cases of acardiac twin pregnancy or in monochorionic multiple pregnancy with a compromised twin, selective feticide may be an ethically acceptable option, aiming to improve the healthy cotwin outcome. As KCl injection cannot be used because of placental anastomosis, fetoscopic cord obliteration may be offered as a safe alternative. Cord occlusion techniques aim mainly to decrease the morbidity and mortality of the surviving twin. It may be performed by cord ligation using two or three ports[51,52] (Figures 35.17–35.20) with the increased risk of side-effects or by a recently described single-port technique using a 2.5-mm bipolar coagulation forceps under ultrasound guidance[62,63]. In terms of results, studies of cord coagulation in 23 and 46 cases, respectively, reported a 71–87% survival rate with 40% and 12% rates of preterm labor[62,63].

Obstructive uropathies

Fetal lower urinary tract obstruction, such as in the case of posterior urethral valve, is associated with a risk of chronic renal failure, oligohydramnios and pulmonary hypopla-

Table 35.2 Survival rate of fetuses with twin-to-twin transfusion syndrome (TTTS) treated by septostomy

	Hubinont et al.[45] (n = 7)	Saade et al.[46] (n = 9)	Moise et al.[49] (n = 73)
Second-trimester TTTS (n)	7	5	73 (below 24 weeks)
Survival rate (%)	57	83	78

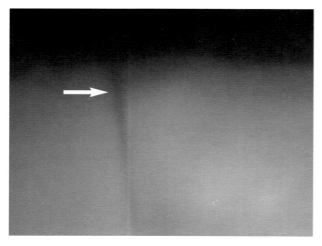

Figure 35.17 Fetoscopically operated cord ligation in abnormal monochorionic twin pregnancy: looping of the cord by a black-colored suture (arrow)

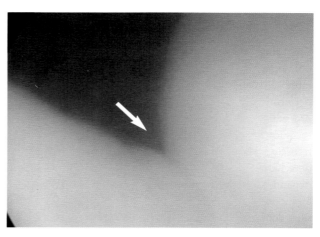

Figure 35.19 Fetoscopically operated cord ligation in abnormal monochorionic twin pregnancy: cord with the knot (arrow)

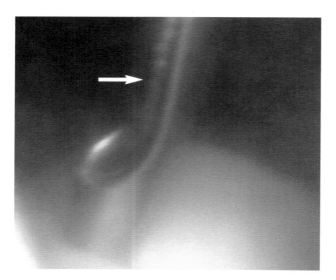

Figure 35.18 Fetoscopically operated cord ligation in abnormal monochorionic twin pregnancy: the knot is tied by using a knot pusher (arrow)

sia[64]. *In utero* therapy may be offered in these pregnancies either by open fetal surgery[64] or, more often, by percutaneous ultrasound-guided vesicoamniotic shunt[65]. The high morbidity associated with open surgery and displacement or obstruction of the catheter has recently opened the door to a third therapeutic alternative: percutaneous fetal cystoscopy with laser fulguration of the urethral valve[66,67]. This procedure improves the diagnosis (visualization of thickened bladder neck, dilated proximal urethra, ureteral orifices) and can exclude other abnormalities such as urethral atresia or persistent cloaca. However, the survival rate and the urological outcome should be studied in a larger series before being routinely applied.

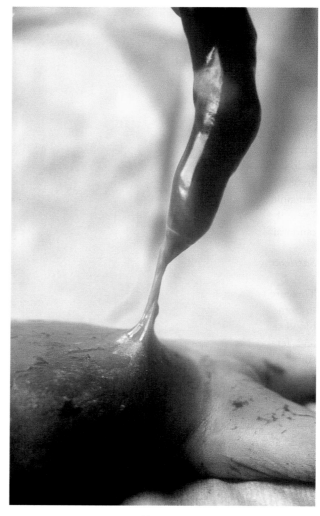

Figure 35.20 Fetoscopically operated cord ligation in abnormal monochorionic twin pregnancy: postmortem aspect of cord ligation

Congenital diaphragmatic hernia

This abnormality is associated with a risk of severe pulmonary hypoplasia and a high neonatal mortality rate[68]. Prenatal surgery based on animal studies involves performing a fetal tracheal occlusion either by an open procedure[69] or, more recently, by fetoscopy[70]. Two techniques have been reported: tracheal occlusion[71] and fetoscopic endoluminal tracheal occlusion using a detachable balloon[72]. This can prevent abnormal lung fluid dynamics and enhances lung growth. Preliminary results of a randomized trial suggest that fetoscopic tracheal occlusion does not increase the survival rate compared with postnatal management[71]. Endotracheal placement of the balloon, performed in 20 cases with bad-prognosis congential diaphragmatic hernia, was technically successful in 65%. Survival rate was 50%, with a normal neurological assessment in ten infants[72]. However, long-term follow-up will be required to confirm the benefits of these new surgical approaches.

Myelomeningocele

This neural tube defect with a prevalence of five cases for every 10 000 births is associated with various degrees of paraplegia, neurogenic sphincter dysfunction and severe mental retardation in the presence of associated hydrocephaly[73]. A recent article reported four second-trimester cases of myelomeningocele, which underwent endoscopic coverage of the defect using a maternal skin graft[74]. Only two of them survived at birth, and these remaining two had a satisfactory neurological outcome. Even if the technique is feasible and seems attractive, randomization and long-term follow-up are needed.

Sacrococcygeal teratoma

This rare tumor is generally treated surgically at birth, but in some cases, large tumors associated with substantial blood sequestration may induce high-output heart failure and fetal hydrops, with a poor prognosis. Several fetal surgical approaches have been reported, including *ex utero* surgery[75], endoscopic laser coagulation[76], cystic decompression by needling[77] and, in our department, a trial of thermocoagulation of the feeding vessels using a needle-sized device introduced transabdominally under ultrasound guidance (unpublished data).

Placental chorioangioma

A case report of a large chorioangioma treated successfully by laser coagulation of the feeding vessel introduces the opportunity to treat this severe complication by fetoscopy[78].

Fetal cardiac surgery

Fetal catheterization has been successfully performed in sheep[79], and could be a potential approach for treating fetal heart-block using a pacemaker, as well as performing valvuloplasty in cases of severe vessel stenosis.

RISKS, SAFETY AND COMPLICATIONS

Before performing a fetoscopy, both the risks and potential benefits should be clearly explained to the patient. Potential risks for maternal and/or fetal injury have been previously reported[6–8]; fetal loss is the most common complication, with an incidence between 3%[5,6] and 9%[8]. In diagnostic fetoscopy, premature rupture of the membranes occurs in approximately 5–7% of cases[6]. It may reach 10% in a group of therapeutic endoscopy procedures (TTTS treated by laser coagulation)[43], and even 30% in fetoscopic cord ligation[61]. Amniotic fluid leakage may be avoided by reducing trocar size and the number of ports, and perhaps by using a gelatin sponge[80] or a collagen plug[81], as demonstrated in animal models. Recently, a trial of closure of iatrogenic membrane defects following fetoscopy, using platelet sealant, fibrin glue and powered collagen injection, was successful in 7/8 cases[82]. The risk of fetal eye injury by endoscopic white light has been excluded in fetal lamb and rat models[83,84].

Quintero *et al.* reported a failure rate of 16% in diagnostic endoscopy, mainly due to early gestation (5th and 6th weeks), obesity and severely retroverted uterus[6].

Maternal risks are not negligible[85], and include hemorrhage (one case in our experience; unpublished data), chorioamnionitis and pulmonary and potential amniotic embolism. Amniotic air insufflation was found to be safe in a sheep model[86].

CONTRAINDICATIONS

Fetal endoscopy should not be performed in pregnant patients with active bleeding, suspicion of premature rupture of the membranes and intrauterine infection[6,8,85].

CONCLUSIONS

Fetoscopy is now a well-established tool in fetal medicine. Embryofetoscopy allows the confirmation of first-trimester prenatal diagnosis of structural anomalies affecting mainly the face and/or limb extremities. It can confirm early ultrasound diagnosis prior to dilatation and curettage, allowing, in some cases, genetic counseling. Early tissue sampling is feasible in early gestation.

Minimally invasive fetal surgery by endoscopy is used routinely in specific fetal conditions. In complicated multiple pregnancies (TTTS, selective cord ligation), these

minimale pour le foetus? Gunaïkeia 1996; 1: 3115–19

60. Robyr R, Lewi L, Salomon LJ, et al. Twin-to-twin transfusion syndrome. Am J Obstet Gynecol 2006 Mar; 194: 796–803

61. Yamamoto M, EI Murr L, Robyr R, et al. Incidence and impact of perioperative complications in 175 fetoscopy-guided laser coagulations of chorionic plate anastomoses in fetofetal transfusion syndrome before 26 weeks of gestation. Am J Obstet Gynecol 2005; 193: 1110–16

62. Yesidaglar N, Zikulnig L, Gratacos E, et al. Bipolar coagulation with small diameter forceps in animal models for in utero cord obliteration. Hum Reprod 2000; 15: 865–8

63. Robyr R, Yamamoto M, Ville Y. Selective feticide in complicated monochorionic twin pregnancies using ultrasound-guided bipolar cord coagulation. Br J Obstet Gynaecol 2005; 112: 1344–8

64. Harrison M. Atlas of Fetal Surgery. London: Chapman & Hall, 1996; Part II: 63–79

65. Goldbus MS, Filly RA, Callen PW, et al. Fetal urinary tract obstruction: management and selection for treatment. Semin Perinatol 1985; 9: 91–101

66. Quintero RA, Morales WJ, Allen MH, et al. Fetal hydrolaparoscopy and endoscopic cystotomy in complicated cases of lower urinary tract obstruction. Am J Obstet Gynecol 2000; 183: 324–30

67. Hofmann R, Becker T, Meyer-Wittkopf M, et al. Fetoscopic placement of a transurethral stent for intrauterine obstructive uropathy. J Urol 2004; 171: 384–6

68. Adzick NS, Nance ML. Pediatric surgery Part two. N Engl J Med 2000; 342: 1726–32

69. Harrison M. Atlas of Fetal Surgery. London: Chapman & Hall 1996; Part II: 93–145

70. Harrison MR, Mychaliska GB, Albanese CT, et al. Correction of congenital diaphragmatic hernia in utero: those with poor prognosis (liver herniation and low lung to head ratio) could be saved by fetoscopic temporary tracheal occlusion. J Pediatr Surg 1998; 33: 1017–22

71. Cass DL. Fetal surgery for congenital diaphragmatic hernia: the North American experience. Semin Perinatol 2005; 29: 104–11

72. Deprest J, Jani J, Gratacos E, et al., FETO Task Group. Fetal intervention for congenital diaphragmatic hernia: the European experience. Semin Perinatol 2005; 29: 94–103

73. Steinbok P, Irvine B, Cochrane DD, Irwin BJ. Long term outcome and complications in children born with meningomyelocoele. Childs Nerv Syst 1992; 8: 92–6

74. Bruner JP, Richards O, Tulipan NB, Arney TL. Endoscopic coverage of fetal myelomeningocoele in utero. Am J Obstet Gynecol 1999; 180: 153–8

75. Chiba T, Albanese CT, Jennings RW, et al. In utero repair of rectal atresia after complete resection of sacrococcygeal teratoma. Fetal Diagn Ther 2000; 15: 187–90

76. Hecher K, Hackelloer BJ. Intrauterine endoscopic laser surgery for fetal sacrococcygeal teratoma. Lancet 1996; 347: 470–2

77. Garcia AM, Morgan WM, Bruner JP. In utero decompression of a cystic grade IV sacrococcygeal teratoma. Fetal Diagn Ther 1998; 13: 305–8

78. Quarello E, Bernard JP, Leroy B, Ville Y. Prenatal laser treatment of a placental chorioangioma. Ultrasound Obstet Gynecol 2005; 25: 299–301

79. Kohl T, Stumper D, Witteler R, et al. Fetoscopic direct fetal cardiac access in sheep: an important experimental milestone along the route to human fetal cardiac intervention. Circulation 2000; 102: 1602–4

80. Luks FI, Deprest JA, Peers KHE, et al. Gelatin sponge plug to seal fetoscopy port sites: technique in ovine and primate models. Am J Obstet Gynecol 1999; 181: 995–6

81. Gratacos E, Wu J, Yesildaglar N, et al. Successful sealing of fetoscopic access sites with collagen plug in a rabbit model. Am J Obstet Gynecol 2000; 182: 142–6

82. Young BK, Roman AS, McKensie AP, et al. The closure of iatrogenic membrane defects after amniocentesis and endoscopic intrauterine procedures. Fetal Diagn Ther 2004; 19: 296–300

83. Deprest J, Luks F, Peers KHE, et al. Natural protective mechanisms against endoscopic white-light injury in the fetal lamb eye. Obstet Gynecol 1999; 94: 124–7

84. Bonnett ML, Quintero RA, Carreno C, Crossland WJ. Effect of endoscopic white light on the developing rat retina. Fetal Diagn Ther 1997; 12: 76–80

85. Gratacos E, Deprest J. Current experience with fetoscopy and the Eurofoetus registry for fetoscopic procedures. Eur J Obstet Gynecol Reprod Biol 2000; 92: 151–9

86. Kohl T, Reckers J, Strumper D, et al. Amniotic air insufflation during minimally invasive fetoscopic fetal cardiac interventions is safe for the fetal brain in sheep. J Thorac Cardiovasc Surg 2004; 128: 467–71

87. Van Schoubroeck D, Lewi L, Ryan G, et al. Fetoscopic surgery in triplet pregnancies: a multi-center case series. Am J Obstet Gynecol 2004; 191: 1529–32

88. Harrison M. Fetal surgery. Am J Obstet Gynecol 1996; 174: 1255–64

89. Papadopoulos NA, Papadopoulos MA, Kovacs L, et al. Foetal surgery and cleft lip and palate: current status and new perspectives. Br J Plast Surg 2005; 58: 593–607

90. Cowan MJ, Goldbus MS. In utero hematopoietic stem cell transplants for inherited diseases. Am J Pediatr Hematol Oncol 1994; 16: 35–42

91. Yang EY, Cass DL, Sylvester KG, et al. Fetal gene therapy: efficacy, toxicity and immunologic effects of early gestation recombinant adenovirus. J Pediatr Surg 1999; 34: 235–41

Laparoscopic abdominal cerclage

R Al-Fadhli, T Tulandi

Recurrent second-trimester pregnancy loss, due to inability of the cervix to hold the pregnancy, is commonly known as cervical insufficiency. Characteristically, it is associated with painless dilatation of the cervix without uterine contraction. The membranes then protrude into the vagina and rupture, leading to rapid and painless delivery of the fetus. In many cases there is a clear history of traumatic injury to the cervix, such as traumatic delivery or a surgical procedure to the cervix, or congenital conditions such as uterine anomaly and diethylstilbestrol (DES) exposure. It is thought that the condition is due to a defect in the strength of the cervical tissue, either congenitally or acquired, resulting in the inability to maintain a pregnancy[1]. The incidence of cervical insufficiency is very difficult to determine because there are no clear clinical criteria for the diagnosis. However, cervical incompetence can be diagnosed in 0.1–1.0% of all pregnancies, and in 8% of women with repeated mid-trimester pregnancy loss[2].

The treatment consists of placing a purse-string suture around the cervix. The conventional method is by placing the sutures vaginally. This was first described by Lash and Lash in 1950[3], whereby they applied the suture in non-pregnant women. Subsequently, Shirodkar described his technique of insertion of a cervical suture in pregnancy[4]. The procedure is performed by first incising the anterior vaginal wall and pushing the bladder upward. The suture is placed under the vaginal wall around the cervix at the level of the internal os. Five women were also operated on in the non-pregnant state: three conceived. McDonald, in 1957, described a simpler purse-string suture around the body of the cervix without burying the sutures under the vaginal wall[5]. Although there is no good randomized study, clinical evidence strongly suggests that cervical cerclage decreases the occurrence of second-trimester pregnancy loss[6–13].

In a small proportion of women, cervical cerclage cannot be performed. In attempts to overcome this problem, several authors have advocated abdominal cerclage[14–16]. The indications to perform abdominal cervical cerclage are: short cervix, preventing adequate application of the suture, or when vaginal cerclage has previously failed.

ABDOMINAL CERCLAGE

Most women requiring cervical cerclage can be managed by a vaginal operation. However, those with an extremely short, deformed, scarred or absent cervix cannot be treated by the vaginal approach. Here, the cerclage has to be placed via an abdominal approach. Benson and Durfee described the first transabdominal cervicoisthmic cerclage (TCC) in 1965[17]. Most series have described TCC placement in pregnancy towards the end of the first trimester. However, preconception or interval placement of TCC has also been described, and many suggest some benefits over TCC placement in pregnancy. Groom et al. reported that preconception transabdominal cervicoisthmic cerclage was associated with a postoperative fetal survival rate of 100% for pregnancies that reached more than 12 weeks of gestation, compared with a preoperative fetal survival rate of 12%[18]. Anthony et al.[15] reported that this procedure increased the successful pregnancy rate from 16 to 86.6%. Nine of their 13 abdominal cerclages were performed in the non-pregnant state. In a review of 111 patients, the success rate was 89%, compared with only 19% before TCC[19].

The procedure is performed under anesthesia through a transverse suprapubic incision. The peritoneum overlying the bladder and uterus is divided, and the bladder is pushed caudally. The uterine vessels are identified and displaced laterally, and a suture is then placed around the cervix at the level of the internal os. The suture is tied posteriorly; this is to allow removal of the suture by posterior colpotomy if necessary[19]. The high anatomic placement of TCC compared with transvaginal cervical cerclage is believed to lead to improved results.

Potential advantages of the abdominal approach include high placement of the suture, no slippage of the suture, lack of a foreign body inside the vagina that could predispose to ascending infection and premature labor and the ability to leave the suture in place between pregnancies[20].

Until recently, abdominal cerclage required a laparotomy. The uterine vessels have to be dissected from the cervix to allow insertion of the suture medially. The technique is more demanding than that by the vaginal approach, and might lead to excessive bleeding from the uterine vessels. Transillumination of the uterine vessels and their branches with a laparoscope, and placing the suture through the avascular area of the paracervical tissue medial to the vessels, have been proposed. However, a laparotomy is still needed[21]. Excessive manipulation of the pregnant uterus could also lead to pregnancy loss. A simpler and less invasive abdominal cerclage would be beneficial.

Contraindications to abdominal cerclage are similar to those of the vaginal approach, including bulging membrane, ruptured membranes, intrauterine infections, fetal death, vaginal bleeding and a life-threatening maternal condition. Specific indications for transabdominal cerclage are: congenital short or absent cervix or extensively amputated cervix, marked scarring of the cervix, deep and jagged multiple cervical defects or previous failed vaginal cerclage. The efficacy of transabdominal cerclage has been established over more than three decades.

LAPAROSCOPIC ABDOMINAL CERCLAGE

A less invasive approach is laparoscopic abdominal cerclage[20,22]. This approach carries the advantages of the laparoscopic procedure, including no hospitalization, less pain and faster recovery. It can be done with minimal uterine manipulation and minimal dissection. Instead of tracking the uterine vessels and creating a window in the broad ligament, we and others[20] have found that the use of a disposable laparoscopic suturing device, piercing the broad ligament medial to the uterine vessels (Endo Close™; Tyco Healthcare, Gosport, UK), facilitates the procedure without the need for vessel dissection. The result of laparoscopic abdominal cerclage is as good as with abdominal cerclage[20,22–28].

Most cases of abdominal cerclage have been performed during pregnancy, usually after 10 weeks of gestation. Abdominal cerclage by laparotomy and by laparoscopy have been performed in the pregnant and non-pregnant states. In the pregnant state, an enlarged uterus and the potential risks to the fetus might be problems. However, some authors have suggested performing cerclage as an interval procedure (before pregnancy). In patients whose need for abdominal cerclage is clear, performing the procedure in the non-pregnant state has some advantages. These include decreased fetal or maternal risks, easy manipulation and exposure, and minimal bleeding.

CONCERNS ABOUT ABDOMINAL CERCLAGE IN NON-PREGNANT STATE

Many concerns have been raised about interval cerclage. One such concern is that the chance of conceiving following abdominal cerclage may be impaired. However, in patients who underwent laparoscopic radical trachelectomy and prophylactic cervical cerclage, the pregnancy rate was 55% by the 36th month of exposure[29]. One of the theoretical concerns relating to cerclage as an interval procedure is when the patient suffers another miscarriage. However, the cervix can easily be dilated to 8 mm, and curettage can be performed in the presence of a cerclage. Alternatively, laparoscopic removal of the cerclage can be performed. A pregnancy of >24 weeks' gestation clearly requires a cesarean delivery.

TECHNIQUE OF LAPAROSCOPIC ABDOMINAL CERCLAGE

The procedure is performed under general anesthesia. The patient is placed in the dorsal lithotomy position followed by insertion of an indwelling catheter. In a non-pregnant state, a uterine manipulator is inserted into the uterine cavity. Laparoscopy is done in the usual fashion, using two secondary trocars at low abdominal quadrants. Depending on the height of the uterus, the secondary trocars are inserted higher than those in the non-pregnant condition, and they should be inserted under direct vision. They are placed higher than the level of the uterine fundus.

The peritoneum of the uterovesical reflection is injected with normal saline to facilitate separation of the bladder from the cervix (Figures 36.1 and 36.2). In contrast to others[22], we identify but do not dissect the uterine vessels.

Cerclage is performed using a 5-mm Mersilene® polyester tape. The tape is first prepared by removing the needles from its ends, and the end of the tape is tapered. The adequate length is about 15 cm. The tape is then passed into the pelvis and positioned behind the uterus.

A disposable Endo Close suturing device is passed into the abdominal cavity suprapubically. Its tip is directed toward the isthmus, medial to the uterine vessels (Figure 36.2). The cardinal ligament and the cervical body are pierced, and the tip can be seen at the posterior leaf of the broad ligament just above the insertion of the uterosacral ligament. The end of the tape is grasped with the device, and the device is withdrawn anteriorly, bringing with it the tape (Figures 36.3 and 36.4). The procedure is then repeated on the opposite side, bringing the other end of the tape anteriorly. Using two laparoscopic needle holders, the two ends of the tape are tied anteriorly with a square knot (Figure 36.5). It is secured by another knot. The excess suture material is trimmed. The presence of the

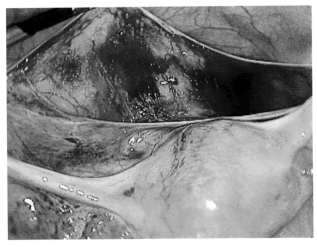

Figure 36.1 The bladder has been separated from the cervix. Reproduced from reference 20, with permission

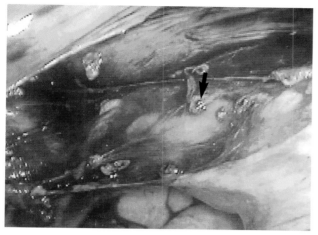

Figure 36.2 An arrow indicates the entry site of the suturing device. Note that the uterine vessels are located medially. Reproduced from reference 20, with permission

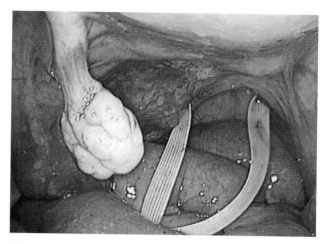

Figure 36.3 Posterior view of the uterus. Note that the suture has been placed around the posterior cervix

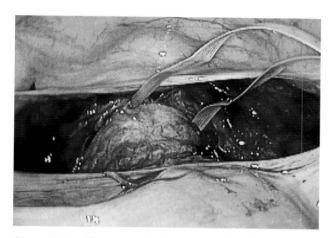

Figure 36.4 The suture has been properly placed

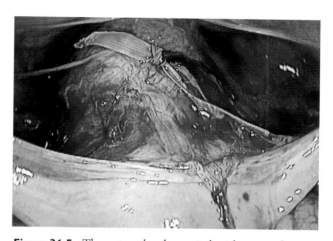

Figure 36.5 The suture has been tied with square knots

uterine manipulator inside the cervix prevents strangulation of the cervix. The abdominal cavity is irrigated with normal saline solution and homeostasis is confirmed.

SUMMARY

In women with an extremely short, deformed, scarred or absent cervix, abdominal cerclage is needed. It is conventionally performed by the laparotomy approach. Laparoscopic abdominal cerclage is a less invasive technique that could replace the laparotomy technique. It should be performed by laparoscopic surgeons with expertise in laparoscopic suturing. The authors have shown that dissection of the uterine vessels is not needed. Laparoscopic abdominal cerclage does not require

hospitalization, is associated with less pain and leads to faster recovery.

In patients whose need for abdominal cerclage is clear, performing the procedure in the non-pregnant state has some advantages. These include decreased fetal or maternal risk, easy manipulation and exposure, and minimal bleeding. Laparoscopic abdominal cerclage is equal to, or may be better than, abdominal cerclage by laparotomy.

REFERENCES

1. Ludmir J. Sonographic detection of cervical incompetence. Clin Obstet Gynecol 1988; 31: 101–9

Table 37.1 Classification of laparoscopic artificial assistance devices

Laparoscope holders: hold the laparoscope only

Static: the surgeon moves the laparoscope holder manually

    Kronner™ (Kronner Prototypes Inc, Roseburg, OR, USA)

    PASSIST

    Tiska® (Karlsruhe Research Center, Karlsruhe, Germany)

Dynamic: the surgeon moves the laparoscope holder by voice, finger or head control

    Aesop (Computer Motion): voice

    ImagTrack™ (Olympus, Tokyo, Japan): finger

    LapMan® (Medsys, Bembloux, Belgium): finger

    EndoAssist™ (Armstrong, Healthcare Ltd, Wycombe, UK): head

Laparoscope holders and instrument manipulators

Zeus™ (Computer Motion, Goleta, CA, USA)

da Vinci™ (Intuitive Surgical, Sunnyvale, CA, USA)

The idea of a dynamic laparoscope holder, able to displace the endoscope along the three axes under the command of an ergonomic control unit, was therefore conceived. This laparoscope manipulator was developed in collaboration with the surgical material firm, Medsys (Gembloux, Belgium).

At the same time, an ergonomic external control unit was developed. The challenge was to find which neuromuscular function could be used to achieve the command of six degrees of freedom, corresponding to displacement in three dimensions. A foot pedal requires eye control and can be uncomfortable in the long run, as noted by Mettler et al.[1]. Besides, the foot is already often used to command coagulation. Voice interface is an attractive idea but limited by two drawbacks: answering the order takes longer, slowing down the operation when the surgeon needs to move about a lot, and it is impossible to move obliquely.

We initially designed a remote control activated by the left fingers of the surgeon, fitting into the palm under the surgeon's glove; the left fingers were chosen because they belong to the surgically minor hand, and their function in dissection is limited to traction, retraction and irrigation, relatively trivial tasks compared with their potential. A variant in the form of a joystick box clipping onto the instrument under the index finger is now also available.

General description

The LapMan® (Figures 37.1 and 37.2) uses inexpensive technology, based on the electromechanical control of brakes regulating the displacement of a series of articulated arms, constructed to cover the three dimensions of space.

The assistant, of low bulk and mobile on motorized wheels, is composed of a rolling base and a sterile autoclavable shaft, which comes connected to the scope through an easy-release system. The machine displaces the shaft in the three dimensions, translating the displacement of the laparoscope connected to it. A laser pointer indicates the geometric center of the assistant.

The first human–machine interface we developed – the hand control (Figure 37.3) – is a small embedded electronic circuit, molded on the palm of one of the authors, to raise the thenar eminence towards the fingers in their natural flexed position. Six knobs corresponding to the six directions are distributed on the pad, which can be disposed along two schemes according to personal preference: three rows of two knobs, using the last three fingers, or two rows of three knobs using the last two. The unit holds to the index finger under a sterile glove. Pressing a button leads to a radiofrequency emission that is recognized by the receiver of the equipment. Pressing several buttons at once, according to a defined scheme, enables set-up actions to be realized during the calibration phase, such as switching on the laser pointer, backward/forward, upward/downward movements of the whole device or placing the arm in the neutral position. This pad is autoclavable, and the batteries allow 1 hour of uninterrupted activation.

We later developed another intuitive interface (Figure 37.4) in the form of a free, radiofrequency-emitting clippable joystick designed to be attached to the edge of the laparoscopic instrument, just under the index finger of the operator. The set-up phase on the right side of the patient is rapid; approximation of the scope holder to the umbilicus requires a 2-minute laser calibration.

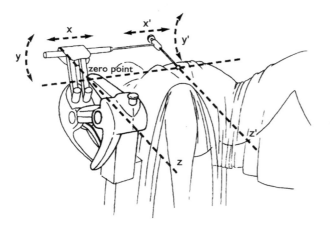

Figure 37.1 LapMan®: principle

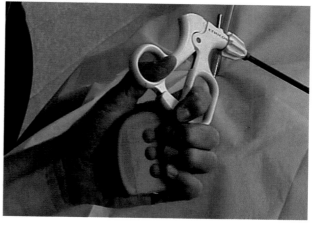

Figure 37.3 LapMan: hand control (under the glove)

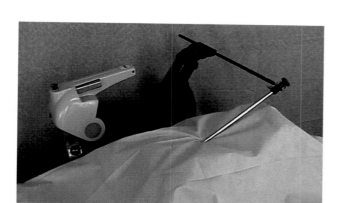

Figure 37.2 LapMan: external view

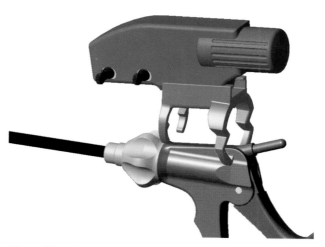

Figure 37.4 LapMan: joystick clipped onto the instrument

As there is a learning curve to familiarize oneself with the position of the buttons on the pad, software was developed allowing navigation in a three-dimensional pelvic environment using a palm-pad joystick, connected to the serial port of the surgeon's office PC; it is then possible to train effectively out of theater.

Advantages

This laparoscopic manipulator has several advantages. It provides the surgeon with a steady image and offers a simultaneous response to the surgeon's commands, positively influencing the fluency of the operation. Steadiness is obviously useful for suturing and helps in orientation. Besides restoring autonomy of vision, it allows work in conditions of reduced personnel; solo surgery for straightforward cases is carried out in very comfortable conditions. Compared with other laparoscopic assistance systems, the LapMan is not cumbersome, is easy to move on its rolling base and, for these reasons, could surely be labeled 'nurse-friendly'. The electromechanical technology is simple and robust; it is also by far the cheapest of all engine-driven

laparoscope holders ever produced. The polyvalence of the LapMan must be emphasized, as it allows one to perform abdominal surgery by rotating the LapMan cranially and permits operation from either side of the patient. In the list of advantages, compared with other modalities, the LapMan has the essential characteristic of answering instantaneously to the surgeon's command, important on two levels: (1) it will probably function better in operative fields with a frequently moving scope; (2) it is safer, as release of the knob stops the move instantaneously.

In common with all laparoscope holders, dynamic scope holders do not cope well with the need to move frequently on the target (as the movements are sequential, not oblique). These situations are encountered in severe adhesiolysis cases, large structures (large uteri, ovarian cysts, etc.) and in operations covering two distant fields (laparoscopic promontofixation).

Indications in gynecological surgery

Considering the first version of the hand control, we initially stated that use of the LapMan was indicated in reduced personnel conditions for straightforward, uncomplicated cases of laparoscopic surgery, which in gynecology represents all adnexal surgery and small- to medium-size uterus surgery (myomectomy, laparoscopic subtotal hysterectomy (LASH), laparoscopic hysterectomy (LH)), and in digestive surgery and gallbladder and hiatal surgery.

The latest developments of the interface, which produced a more sophisticated joystick by increasing the ergonomics and intuitiveness, definitely enable the surgeon to operate on more complex pathologies in restricted personnel conditions and yield increased satisfaction from being able to reoperate bimanually with visual operative field control.

The concept of solo surgery: response to lack of operating room staff (Figure 37.5)

The development of surgeon-controlled laparoscope holders has an interesting implication: it allows the surgeon to operate in restricted personnel conditions for straightforward, uncomplicated procedures. Adnexal surgery of moderate size (5–6 cm) and subtotal hysterectomy cases of (sub) normal size are ideally suited to laparoscopic solo surgery, because the target organ is mobile and the range of scope manipulation is somewhat limited. In the event of reduced personnel resources, these artificial arms render these procedures possible; solo surgery sessions can therefore be performed in emergency cases (bleeding ectopic pregnancy, acute adnexal pathology) or planned on an elective basis, grouping, for example, trans-hysteroscopic resections and simple laparoscopic surgery cases. Table 37.2 lists the procedures which may be performed in these conditions.

OTHER LAPAROSCOPE HOLDERS[2]

Passive laparoscope holders

Several laparoscope holders are available on the market today (Table 37.2). They attach to the rail side of the oper-

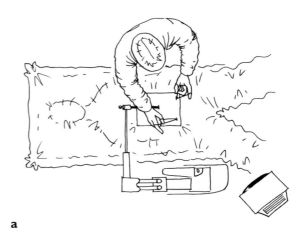

a

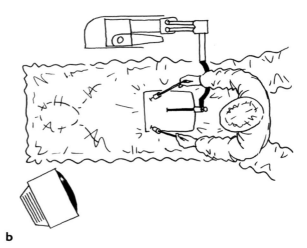

b

Figure 37.5 Solo surgery with the LapMan: (a) in gynecology, (b) in abdominal surgery

ating table. Their use depends essentially on the resistance to movement that they can provide and the facility to change position comfortably. These holders can also be used to hold instruments. The Tiska® endoarm[3,4] has been widely investigated, and gives surgeons a great deal of satisfaction. Also worthy of note is the Kronner telescopic arm laparoscope holder (Figure 37.6); pressing an electronic control attached to the camera releases the joints for quick

Table 37.2 Indications for the LapMan in laparoscopic solo surgery

Adnexal surgery (ovariectomy, adnexectomy, salpingotomy, salpingectomy, ectopic pregnancy, ovarian cystectomy)

Small- to mid-size laparoscopic hysterectomy (LH, LASH)

Myomectomy (subserosal)

LH, laparoscopic hysterectomy; LASH, laparoscopic subtotal hysterectomy

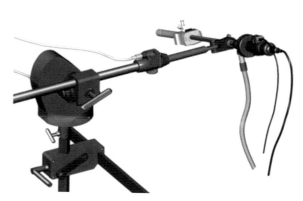

Figure 37.6 Kronner laparoscope holder

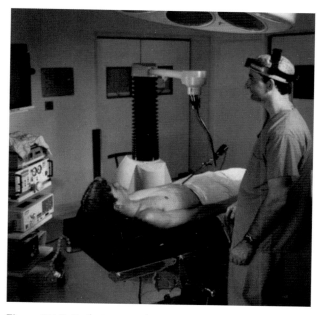

Figure 37.8 EndoAssist™ laparoscope holder (interface: head tilt)

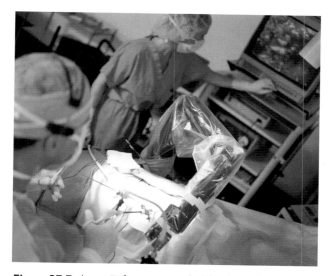

Figure 37.7 Aesop™ laparoscope holder (interface: voice)

position changes. The position is held by gas pressure available in the operating room.

Passive laparoscope holders offer image steadiness and a substitution for human assistance, when necessary.

Active laparoscope holders

To move in the operative field, passive laparoscope holders need to be moved by the surgeon's hand; this interrupts his concentration and limits eye–hand coordination. Besides providing steadiness and a substitute for human assistance, active laparoscopic holders (see Table 37.1) have been developed to offer simultaneous vision and instrument control, as is the case in classic surgery.

Active machines differ in technology, some being much more expensive than others, and the interface used for command. The ideal characteristics should take into account cost, robustness, cumbersomeness, set-up time, user-friendliness of the control unit and response time.

Aesop™ 3000 (Computer Motion)

Aesop (Figure 37.7) has come up with several control units: foot, hand and voice operated. Comparative studies tend to consider voice control as being preferable to the other options[1,4–6]. The Aesop 3000 is a voice-controlled surgical robot imitating the form and function of the human arm. By orally introducing simple spoken commands, the robotic arm moves the scope in the three dimensions of space. The response is almost instantaneous. Speech-recognition technology requires the surgeon to familiarize the system with his voice. Each order must be specifically introduced, for the machine not to become confused with background theater noise. The displacement in space is the sum of simple displacements, and obliquity is not achieved. This model was inspired by robotic technology, which makes it the most expensive in its category, although cost-effectiveness has been demonstrated[7].

EndoAssist™ (Armstrong)

This system (Figure 37.8) holds a conventional laparoscope and camera, and moves them in accordance with the surgeon's head, which it tracks using a headband pointer. Thus, a glance at the right-hand side of the monitor causes the camera to pan in that direction. The robot only moves if the surgeon presses a foot switch, but allows different head movements at other times[5].

FIPS

The FIPS (Figure 37.9)[4,8] is a remote-controlled arm capable of moving a rigid endoscope with about four

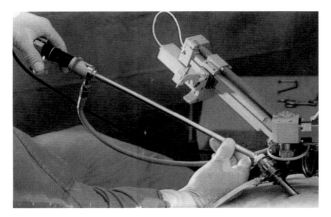

Figure 37.9 FIPS laparoscope holder (interface: voice or finger)

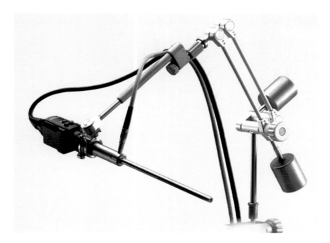

Figure 37.10 ImagTrack laparoscope holder (interface: finger)

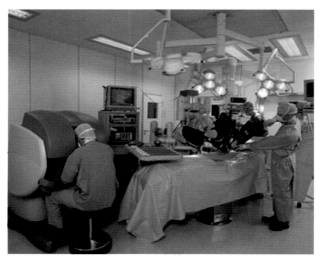

Figure 37.11 da Vinci™ robot

degrees of freedom, while maintaining an invariant point of constrained motion coincident with the trocar puncture site through the abdominal wall. The system is driven by means of speaker-independent voice control or a finger-ring joystick clipped onto the instrument shaft close to the handle. When the joystick is used, the motion of the endoscope is controlled by the fingertip of the operating surgeon, which is inserted into the small ring of the controller in such a way as to make the motion of the fingertip correspond directly to the motion of the tip of the endoscope.

ImagTrack (Olympus)

A 13-mm integrated camera/laparoscope (Figure 37.10)[9,10] with an 80° visual field is inserted intraumbilically. Inside this immobile field (the laparoscope stands still), a mobile charge coupled device (CCD) chip is displaced in an *x–y* axis, under voice or fingertip control, through a unit attached to the handle of the left instrument. In/out is obtained by a zooming effect. This system has already proved its feasibility in simple laparoscopic surgery. The main advantage is rapid manipulation of the lens displacement, but the inability to approach organs physically could result in a reduced sense of depth perception. The integrated aspect of the camera/scope makes multiuse of the camera for other forms of surgical endoscopy impossible.

Others

There has been very active interest in this field, and other systems have been conceived, some still under development. A self-guided robotic camera control system (SGRCCS)[11] is based on color tracking. The tip of one instrument is marked with a specific color and the camera is programmed to follow this unnatural dye, moving the laparoscope holder so that the color always stays in the operative field. Blood does not significantly interfere. The inconvenience is that this instrument must always remain in the field.

INSTRUMENT MANIPULATION

With the manipulation of instruments by fully integrated robots (Figure 37.11) a new dimension is reached compared with simple laparoscope holders, and these robots will serve different purposes. This development responds to the need to refine the precision of movements, essentially microsuturing, but not the concept of solo surgery, as the set-up and change of instruments nevertheless requires the presence of an assistant at the side of the patient.

Indeed, associated with the automated scope holder, there has been extensive development in the robotic enhancement of instrument manipulation itself. The

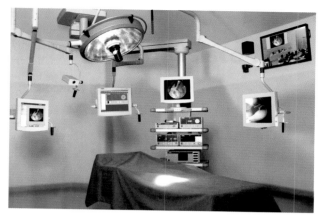

Figure 37.12 Karl Storz OR1™

instruments are supported by robotic arms and no longer by the human hand; the surgeon operates from a console at a distance from the patient, in the same or another room, in the same hospital or even from another country, through Internet connections.

A description of these fully integrated robots and their performance in the field of laparoscopic gynecological surgery is presented in Chapter 38.

FULLY INTEGRATED OPERATING ROOM

Several companies are now integrating the management of the operative laparoscopic surgery theater suite into a fully surgeon-controlled environment[12]. Surgical robotic companies are adapting their robot products to this type of technology, maximizing, more than ever, the concept of surgical ergonomics. Karl Storz is among those leading the way in this integration process. The main idea behind the Karl Storz OR1™ (Figure 37.12) integration concept is a standardized communication bus (SCB). This interface forms the basis for the entire system. Endoscopic devices, such as video cameras, cold light sources, insufflators and suction and irrigation pumps, as well as the operating table, blinds and operating light, are controlled via the SCB.

An integrated digital recording system simplifies the archiving of image, video and audio data of important surgical steps and results. This information can be used for both patient documentation and scientific evaluations. Connection to the hospital information system (HIS) and picture archiving and communication system (PACS) optimizes quick access to patient and image data.

In addition, telemedicine applications, such as video conferences and live operations for teaching and training purposes, can be controlled directly from the operating area, owing to the integration of state-of-the-art audio and video technology. This also allows the 'virtual presence' of a remotely placed expert, who would be able to provide a second opinion to an ongoing live operative procedure.

There is no doubt that working conditions in laparoscopic surgery will evolve in the future towards better comfort. It is difficult to believe that basic straightforward laparoscopic cases will always need two operators; staff shortages should not be an obstacle to performing endoscopic surgery. In this respect, future developments in the field of artificial assistance need to be followed with the greatest interest.

REFERENCES

1. Mettler L, Ibrahim M, Jonat W. One year of experience working with the aid of a robotic assistant (the voice-controlled optic holder AESOP) in gynaecological surgery. Hum Reprod 1998; 13: 2748–50
2. Jaspers JE, Breedveld P, Herder JL, Grimbergen CA. Camera and instrument holders and their clinical value in minimally invasive surgery. Surg Laparosc Endosc Percutan Tech 2004; 14: 145–52
3. Shurr MO, Arezzo A, Neisius B, et al. Trocar and instrument positioning system TISKA. An assist device for endoscopic solo surgery. Surg Endosc 1999; 13: 528–31
4. Arezzo A, Ulmer F, Weiss O, et al. Experimental trial on solo surgery for minimally invasive therapy. Comparison of different systems in a phantom model. Surg Endosc 2000; 14: 955–9
5. Yavuz Y, Ystgaard B, Skogvoll E, Marvik R. A comparative experimental study evaluating he performance of surgical robots Aesop and Endosista. Surg Laparosc Endosc Percutan Tech 2000; 10: 163–7
6. Mettler L. Robotics versus human golden fingers in gynaecological endoscopy. Presented at the First World Congress on Controversies in Obstetrics, Gynecology and Infertility, Prague, Czech Republic, 1999
7. Dunlop KD, Wanzer L. Is the robotic arm a cost-effective surgical tool? AORN J 1998; 68: 265–72
8. Buess GF, Arezzo A, Schurr MO, et al. A new remote-controlled endoscope positioning system for endoscpoic solo surgery. The FIPS endoarm. Surg Endosc 2000; 14: 395–9
9. Niebuhr H, Born O. Image tracking system. A new technique for safe and cost-saving laparoscopic operation. Chirug 2000; 71: 580–4
10. Kimura T, Umehara Y, Matsumoto S. Laparoscopic cholicystectomy performed by a single surgeon using a visual field tracking camera: early experience. Surg Endosc 2000; 14: 825–9
11. Omote K, Feussner H, Ungeheuer A, et al. Self-guided robotic camera control for laparoscopic surgery compared with human camera control. Am J Surg 1999; 177: 321–4
12. Berci G, Phillips EH, Fujita F. The operating room of the future: what, when, and why? Surg Endosc 2004; 18: 1–5

expert care without requiring patients to travel. The main difficulty with telesurgery has been the lack of a rapid and secure means of transmitting signals between the surgeon and the operating room, as the signal latency must be less than 330 ms to prevent perceptible delay. Anvari *et al.* recently reported performing 21 telesurgical procedures between two hospitals in Canada, 250 miles apart, using an existing commercial Internet fiberoptic network, with the goal being to provide telementoring and telesurgery between eight teaching hospitals and 32 rural communities in Canada over the next 3 years[10]. Ultimately, a wireless system could allow telesurgery to be performed on ships, or even in space.

SURGICAL TRAINING AND PREOPERATIVE PLANNING

Virtual reality trainers could augment operative experience by enabling physicians to practice both basic skills and actual surgical procedures of varying degrees of difficulty, as well as with variations in anatomic and pathological states. The movements and forces of the instruments can be tracked and recorded for later review by a mentor as a more efficient, less costly and safer way to educate and credential physicians.

Virtual surgical planning would involve planning, practicing and viewing the outcome of a procedure using a virtual three-dimensional (3D) model of the patient generated by preoperative imaging studies, anatomic atlases and other data, such as organ deformation with surgical manipulation. The next step would be to superimpose this model over the 3D image of the patient on a monitor or head-mounted display in the operating room, such that deep structures could be 'seen'. It may even be possible to record the movements of the instruments from the surgical planning session and program them into the robot, which could then carry out the process with greater precision.

TECHNIQUE

The procedure described is a robotically assisted reversal of a tubal ligation. The advantage of robotic access is the ability of the robot to perform precise, fine movements required for tubal surgery.

Specific equipment

The only robotic system that is still marketed for gynecological surgery is the da Vinci system. The basic robotic set-up consists of a console, a video cart and a robotic tower (Figure 38.1). The surgeon sits at a console away from the surgical field (Figure 38.2). In the da Vinci procedure, the surgeon looks into a console that has a dual lens system within the 12-mm laparoscope. The system provides true

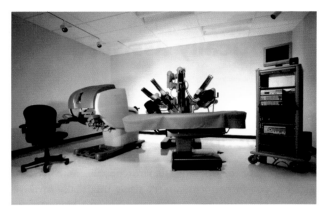

Figure 38.1 The complete robotic unit consists of a console, the robotic tower and the video cart. Courtesy of Intuitive Surgical

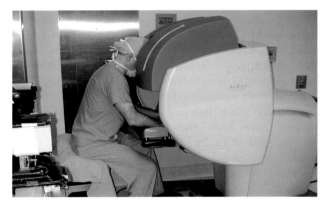

Figure 38.2 The surgeon is seated at the console to perform the surgery. Courtesy of Intuitive Surgical

binocular 3D vision that is seen with the use of a microscope. Movement of the laparoscope is accomplished through movement of the handles at the console. Movement of the handles at the console allows movement of the robotic arms at the operative site. Motion scaling, the ability to reduce the motion of the surgeon's hands at the surgical site, allows fine, delicate movements. For example, a scaling ratio of 10 : 1 means that for every 1 cm the surgeon moves the handles at the console, the robotic surgical instruments would move 1 mm at the surgical site. The console has infrared beams to deactivate the robotic arms when the surgeon's head is out of the console.

The console is connected by a cable to the video cart and robotic tower (Figure 38.1 and 38.3). The video cart includes the equipment to attach the laparoscope and light sources. The robotic tower supports three or four robotic arms (Figure 38.3). The robotic arms hold the specifically designed instruments that perform the surgery. The instruments have an intra-abdominal articulation 2 cm from the tip. This articulation serves the same function as a human wrist (Figure 38.4). The movement of the instrument tip is intuitive and requires minimal training.

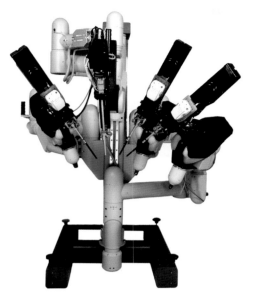

Figure 38.3 The robotic tower has three or four arms that hold instruments or the laparoscope. Courtesy of Intuitive Surgical

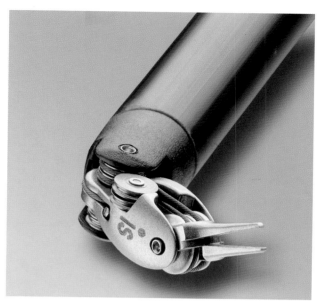

Figure 38.4 The special feature of the robotic arm is the ability for seven degrees of freedom at the effector tip. Courtesy of Intuitive Surgical

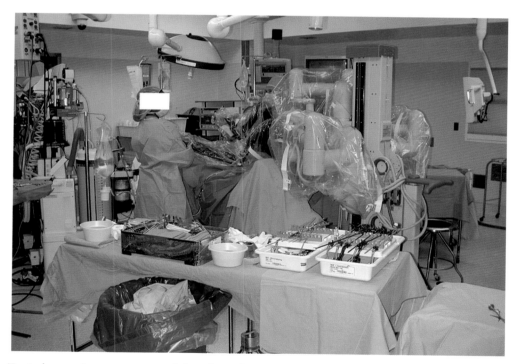

Figure 38.5 Typical operating room set-up of the robot. The tower is placed between the patient's legs and the robotic arms are attached to the instruments in the lateral ports

There are several disadvantages of the surgical robot that warrant mention. Weighing 1200 lb, the da Vinci robot is large and very cumbersome. The operating table cannot be repositioned once the robot is in place. The surgical assistant's access to ancillary ports and the uterine manipulator are severely compromised (Figure 38.5). There is no haptic feedback, and therefore the surgeon will need to use visual cues to assess the limit to which a tissue or suture can be pulled. During initial experience, sutures can be broken, adding to operating time. Port placement for the

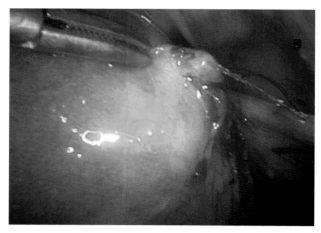

Figure 38.6 The proximal anastomosis site has been prepared and patency is demonstrated

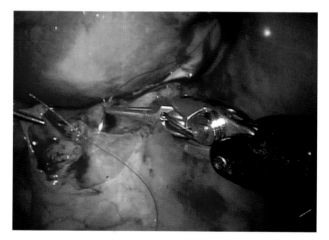

Figure 38.7 The robotic arm is about to drive the needle into the distal mesosalpinx. This is the first stitch

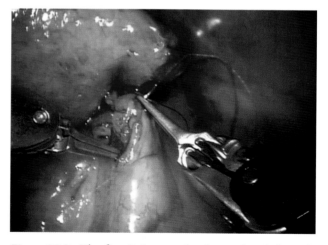

Figure 38.8 The first 8-0 suture has been placed through the muscularis and through the mucosa of the distal anastomosis site. The needle tip is seen through the lumen. The subsequent stitch will be through the proximal site

robotic arms is necessarily higher on the abdomen and is less cosmetic. Experience is required to place these ports for the robotic arms properly so that access to different areas of the pelvis is possible. If for some reason, the surgeon needs to convert to conventional laparoscopy the robotic port sites may not be useful.

Procedure

For a tubal reversal procedure, a four-puncture technique is utilized. The patient is placed in the lithotomy position. A 12-mm trocar is required at the umbilicus for the laparoscope. Two specially designed 8-mm trocars are placed in the right and left lateral abdominal areas. These sites are typically lateral to the rectus muscle and 3–4 cm below the level of the umbilicus. These trocars attach directly to the arms that come off the robotic cart. A fourth 5-mm trocar that serves as an accessory port is placed just suprapubically. This allows introduction of the fine 6-0 and 8-0 suture into the peritoneal cavity with minimal movement of the panoramic view of the laparoscope. Once peritoneal access is gained with all four trocars, the patient is placed in steep Trendelenburg position. The robotic cart is placed between the legs and the robotic arms are attached to the instruments in the lateral ports (Figure 38.5).

The proximal and distal anastomosis sites are prepared. Microscissors and cautery are available on the robot, or this can be accomplished conventionally before attaching the robot (Figure 38.6). The next step is to approximate the mesosalpinx using a Vicryl® 6-0 suture (Figure 38.7). Once the proximal and distal site are closely aligned, Vicryl 8-0 is used for the classical two-layered closure. The first layer is the mucosal–muscularis layer and the second is the serosal layer. Three to four interrupted stitches are used for each layer. The first is placed at 6 o'clock, so as to tie the knot outside the lumen (Figure 38.8). The next step is to place the 12 o'clock stitch. Typically it is not tied, to allow continued visibility of the lumen. The individual stitches are tied using the standard 'instrument' tie technique (Figure 38.9). A few final serosal stitches are placed (Figure 38.10), and patency of the anastomosis is confirmed by visualizing spill of transcervically injected indigo carmine dye through the fimbriated end of the tube.

CONCLUSION

The da Vinci system can enable the less experienced laparoscopic surgeon to operate on more advanced cases. In situations where fine motor skills are required, such as tubal reversal, there may be an immediate role. Randomized studies looking at short- and long-term outcome data are required to assess the current role of the surgical robot.

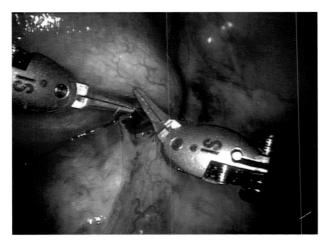

Figure 38.9 The left robotic needle holder is about to circle around the right needle holder to tie the stitch

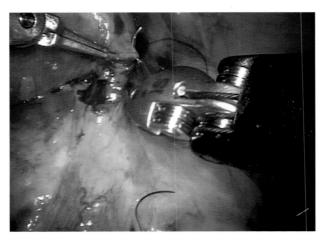

Figure 38.10 This image shows the capability of the robot to place easily the stitch in a reverse direction

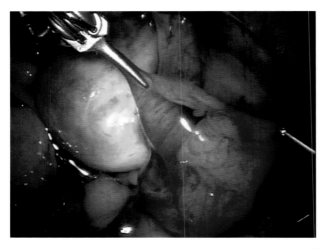

Figure 38.11 The completed anastomosis shows spill of indigo carmine dye through the fimbriated end of the tube

REFERENCES

1. Dharia SP, Falcone T. Robotics in reproductive medicine. Fertil Steril 2005; 84: 1–12
2. Mettler L, Ibrahim M, Jonat W. One year of experience working with the aid of a robotic assistant (the voice-controlled optic holder AESOP) in gynecologic endoscopic surgery. Hum Reprod 1998; 13: 2748–50
3. Dakin GF, Gagner M. Comparison of laparoscopic skills performance between standard instruments and two surgical robotic systems. Surg Endosc 2003; 17: 574–9
4. Falcone T, Goldberg JM, Margossian H, Stevens L. Robotically assisted laparoscopic microsurgical anastomosis: a human pilot study. Fertil Steril 2000; 73: 1040–2
5. Degueldre M, Vandromme J, Huong PT, Cadiere GB. Robotically assisted laparoscopic microsurgical tubal reanastomosis: a feasibility study. Fertil Steril 2000; 74: 1020–3
6. Goldberg JM, Falcone T. Laparoscopic microsurgical tubal anastomosis with and without robotic assistance. Hum Reprod 2003; 18: 145–7
7. Diaz-Arrastia C, Jurnalov C, Gomez G, Townsend C Jr. Laparoscopic hysterectomy using a computer-enhanced surgical robot. Surg Endosc 2002; 16: 1271–3
8. Advincula AP, Song A, Burke W, Reynolds RK. Preliminary experience with robot-assisted laparoscopic myomectomy. J Am Assoc Gynecol Laparosc 2004; 11: 511–18
9. Elliott DS, Frank I, Dimarco DS, Chow GK. Gynecologic use of robotically assisted laparoscopy: sacrocolpopexy for the treatment of high-grade vaginal vault prolapse. Am J Surg 2004; 188 (Suppl 4A): 52–6S
10. Anvari M, McKinley C, Stein H. Establishment of the world's first telerobotic remote surgical service: for provision of advanced laparoscopic surgery in a rural community. Ann Surg 2005; 241: 460–4

Two weeks after surgery, the patient mentioned loss of stools vaginally. Conservative treatment (antibiotics and a diet with no fiber) was applied for several weeks. Three months later, a control X-ray of the bowel with contrast injection confirmed complete healing. This lesion was probably due to a thermal injury.

In this same series, one case of fecal peritonitis occurred 10 days after adenomyotic nodule resection. A bowel enema (with Gastrografin®) revealed a large lateral defect 8–10 cm from the anal margin. A first treatment involving insertion of a drain through the vagina was insufficient (Figure 39.6). A laparotomy was carried out for peritoneal lavage and drainage, and to perform a colostomy.

Since the publication of this first series, the number of laparoscopies performed for adenomyotic rectovaginal nodules increased up to 2147 cases in the series completed in August 2005. Six rectal injuries occurred during 'shaving' of the rectum, and were diagnosed immediately during laparoscopy (Figure 39.7). As all the patients received a prior bowel preparation, immediate laparoscopic suture could be performed in one or two layers (Figure 39.8). Tissucol® was applied to aid healing (Figure

39.9). All the patients ate a fiberless diet for 3 weeks and recovered without any further complications.

We recommend avoiding laser or electrosurgery when performing adhesiolysis of the bowel (Figure 39.10). Indeed, injuries caused by scissors can be more easily managed, with a lower risk of secondary perforation due to necrosis.

Diagnosis In some cases, diagnosis is delayed, and patients present with signs of peritonitis or bowel occlusion. Intraoperatively, the diagnosis is made by direct visualization of the damage.

Management Management of perforations of the bowel is related to the site and extent of the damage, and to when the injury is discovered. For large perforations provoked by the laser beam or an electrosurgical device and diagnosed intraoperatively, a laparotomy with resection of the necrotic zone could be necessary, especially if the endoscopist is not trained for this type of surgery. If the patient has had a preoperative bowel preparation, repair by laparoscopic suture is possible for an experienced surgeon[66]. The bowel must be repaired with two-layer sutures. This type of closure is appropriate only if the damage is limited and superficial. In the presence of a

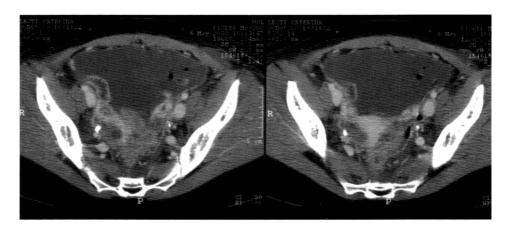

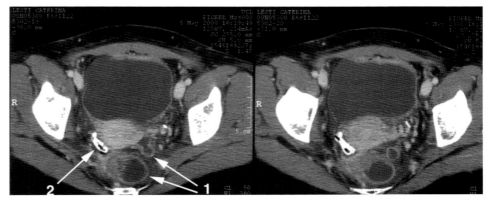

Figure 39.6 Liquid collection in the abdominal cavity, 10 days after adenomyotic nodule resection. Diagnosis of fecal peritonitis was made. 1, 3-cm collection in the left pararectal space; 2, vaginal drain

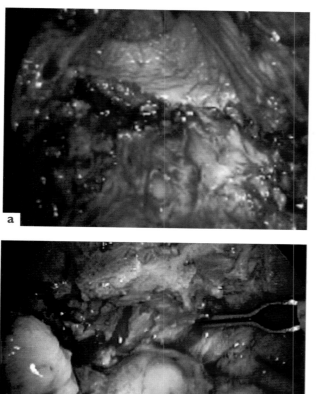

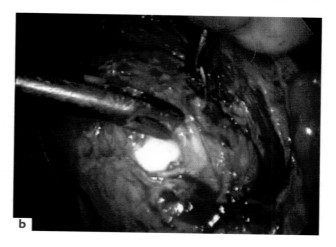

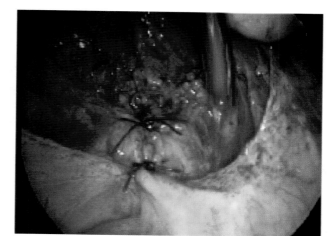

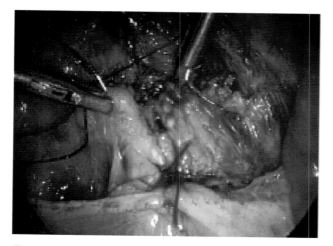

Figure 39.7 Rectal perforations. (a) and (b) The rectal cannula is seen through the rectal lesion. (c) Rectal mucosa

Figure 39.8 Laparoscopic rectal suture in two layers

significant bowel lesion or peritonitis, a timely intraoperative consultation with the general surgeon is mandatory to decide how to handle the damage.

Prevention Surgery must only be carried out by an experienced surgeon, with adequate instruments[67], especially when bowel adhesiolysis is required. Care must be taken when using monopolar electrosurgery to ensure that the patient's return plate is properly attached, the instruments are well insulated and the bowel is out of the field of energy application. With bipolar coagulation, the

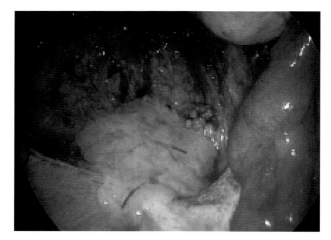

Figure 39.9 Tissucol® applied to rectal suture

forceps must not come into contact with the bowel when activated or immediately after inactivation.

In our department, if difficult laparoscopic surgery (resection of a rectovaginal adenomyotic nodule, suspicion of numerous adhesions) is to be performed, the patient receives a bowel preparation. Thus, in the case of bowel lesions diagnosed during surgery, direct suture can be performed. This technique avoids the temporary colostomy that is normally indicated in this type of complication without a bowel preparation.

Bladder injury during surgical procedures

This complication occurs more frequently in the case of patients who have a history of cesarean section or previous surgery, or whose bladder is not empty before surgery. The injury can happen during the installation phase (insertion of the insufflation needle or trocars) or during the operative procedure, by thermal injury (electrocoagulation, laser) and blunt dissection.

Mode of diagnosis   Urine may be seen in the pelvis, usually secondary to an extraperitoneal perforation or laceration. If an injury is suspected but no definitive urine is seen, two tests for diagnosis are possible. First, 5 ml of indigo carmine or methylene blue can be administered intravenously. Another possibility is to inject methylene blue, diluted in 500 ml of saline solution, retrogradely through a urine catheter, so that the bladder can be checked laparoscopically for leakage. Because the bladder is hidden within the true pelvis, injuries to the lateral and posterior wall may be missed visually. Therefore, if bladder damage is suspected postoperatively, a gravity cystogram should be performed immediately. Approximately 250 ml of contrast medium is infused into the bladder by gravity drainage, and an X-ray film is obtained. If a rupture is seen, a catheter is inserted to allow gravity drainage, which starts immediately. Small bladder perforations may be seen on the lateral, oblique or drain-out films. Radiographically,

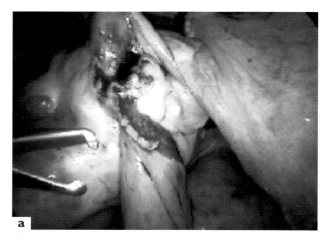

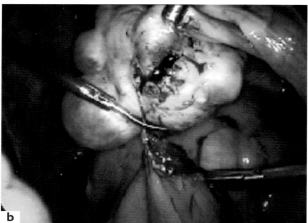

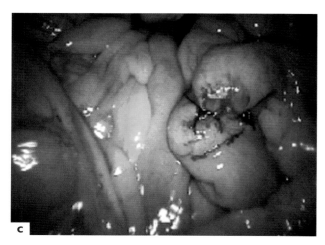

Figure 39.10 (a) and (b) Adhesiolysis of the small intestine with scissors. (c) Sutured bowel

intraperitoneal injuries will allow contrast medium to fill the cul-de-sac, outline loops of bowel and extend along the pericolic gutter.

Suprapubic pain and fullness, with or without diminished urine output, may suggest bladder injury. If an intraperitoneal bladder injury has been missed, a dramatic increase in blood urea nitrogen (BUN), due to urinary contact with the peritoneum, is observed. The definitive diagnosis is made by cystography.

Thermal injuries to the bladder may not manifest themselves initially. Sudden hematuria, well into the post-operative period, may be a sign of thermal damage. A true perforation may not yet be present and, therefore, a negative cystogram may be misleading. Cystoscopy should be performed to identify any areas of devitalized tissue.

Management   The first rule in the treatment of a bladder injury is a 10-day drainage. In the case of small leaks (< 1 cm) or extraperitoneal damage, drainage may be sufficient. A gravity cystogram is performed on day 8–10, and, if no extravasation is noted, the catheter is removed.

In other cases, immediate surgical repair is necessary.

In a case of significant bladder laceration, open surgery may be required to identify the lesion clearly and close the perforation carefully in one or two layers, with Vicryl® 2-0. In most cases, laparoscopic repair can be easily performed. A one- or two-layer suture must be carried out. The bladder catheter is left in place for 10 days. Prior to catheter removal, a cystogram can be performed. If the leak persists, drainage is prolonged for up to 20 days before repeating the cystogram.

In the case of bladder laceration in our first series, the diagnosis was made during the vaginal approach in laparoscopy-assisted vaginal hysterectomy. The closure of the laceration was performed vaginally, using 2-0 chromic catgut.

In the case of delayed diagnosis, bladder injuries are handled in the same way as for other traumatic ruptures. Intraperitoneal leaks are repaired and drained.

Prevention   The first step before inserting the suprapubic trocar is to check that the bladder is well catheterized. After emptying the bladder, the second step to prevent trocar damage is visualization of the dome of the bladder when inserting the trocar. Patients who have had a previous cesarean section, or who have undergone multiple pelvic surgery, could present with an anatomic distortion in peritoneal bladder repair; thus, the anatomy has to be taken into consideration.

Ureteral injury during surgical procedures

The incidence of this type of injury has risen during the past 10–15 years, essentially due to three different factors. The increasing number of surgeons using these techniques and the use of new instruments inevitably contribute to the growing incidence. But another important reason is the increased use of laparoscopy for complicated surgical procedures such as hysterectomy, lymphadenectomy and extensive endometriotic lesions of the uterosacral ligaments and rectovaginal septum.

In 1994, we published a review of the literature and personal cases before that year[68]. Ureteral lesions occurred during surgery for sterilization and endometriosis.

In our personal series from 1986 to 2000[69], ten ureteral lesions were encountered (Table 39.3) in more than 19 000 gynecological laparoscopies, giving an incidence of 0.05%. The prevalence was 2/12 000 (0.016%) until 1992, and then 8/7000 (0.11%), i.e. 6.8 times higher than in the first series. In this second series, injuries were sustained during hysterectomies and laparoscopies for severe endometriosis.

In our series of 2147 laparoscopic surgical procedures performed for deep nodular lesions, the rate of ureteral lesions was 0.4%. Indeed, three cases of ureteral transection and three cases of ureteral fistula due to thermal damage occurred in our series. The three cases of ureteral transection were diagnosed on the first or second day postoperatively due to the presence of urine in the abdominal drain. In one case, ureteral catheterization could be performed by cystoscopy. In the other two cases, cystoscopic catheterization failed and nephrostomy was performed. The patients were scheduled for surgery involving reimplantation of the ureter into the bladder 3 months later. In the first patient, in whom cystoscopic ureteral catheterization was successful, pyelography after 3 months of catheterization showed spontaneous healing, and no surgery was required. The other two patients underwent laparotomy and reimplantation of the ureter into the bladder. Recovery was uneventful. The three ureteral fistulas were diagnosed on days 7 and 8 postoperatively. The patients presented with abdominal pain and fever. Abdominal examination revealed peritoneal irritation and a computed tomography (CT) scan showed the presence of contrast medium in the retroperitoneal space after injection of a contrast medium. Intravenous pyelography confirmed the presence of a ureteral fistula. In all patients, cystoscopic ureteral catheterization could be performed. Intravenous pyelography after 3 months showed complete healing with an absence of fistulas. The ureteral catheters were removed.

In the literature, the incidence ranges from 0.12 to 0.25%[1,70,71].

A recent review by Ostrzenski *et al.*[73] of 70 ureteral injuries that occurred during laparoscopy reports incidences ranging from < 1 to 2%. Ureteral injuries reported in peer-reviewed journals often lack detailed presentation of the initial laparoscopic surgery, or of the location, type and instrumentation involved in the ureteral injury. Laparoscopy-assisted vaginal hysterectomy was the procedure during which most injuries occurred, and instruments involved in electrocoagulation were the main offenders.

Ureteral injury is often not due to the actual transection, but to the application of thermal energy near the ureter, causing tissue necrosis with subsequent stenosis and fistulas. Therefore, symptoms do not usually appear before 7 days after surgery. Indeed, a period of 7 days is generally required for the development of a ureteral fistula.

SECTION II
Operative hysteroscopy

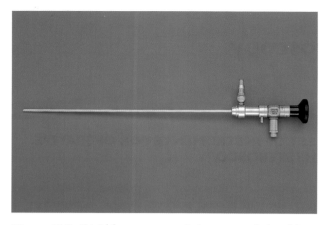

Figure 40.2 Rigid hysteroscope (telescope and sheath)

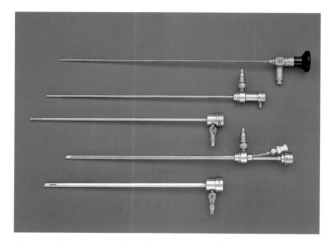

Figure 40.3 Bettocchi hysteroscope®. From top to bottom: telescope (diameter 2.9 mm), diagnostic sheaths single/continuous flow, sheaths with working channel instruments size 5F

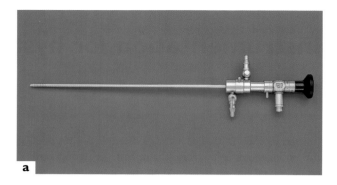

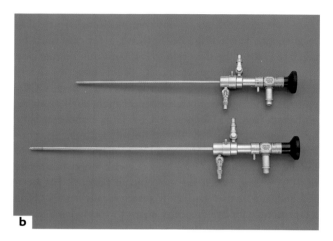

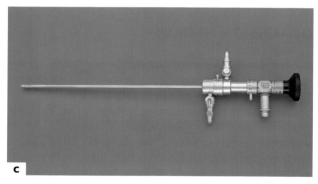

Figure 40.4 (a) Bettocchi hysteroscope, telescope (diameter 2.9 mm) with continuous flow sheath, outer diameter 4.5 mm. (b) Bettochi hysteroscopes in different diameters. (c) Bettochi hysteroscope, telescope (diameter 2.0 mm) with continuous flow sheaths, outer diameter 3.6 mm

light transmission and a sheath diameter between 3.5 and 4 mm (Figure 40.3). This allows direct access to the uterine cavity in almost all cases, and is associated with significantly fewer complaints in comparison with 5-mm instruments. The field of view and brightness are reduced in these hysteroscopes owing to the smaller diameter of the telescope, and this can cause occasional difficulties in a large, bleeding uterine cavity.

Some manufacturers offer hysteroscopes which allow the optional use of an additional inner sheath that is inserted into the outer sheath (Figure 40.4). By assembling both sheaths, it is possible to create a continuous flow system which can be used for controlled irrigation of the uterine cavity (Figures 40.5 and 40.6). The entire outer diameter can then be extended to 4.5–5 mm.

Resectoscope (Figure 40.7)

The resectoscope is an instrument borrowed from urology, where it has been used for transurethral prostate resection and the removal of biopsy specimens from the bladder wall. It has a 0°, 12° or 30° rod lens telescope with integrated fiberoptic light transmission.

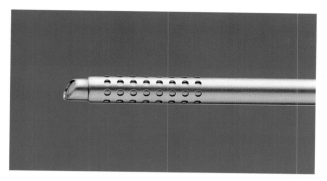

Figure 40.5 Bettochi hysteroscope: close-up with 3.8 mm and 4.5 mm outer sheath system

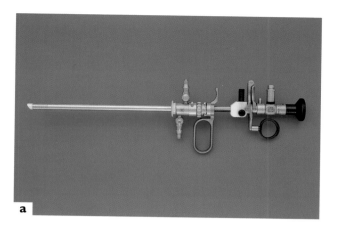

a

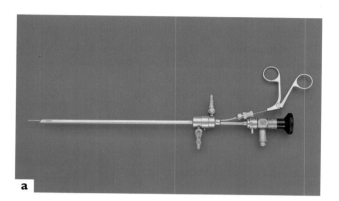

a

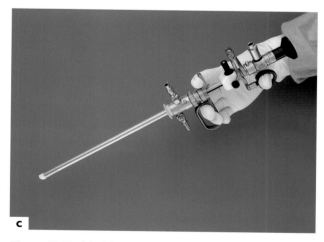

b

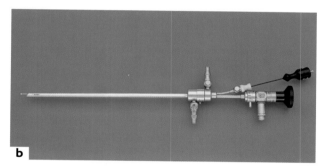

b

Figure 40.6 (a) Bettochi hysteroscope, telescope (diameter 2.9 mm), sheaths with working channel (size 5 mm) with (a) grasping forceps size 5 F and (b) bipolar needle size 5 F

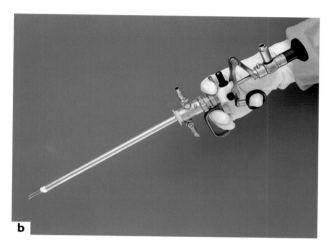

c

Figure 40.7 (a)–(c) Resectoscope (monopolar system)

Working elements (Figure 40.8)

Various elements, such as resection loops, rollerballs, roller cylinders, dissection needles and vaporization electrodes, are available as working elements. The loop is used in myoma, polyp and endometrial resections. Rollerballs and roller cylinders are applied during endometrial destruction by means of coagulation technology. The vaporization electrode is generally an oblong electrode with three or four relatively small recesses, equally distanced. It is operated with a very high-performance cutting current.

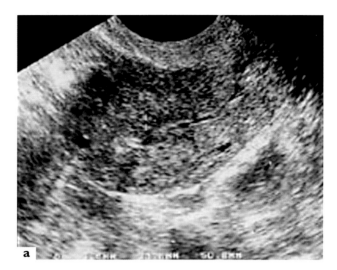

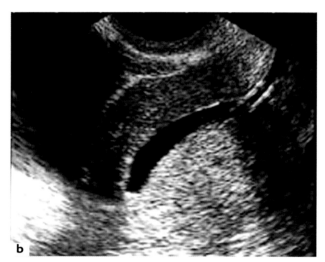

Figure 41.2 (a) Transvaginal sonography provides a sagittal view of the uterus; (b) with saline infusion sonohysterography, after saline infusion, the endometrium appears normal, without pathology

pedicle that is more heterogeneous and with peripheral vascularity.

Certain problems can occur, however. Sometimes, SIS may be impossible to perform because of cervical stenosis, but, in experienced hands, this technique has been carried out in more than 98% of women. In most cases, it takes no longer than 3–5 min.

There have been no reported cases of infection, although, in our series, one woman developed pelvic inflammatory disease after SIS; however, she had undergone hysterosalpingography some days earlier. We do not prescribe antibiotics routinely. In a case of suspected pelvic inflammatory disease or hydrosalpinx, hysterosonography is not performed. The possibility has been raised of retrograde seeding of adenocarcinoma cells in cases of

intrauterine neoplasia. Alcazar et al.[2] observed one case out of 14 in which malignant cells were present in the spilled fluid after SIS in a case of endometrial carcinoma. This observation has already been previously reported after diagnostic dilatation and curettage (D&C) or after hysterosalpingography, and does not appear to have any deleterious impact on the prognosis (in this pathology) of the neoplasia. In the case of cervical incompetence, such as reflux, a Foley catheter can be used.

Indications

Saline infusion sonohysterography is indicated in the following situations:

- Infertility investigation of uterine malformations, submucosal fibroids, polyps or synechiae

- Menorrhagia unsuccessfully treated with medication (Figures 41.3–41.5)

- Metrorrhagia (Figure 41.6)

- Follow-up of endometrial tissue at high risk of neoplasia, such as in patients with high blood pressure or diabetes, tamoxifen-treated patients or the obese (Figure 41.7)

- Endometrial thickness >5 mm in menopausal women (Figure 41.8)

- Poor imaging quality arising from the aspect axis or echogenicity of the endometrium

Transvaginal sonography can be an accurate diagnostic tool in evaluating women with abnormal vaginal bleeding. The endometrial thickness can be measured, and the ovulatory and hormonal status observed. Transvaginal sonography can detect endometrial thickening and heterogenicity and suggest possible masses; however, it is not as useful in determining the exact location of the masses. Saline infusion sonohysterography can enhance visualization of the endometrial lining and possible intracavitary masses.

Contraindications

Saline infusion sonohysterography should not be used in women with:

- Pelvic inflammatory disease

- A positive pregnancy test

- Suspected endometrial neoplasia

Results

Sonohysterography is a highly sensitive, specific and accurate screening procedure for evaluation of the uterine cavity in abnormal uterine bleeding (menorrhagia or metrorrhagia). Chittacharoen et al.[3] observed a specificity of 83%, a sensitivity of 97%, a positive predictive value of 97% and a negative predictive value of 83% in a study in

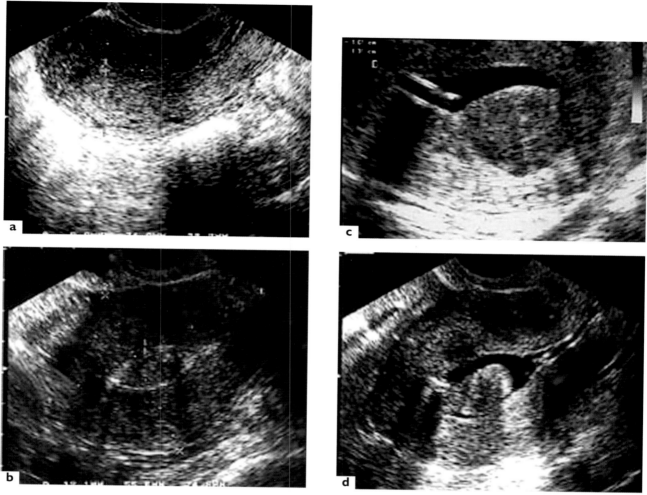

Figure 41.3 A 40-year-old patient with menorrhagia. Transvaginal sonography shows (a) a sagittal view of the endometrium of 6-mm thickness; and (b) endometrial thickness with a small focus at 12 mm; (c) and (d) saline infusion sonohysterography gives visualization of a polyp

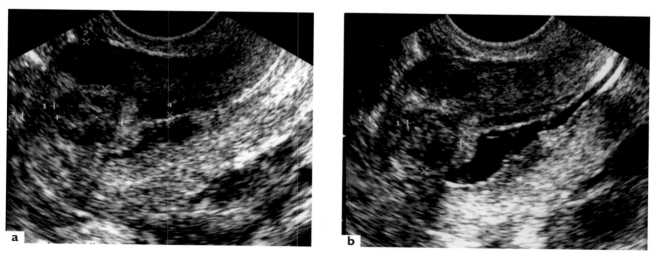

Figure 41.4 A 40-year-old patient with menorrhagia. (a) Transvaginal sonography, sagittal view, shows a normal endometrium and an intramural myoma of 16 mm; (b) deformation of the endometrium by the myoma is visualized with saline infusion sonohysterography. Saline infusion sonohysterography shows that a part of the myoma is submucosal and can be removed by hysteroscopy

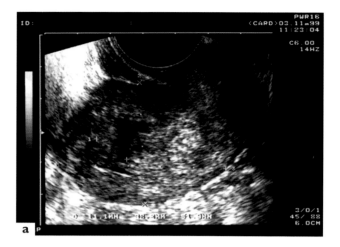

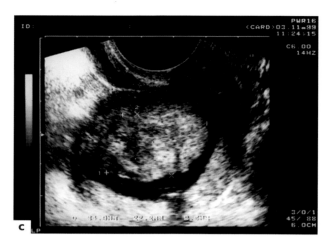

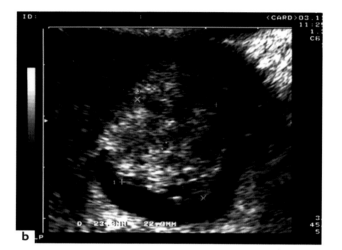

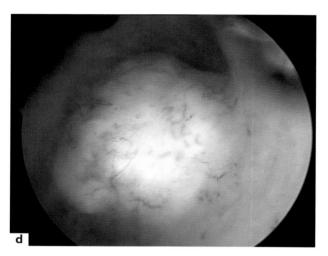

Figure 41.5 A 40-year-old patient with menorrhagia. (a) Transvaginal sonography, sagittal view, shows the normal uterine size, and suspicion of a mass effect inside the uterus with irregular limits; (b) and (c) saline infusion sonohysterography provides visualization of a pure submucosal myoma of 22×22 mm; (d) hysteroscopic view (note atrophic endometrium due to gonadotropin releasing hormone (GnRH) agonist treatment)

which SIS was compared with pathological findings in 52 women (mean age 41 years, range 29–58 years). Adenocarcinomas were excluded, and SIS correctly diagnosed two-thirds of cases of endometrial hyperplasia. Clevenger-Hoeft et al.[4] observed that premenopausal women with abnormal bleeding had a higher prevalence of polyps (43%), intracavitary myomas (21%) and intramural myomas (58%) than did premenopausal women without abnormal bleeding (respectively, 10%, 1% and 13%). It is essential that uterine pathologies are diagnosed, and, therefore, if a patient presents with abnormal bleeding, she must undergo the most thorough investigation in order to have the correct treatment. We suggest that women with multifocal or sessile lesions should undergo a guided biopsy procedure (hysteroscopy), and that polyps of

benign appearance should also be removed to control bleeding and eliminate the risk of intraepithelial neoplasia, especially in older women.

In 1998, Schwarzler et al.[5] evaluated the use of transvaginal sonography, sonohysterography and diagnostic hysteroscopy for the preparatory assessment of the uterine cavity. The end-points were uterine abnormalities detected by operative hysteroscopy and histology. More than 100 patients with abnormal uterine bleeding were recruited. Uterine abnormalities were present in 53% of cases. The overall sensitivity of transvaginal sonography improved after sonohysterography (from 67 to 87%), as did the specificity (from 89 to 91%). The positive predictive value increased from 88 to 92% and the negative predictive value from 71 to 86%. The use of SIS also improved the

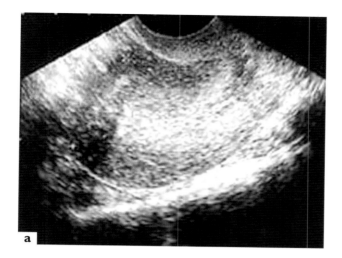

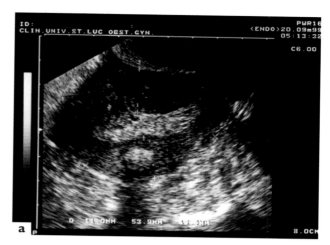

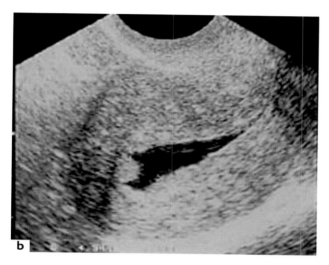

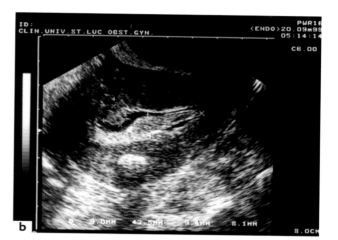

Figure 41.7 A 60-year-old patient taking tamoxifen. (a) Transvaginal sonography: endometrial thickness of 11 mm; (b) saline infusion sonohysterography shows two polyps, anterior 8 mm and posterior 9×20 mm (note atrophic endometrium)

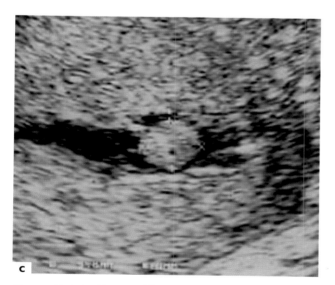

Figure 41.6 A 45-year-old patient with metrorrhagia. (a) Transvaginal sonography shows a normal appearance and thickness of the endometrium; (b) and (c) saline infusion sonohysterography provides visualization of a small fundal polyp

quality of information about the localization and size of polyps and submucosal fibroids.

The use of saline infusion to enhance visualization of the endometrium increased the diagnostic accuracy of transvaginal sonography, and also provided some additional information. Thus, SIS is a simple, non-invasive and effective tool which may be used in the evaluation of patients, instead of diagnostic hysteroscopy.

Infertility and *in vitro* fertilization

Soares *et al.*[6] evaluated the diagnostic accuracy of sonohysterography in uterine cavity diseases in infertile patients. Each patient underwent SIS, conventional transvaginal sonography, hysterosalpingography and hysteroscopy.

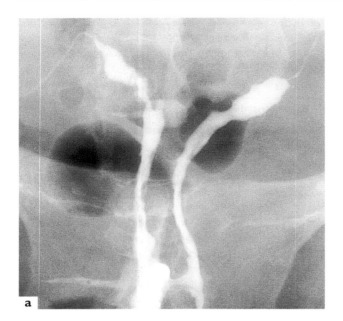

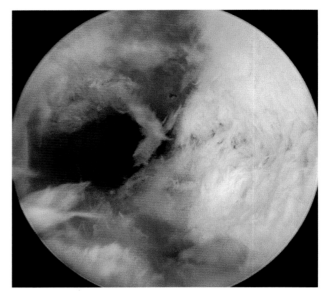

Figure 41.11 Intrauterine adhesions

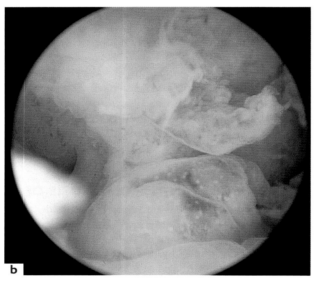

Figure 41.10 Müllerian abnormalities. (a) Hysterography reveals the presence of a complete uterine septum. Note the presence of fistula between the two cervical canals and of endometrial polyps. (b) Hysteroscopy confirms the diagnosis of both septum and polyps

Müllerian anomalies

Müllerian anomalies may be associated with normal fertility, infertility or recurrent abortion. The extent of the anomaly can range from complete agenesis of the Müllerian system to minimal deformities of the uterine form. Diagnosis usually requires combined hysteroscopy and laparoscopy. The presence of a uterine filling defect at hysterosalpingography or at hysteroscopy should be further evaluated by laparoscopy. The defect may represent a uterine septum (Figure 41.10), a bicornuate uterus or a submucous myoma. Rudimentary uterine horns, another form of Müllerian anomaly, can be detected laparoscopically and their relationship with the main cavity evaluated hysteroscopically.

Intrauterine synechiae

Traumatic intrauterine adhesions (Asherman's syndrome) (Figure 41.11) usually result from manipulation of the endometrial cavity following pregnancy. Curettage performed postpartum or following an abortion may cause scarring and synechiae secondary to destruction of the basal layer of the endometrium. Patients may present with hypomenorrhea, amenorrhea, infertility or spontaneous pregnancy loss. Recurrent abortion and abnormalities of implantation and placental development have also been described in association with this condition.

Intrauterine synechiae can be diagnosed by hysterosalpingography or hysteroscopy. The hysterosalpingogram shows a small, fragmented and distorted uterine cavity. The hysteroscopic image consists of pale endometrial patches and fibrotic strands, crossing the endometrial cavity. The adhesions are paler than the surrounding endometrium.

A hysteroscopic diagnosis of intrauterine adhesions is essential, as the disease can be missed or mistakenly diagnosed by hysterosalpingography. Hysteroscopy also permits better assessment of the extent of adhesions, an important factor in determining therapy and prognosis.

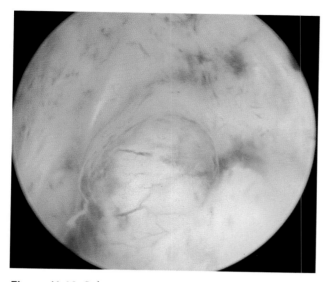

Figure 41.12 Submucous myoma

Submucous myomas

Uterine myomas can be found in a variety of locations. Those protruding into the uterine lumen are a common cause of abnormal uterine bleeding and may lead to infertility. Submucous myomas cause infertility by a variety of mechanisms related to embryo implantation. They can also cause preterm or dysfunctional labor. Submucous myomas are suspected in patients with enlarged uteri and those in whom filling defects are detected by hysterosalpingography. The hysterosalpingographic suspicion of the lesions should be confirmed by hysteroscopy. At hysteroscopy, the tumor is seen to protrude into the uterine cavity (Figure 41.12) and is covered with pale endometrium. Submucous myomas can be distinguished from endometrial polyps. In addition to providing a definitive diagnosis, hysteroscopy can reveal more accurately the localization of the tumor and permit better assessment of its size. The degree of intramural involvement cannot be determined.

Tubal disease

Involvement and occlusion of the intramural portion of the Fallopian tubes may be detected hysteroscopically. The significance of these lesions and their relationship to infertility has not been clearly established. Transuterine evaluation of tubal status prior to tuboplasty has been recommended[16]. The value of this method is debatable, however, as it is difficult to perform, and the same information can be obtained from a simple hysterosalpingogram.

Endometritis

Endometritis is a potential cause of infertility and recurrent pregnancy loss.

Sperm migration test

Hysteroscopy has been used to assess the survival of spermatozoa in the upper genital tract. Using a CO_2 hysteroscope, spermatozoa are obtained from the uterine cavity and the tubal ostia following intercourse, and their motility is assessed.

Gamete intrafallopian transfer and zygote intrafallopian transfer

Because the hysteroscope provides an excellent means of delivering instrumentation or substances to the Fallopian tubes from the uterine side, several techniques of intratubal manipulation have been attempted, such as tubal insemination and the postcoital test. More recently, hysteroscopy has been used with the techniques of gamete intrafallopian transfer (GIFT) and zygote intrafallopian transfer (ZIFT) to transfer the gametes or the zygote into the Fallopian tubes from the uterine side, rather than from the fimbriated end by laparoscopy or minilaparotomy.

It is possible that, with experience and the simplification of outpatient hysteroscopy, this may become a routine study for candidates for IVF, to evaluate the maturity or dysmaturity of the endometrium and predict the likelihood of implantation[17]. Furthermore, transfer of the early embryo can be accomplished under visual control.

Abortion

In cases of abortion, hysteroscopy is useful to check the presence or absence of trophoblastic tissue (Figure 41.13). Echography, computed tomography, magnetic resonance imaging and hysteroscopy can help in the diagnosis of a suspected hydatidiform mole (Figure 41.14).

Abnormal uterine bleeding

The common causes of abnormal uterine bleeding differ with age. In the early pubertal years, abnormal bleeding is usually dysfunctional, and is only rarely associated with an organic lesion. Dysfunctional bleeding often responds favorably to hormonal manipulation, and hysteroscopy is not usually needed. On occasion, however, persistent or severe bleeding may signal uterine pathology, such as endometrial polyps (Figure 41.15), myomas or adenomyosis (Figure 41.16). In the reproductive years, pregnancy-related complications are the most common cause of abnormal bleeding. Hysteroscopy is of value in some patients with retained products of conception following a spontaneous or induced abortion, which can be

465

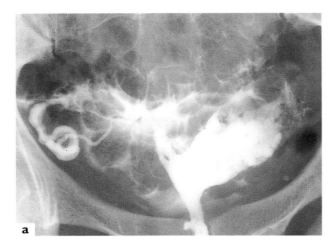

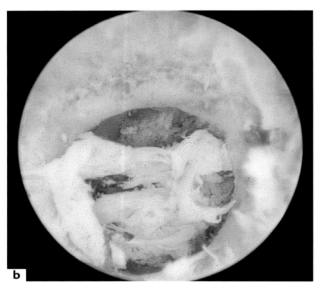

Figure 41.13 Uterine septum with residual trophoblastic tissue in the left horn: (a) hysterography; (b) hysteroscopy

difficult to locate by dilatation and curettage. Uterine myomas and endometrial and cervical polyps are also a common cause of abnormal bleeding in this age group. Polyps tend to move with the flow of the distension medium, whereas submucous myomas, which may have a similar appearance, do not. Evaluation should consist of endometrial sampling, hysterosalpingography and hysteroscopy.

In postmenopausal women with abnormal uterine bleeding, uterine and cervical neoplasia must be excluded. Hysteroscopy can serve as an adjunct to other diagnostic methods in patients in whom abnormal bleeding persists. Atrophic endometrium, another common cause of bleeding in this age group, can easily be diagnosed at hysteroscopy. Endometrial polyps can sometimes also be detected in these patients.

Historically, dilatation and curettage (D&C) has been used as a diagnostic and, often, therapeutic tool. The diagnostic accuracy of D&C has been scrutinized in efforts to determine the sensitivity and specificity of the technique. Advantages of the hysteroscope in the evaluation of abnormal uterine bleeding include, most notably, the ability to see lesions and to evaluate the endometrial cavity more objectively[18]. Indeed, comparisons have been made between the results of hysteroscopically directed biopsy and D&C in treating patients. Valle[18], Mohr[19] and Gimpelson[20] all concluded that panoramic hysteroscopy, especially with directed biopsy, is superior to D&C in patients with uterine bleeding. Alternatively, Goldrath and Sherman combined out-patient panoramic hysteroscopy with suction curettage, and suggested the superiority of this technique to D&C in terms of diagnostic accuracy, cost, safety and convenience[21].

Endometrial and cervical cancer

Hysteroscopy for abnormal bleeding can detect suspicious areas in the uterus and the cervix. The hysteroscopic appearance of endometrial carcinoma consists of exophytic or endophytic lesions. Polypoid or whitish areas may indicate necrosis within the tumor. The concern about cancer spread secondary to the hysteroscopic procedure has been addressed by various authors, and no evidence for its occurrence has been found[22,23]. Hysteroscopic examination has been found to be reliable, particularly when difficulties are encountered in assigning the tumor to stage I or II.

The instrument may also be used in detecting premalignant endometrial lesions, such as polypoid or adenomatous lesions with dystrophic or dyplastic hyperplasia. The microhysteroscope can be of great value in detecting such early changes in patients with a known high risk of endometrial cancer, such as diabetics and obese individuals. Hysteroscopy can also provide an excellent view of the cervical canal, and can thus be used in the diagnosis of cervical neoplasia[24].

Assessing the extent of involvement

Joelsson *et al.* in 1971, used hysteroscopy to try to distinguish cervical infiltration by tumors[25]. Clearly, if a tumor is seen growing within the endocervix, the endocervix is involved. However, the diagnosis of stage II carcinoma of the endometrium should be based on the histological contiguity of the endometrial carcinoma to normal cervical tissue (glands and stroma). This is not difficult if cervical glands or even the cervical squamous epithelium are contiguous to the cancer. However, this may be difficult if there is only stromal tissue with cancer, or if there is only cancer and no cervical tissue at all. To make a diagnosis of stage II endometrial cancer in both these cases, the specimen must come from the endocervix.

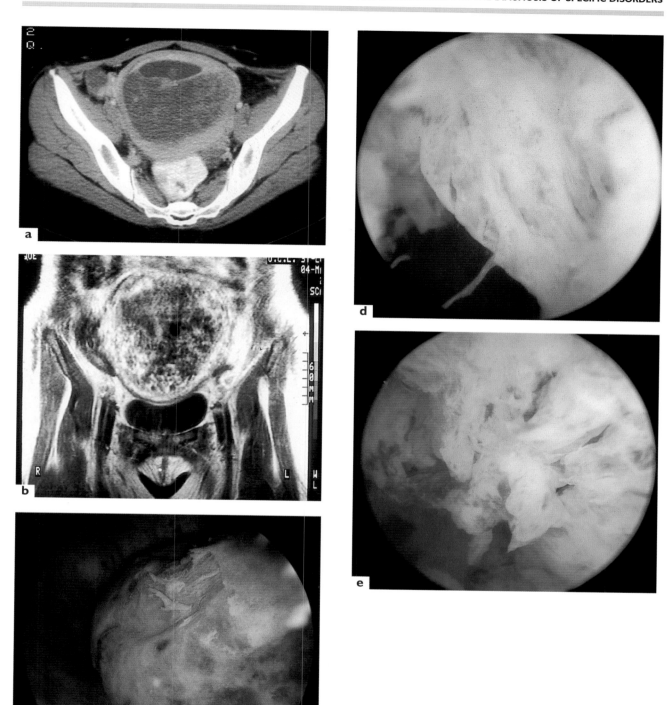

Figure 41.14 Hydatidiform mole: (a) computed tomography; (b) magnetic resonance imaging; (c)–(e) hysteroscopy

Such a biopsy requires experience rather than direct visualization of the biopsy site, because the small cup of even the Storz instrument will not yield sufficiently deep tissue. The most tantalizing aspect of this problem is that the more anaplastic adenocarcinomas and serous uterine papillary tumors may infiltrate the stroma of the endocervix, but the endocervical canal may appear quite normal. A deep endocervical biopsy may be better than the hysteroscope for detecting such cases of endometrial cancer. In patients with superficial infiltration of the upper endocervix by endometrial cancer, hysteroscopy will certainly provide a precise topographic description of the

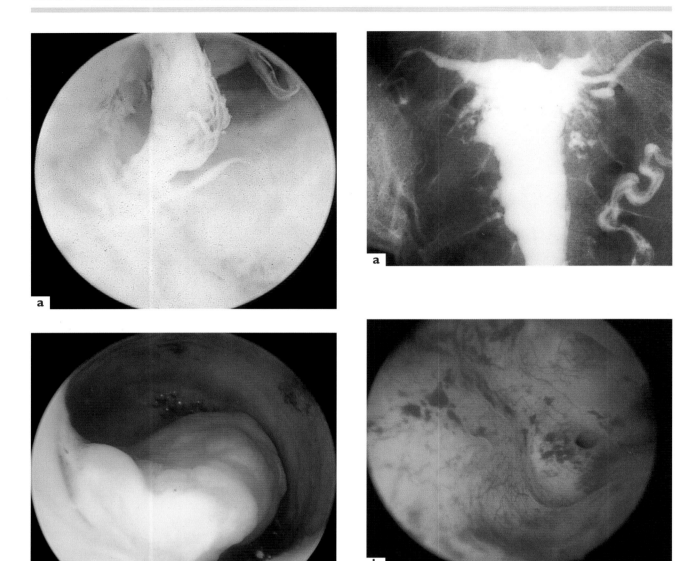

Figure 41.15 (a) Small endometrial polyp in the left uterine horn; (b) larger polypoid structure

Figure 41.16 Adenomyosis: (a) hysterography; (b) hysteroscopy reveals holes in the uterine cavity

lesion. Magnetic resonance imaging allows suspicion or diagnosis of the myometrial infiltration, but the final diagnosis, however, still needs to be histological. Furthermore, such early superficial spread to the endocervix probably carries no worse a prognosis than a stage I lesion. Deep cervical infiltration is a danger signal for deep myometrial invasion and lymph node involvement[26]. The danger of tumor cell dissemination by Hyskon® or saline solution or even by the flow of CO_2 into the uterine veins is probably not great. Data from hysterographies showed that there was no greater frequency of metastases among patients who had undergone hysterography than among those who had not[27].

Intrauterine foreign bodies

Until recently, foreign bodies within the uterine cavity were not uncommon. The most common offender is still the intrauterine device (IUD), which often becomes misplaced, making retrieval desirable. Several papers have described the usefulness of hysteroscopy in locating displaced IUDs[27–29]. Four patients with retained intrauterine fetal bones examined hysteroscopically have been described[30]. The bones were removed with hysteroscopic instruments in all patients. Other uncommon uses of the hysteroscopic approach include the removal of a Heyman capsule[31] and the broken tip of a plastic suction curette[32].

REFERENCES

1. Deichert U, van de Sandt M, Lauth G, et al. Transvaginal contrast hysterosonography. A new diagnostic procedure for the differentiation of intrauterine and myometrial findings. Geburtshilfe Frauenheilkd 1988; 48: 835–44

2. Alcazar JL, Errasti T, Zornoza A. Saline infusion sonohysterography in endometrial cancer: assessment of malignant cells dissemination risk. Acta Obstet Gynecol Scand 2000; 79: 321–2

3. Chittacharoen A, Theppisai U, Linasmita V, et al. Sonohysterography in the diagnosis of abnormal uterine bleeding. J Obstet Gynecol Res 2000; 26: 277–81

4. Clevenger-Hoeft M, Syrop CH, Stovall DW, et al. Sonohysterography in premenopausal women with and without abnormal bleeding. Obstet Gynecol 1999; 94: 516–20

5. Schwarzler P, Concin H, Bosch H, et al. An evaluation of sonohysterography and diagnostic hysteroscopy for the assessment of intrauterine pathology. Ultrasound Obstet Gynecol 1998; 11: 337–42

6. Soares SR, Barbosa dos Reis MM, Camargos AF. Diagnostic accuracy of sonohysterography, transvaginal sonography, and hysterosalpingography in patients with uterine cavity diseases. Fertil Steril 2000; 73: 406–11

7. Gronlund L, Hertz J, Helm P, et al. Transvaginal sonohysterography and hysteroscopy in the evaluation of female infertility, habitual abortion or metrorrhagia. A comparative study. Acta Obstet Gynecol Scand 1999; 78: 415–18

8. Ayida G, Chamberlain P, Barlow D, et al. Uterine cavity assessment prior to in vitro fertilization: comparison of transvaginal scanning, saline contrast hysterosonography and hysteroscopy. Ultrasound Obstet Gynecol 1997; 10: 59–62

9. Cohen MA, Sauer MV, Keltz M, et al. Utilizing routine sonohysterography to detect intrauterine pathology before initiating hormone replacement therapy. Menopause 1999; 6: 68–70

10. O'Connell LP, Fries MH, Zeringue E, et al. Triage of abnormal postmenopausal bleeding: a comparison of endometrial biopsy and transvaginal sonohysterography versus fractional curettage with hysteroscopy. Am J Obstet Gynecol 1998; 178: 956–61

11. Twu NF, Chen SS. Five-year follow-up of patients with recurrent postmenopausal bleeding. Chung Hua I Hsueh Tsa Chih (Taipei) 2000; 63: 628–33

12. Elhelw B, Ghorab MN, Farrag SH. Saline sonohysterography for monitoring asymptomatic postmenopausal breast cancer patients taking tamoxifen. Int J Gynecol Obstet 1999; 67: 81–6

13. Cohen I, Beyth Y, Tepper R. The role of ultrasound in the detection of endometrial pathologies in asymptomatic postmenopausal breast cancer patients with tamoxifen treatment. Obstet Gynecol 1998; 53: 429–38

14. Taylor PJ. Correlations in infertility: symptomatology, hysterosalpingography and hysteroscopy. J Reprod Med 1983; 8: 339–42

15. Lindemann HJ. Hysteroscopy for the diagnosis of intrauterine causes of sterility. Presented at the World Congress on Fertility and Sterility, Kyoto, Japan, October 1971

16. Quinones GR, Alvarado DA, Aznar RR. Tubal catheterization: applications of a new technique. Am J Obstet Gynecol 1974; 114: 674–9

17. Bordt J, Belkien L, Vancaillie T, et al. Ergebnisse diagnosticher Hysteroskopien in einem IVF/ET Program. Geburtschilfe Frauenheilkd 1984; 44: 813–15

18. Valle RF. Hysteroscopic evaluation of patients with abnormal uterine bleeding. Surg Gynecol Obstet 1981; 153: 521–6

19. Mohr JW. Hysteroscopy as a diagnostic tool in postmenopausal bleeding. In Philips JM, ed. Endoscopy in Gynecology. Downey, CA: American Association of Gynecologic Laparoscopists, 1978: 347–50

20. Gimpelson RJ. Panoramic hysteroscopy with directed biopsies vs. dilatation and curettage for accurate diagnosis. J Reprod. Med 1984; 29: 575–8

21. Goldrath MH, Sherman AI. Office hysteroscopy and suction curettage: can we eliminate the hospital diagnostic dilatation and curettage. Am J Obstet Gynecol 1984; 152: 220–9

22. Johnson JE. Hysterography and diagnostic curettage in carcinoma of the uterine body. Acta Radiol 1973; 326 (Suppl 1): 1–79

23. Sugimoto O. Hysteroscopic diagnosis of endometrial carcinoma: a report of fifty-three cases examined at the Women's Clinic of Kyoto University Hospital. Am J Obstet Gynecol 1975; 121: 105–13

24. Hamou J. Microhysteroscopy: a new procedure and its original applications in gynecology. J Reprod Med 1981; 26: 375–82

25. Joelsson I, Levine RU, Moberger G. Hysteroscopy as an adjunct in determining the extent of carcinoma of the endometrium. Am J Obstet Gynecol 1971; 111: 696–702

26. Anderson B. Hysterography and hysteroscopy in endometrial cancer. In Sciara JJ, Buchsbaum HJ, eds. Gynecology and Obstetrics. New York: Harper & Row, 1980: 850–5

27. Siegler AM, Kemmann E. Location and removal of misplaced or embedded intrauterine devices by hysteroscopy. J Reprod Med 1976; 16: 139–44

28. Taylor PJ, Cumming DC. Hysteroscopy in 100 patients. Fertil Steril 1979; 31: 301–4

29. Valle RF, Sciarra JJ, Freeman DW. Hysteroscopic removal of intrauterine devices with missing filaments. Obstet Gynecol 1977; 49: 55–60

30. Chervenak FA, Amin HK, Neuwirth RS. Symptomatic intrauterine retention of fetal bones. Obstet Gynecol 1982; 59: 58–61S

31. Zipkin B, Rosenfeld DL. Hysteroscopic removal of a Heyman radium capsule. J Reprod Med 1979; 22: 133–4

32. Sciarra JJ, Valle RF. Hysteroscopy: a clinical experience with 320 patients. Am J Obstet Gynecol 1977; 127: 340–8

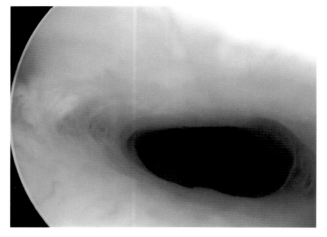

Figure 42.14 The external cervical oritice

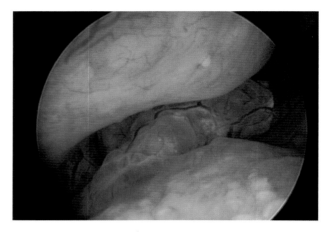

Figure 42.17 Cystic polyp

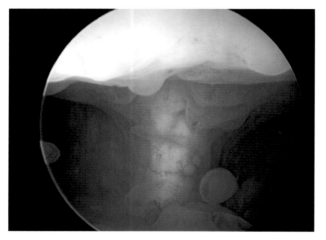

Figure 42.15 Uterine septum

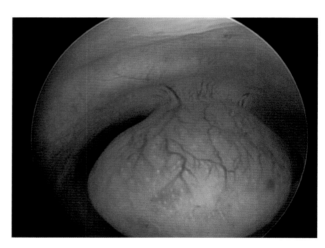

Figure 42.18 Pedunculated endometrial polyp

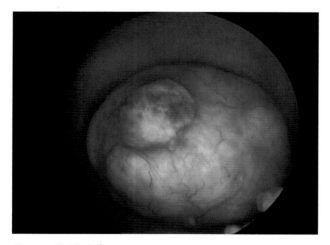

Figure 42.16 Submucous myoma

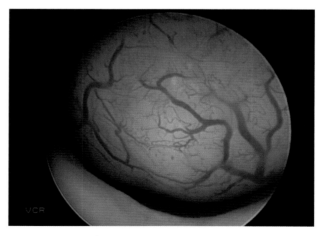

Figure 42.19 Submucous myoma

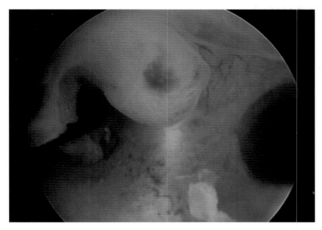

Figure 42.20 Uterine septum and an endometrial polyp

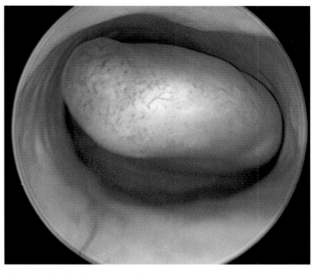

Figure 42.23 Endometrial polyp

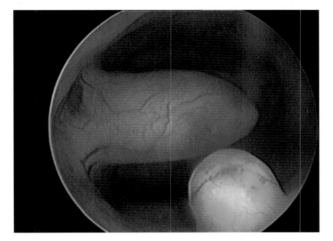

Figure 42.21 Endometrial polyps

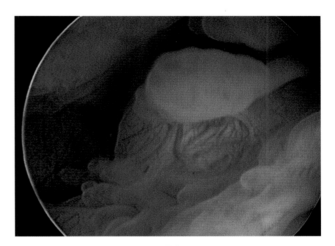

Figure 42.24 Mucous cyst of the cervix

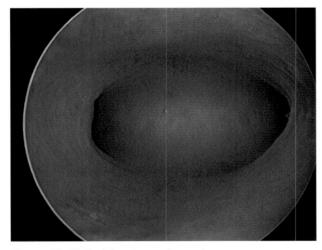

Figure 42.22 Proliferative endometrium

criteria for the diagnosis and classification of endometrial hyperplasia and its overlapping pattern with the normal late secretory endometrium, mainly in premenopausal women, is a drawback that still raises some doubt as to the reliability of this endoscopic procedure if based only on 'visualization' of the uterine cavity[20].

Considering the potential malignant evolution of endometrial hyperplasia, early hysteroscopic diagnosis of this condition may represent an important advance for the gynecologist only if associated with THB.

TARGETED HYSTEROSCOPIC BIOPSIES

The opinion that D&C does not ensure adequate, representative sampling of the endometrial cavity for the

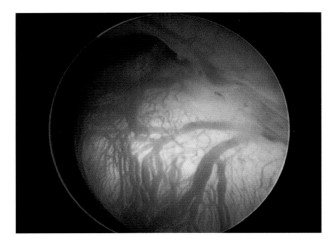

Figure 42.25 Hypervascularized polyp

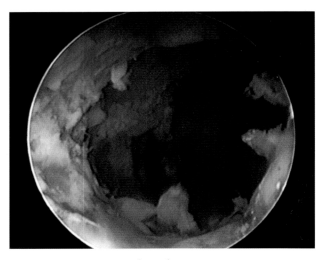

Figure 42.28 Uterine tuberculosis

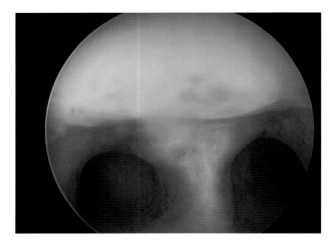

Figure 42.26 Uterine septum

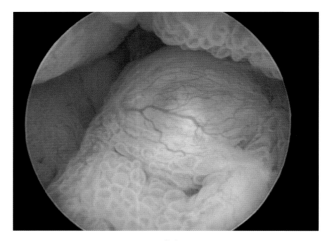

Figure 42.27 Mucous cyst of the cervix

detection of intrauterine pathologies is widely supported in the literature[2,21–24]. Furthermore, endometrial lesions such as focal endometrial hyperplasia and adenocarcinoma can easily be missed with this technique[23–26], as reported above. Endometrial sampling devices such as the Vabra, Pipelle or Novak® lead to the same problems owing to their 'blind' nature[26].

The availability of the new smaller hysteroscopes, including a 5F operative channel, has enabled physicians to perform a THB to confirm the endoscopic 'visual' diagnosis.

A number of papers have reported the reliability of such biopsies compared with blind procedures[21,22,24,26,27]. The 'standard' technique widely used is defined as a 'punch' biopsy: the biopsy forceps bite into the endometrium and are then closed. The mucosa remains inside the jaws and partly around them. The instrument is then extracted through the operative channel while the hysteroscope remains inside the uterine cavity. For this reason, the small diameter of the operative channel shaves the surrounding material away from around the tip of the forceps, and, consequently, the final amount of tissue to be sent to the pathologist is strictly related to the internal volume of the two jaws of the forceps. The critical point in this procedure is the difficulty in obtaining an adequate amount of tissue for histological diagnosis: using small 5F biopsy forceps and the 'punch' technique, Colafranceschi et al.[28] and Bakour et al.[29] calculated an adequate amount of tissue to be not less than 0.8 mm².

In order to obtain enough material routinely for histological diagnosis, the 'standard' technique has been modified[30], adopting the so-called 'grasp' biopsy: the biopsy forceps are placed, with the jaws open, against the endometrium to be biopsied. Then the forceps are pushed into the tissue and along it for 0.5–1 cm, avoiding touching the muscle fibers. Once a large portion of mucosa has been detached, the two jaws are closed and the whole hysteroscope is pulled out of the uterine cavity, without pulling the tip of the instrument back into the channel. In this way, not only the tissue inside the forceps jaws but also the surrounding tissue protruding outside the jaws can be retrieved, thus providing the pathologist with a large amount of tissue.

Moreover, the endoscopist has the chance to perform targeted biopsies of suspicious focal lesions[26]. In some cases, the hysteroscopic visual diagnosis may not correlate with the final histologic diagnosis; it is therefore prudent to carry out endometrial sampling in all doubtful cases.

OPERATIVE TECHNIQUES

Mechanical surgery

Cervical polyps can be treated using sharp scissors; the fibrotic base of these polyps precludes the use of grasping forceps because of the risk of regrowth of the pathology. Endometrial polyps, in menstruating women, can be treated using the 5F 'crocodile' grasping forceps: the base of the polyp is grasped with the open forceps and then gently detached from its implant in the myometrium. In menopausal and perimenopausal women, we prefer to use scissors to separate the polyp from the myometrium, due to the fibrotic or fibrocystic nature of the pathology at that age. In both cases the main problem could be the size of the pathology. If it corresponds to the diameter of the ICO (or is just a little bigger), the detached polyp is easily extracted from the uterine cavity using the crocodile grasping forceps. Bigger polyps have to be brought out of the cavity in pieces, by grasping the polyp with the forceps and pulling, thus tearing off fragments: an arduous, lengthy process.

Anatomic impediments, frequently found in perimenopausal and menopausal women, are widely considered to be an obstacle to correct execution of the hysteroscopic procedure. The use of a small-diameter operative hysteroscope can certainly be a great advantage for the physician, who can now reverse the usual process, by treating the problem before gaining a 'diagnostic' view of the uterine cavity, i.e. first performing an operative procedure and then going into the cavity, to be able to make a diagnosis. All anatomic obstacles, usually fibrotic processes involving the ECO as well as the ICO and resulting in a reduction of the diameter, can easily be treated by cutting the 'fibrotic ring' at two or three points (at 3 and 9 o'clock, for example). The most difficult part of the job is making a correct distinction between fibrotic and muscular tissue, to avoid causing pain.

Intrauterine synechiae are treated using scissors, by cutting them in the middle.

Bipolar surgery

We use the Versapoint® bipolar electrosurgical system (Gynecare, Ethicon, NJ, USA), consisting of a dedicated bipolar electrosurgical generator and two types of electrodes: the 'twizzle', specifically for precise and controlled vaporization (resembling cutting), and the 'spring', indicated for diffuse tissue vaporization. Each electrode consists of an active electrode located at the tip and a return electrode located on the shaft, separated by a ceramic insert. Only tissue in contact with the active electrode in the electrical path circuit will be desiccated or vaporized. The generator provides different modes of operation (waveform): the vapor cut waveform, resembling a cut mode (acronyms are VC1, VC2 and VC3, where VC3 corresponds to the mildest energy flowing into the tissue), the blend waveform (BL1, BL2) and the desiccation waveform, resembling a coagulation mode (DES). The generator is connected to the 5F electrode via a flexible cable. Once connected, the generator automatically adjusts to the default setting (VC1 and 100 W).

Instrument settings

After a test period, we concluded that the default settings of the Versapoint bipolar electrical generator were incompatible with our techniques performed without any type of anesthesia or analgesia, and therefore decided to use the mildest vapor cutting mode (VC3) and to reduce the power setting by half (50 W). For the same reason, we chose the 'twizzle' electrode over the 'spring', as in our experience the 'twizzle' electrode is a more precise 'cutting' instrument, and with lower power settings it can work closer to the myometrium with less discomfort.

Operative technique

Polyps are removed intact with the Versapoint 'twizzle' electrode only if the internal cervical os size is wide enough for their extraction. Otherwise, they are sliced, from the free edge to the base, into two or three fragments small enough to be pulled out through the uterine cavity using 5F grasping forceps with teeth. To remove the entire base of the polyp without going too deep into the myometrium, in some cases the 'twizzle' electrode can be bent by 25–30°, sufficient to obtain a kind of hook electrode. A similar technique has been applied on submucosal myomas, but with the difference that, owing to their higher tissue density, they must first be divided into two half-spheres and then each of these must be sliced as described above. Particular attention is paid to the intramural part of the myoma, if present. To avoid any myometrial stimulation or damage, the myoma is first gently separated from the capsule using mechanical instruments (grasping forceps or scissors) as already described for resectoscopic myomectomy[31]. Once the intramural section becomes submucosal it is sliced with the Versapoint 'twizzle' electrode.

CONCLUSIONS

Diagnostic hysteroscopy has long paid the price of being a purely visual investigation method. On the one hand, the possibility of viewing the uterine cavity after decades of blind procedures aroused considerable enthusiasm, while on the other, the impossibility of taking a biopsy of suspicious tissue under direct visualization limited the diagnostic accuracy of this procedure. Bearing in mind that the anatomy of the cervical canal does not allow the introduction of instruments with an outer diameter greater than 5 mm, the impossibility of performing guided biopsies without the need for dilatation of the cervix (and hence anesthesia) was related to technological problems that, for a long period, precluded the creation of miniaturized hysteroscopes equipped with an instrument channel.

Today, owing to recent advances in instrumentation, operative hysteroscopes with the same outer diameter as that of the previous diagnostic ones are finally available. A new generation of hysteroscopists, familiar with these hysteroscopes and with the modified techniques related to simultaneous use of the scope and the instruments, is finally bringing the hysteroscopic procedure to realization of the full accuracy that has been awaited for the past 20 years.

In the past, we would have been unable to perform these procedures in a 'see and treat' fashion in an outpatient setting without any anesthesia. Improved technology now enables us to perform many operative procedures in an office setting, without significant patient discomfort, reserving operating room time for the resectoscopic treatment of the less common, larger intrauterine pathologies.

There is no longer a distinction between the diagnostic and the operative procedure, but rather a single technique whereby the use of small-diameter operative hysteroscopes together with miniaturized instruments can ensure a final, correct, diagnosis.

REFERENCES

1. Gimpelson RJ, Rappold HO. A comparative study between panoramic hysteroscopy with directed biopsies and dilatation and curettage. A review of 276 cases. Am J Obstet Gynecol 1988; 158: 489–92
2. Loffer FD. Hysteroscopy with selective endometrial sampling compared with D&C for abnormal uterine bleeding: the value of a negative hysteroscopic view. Obstet Gynecol 1989; 73: 16–20
3. Siegler AM. Therapeutic hysteroscopy. Acta Eur Fertil 1986; 17: 467–71
4. Bettocchi S, Ceci O, Di Venere R, et al. Advanced operative office hysteroscopy without anaesthesia: analysis of 501 cases treated with a 5 Fr. bipolar electrode. Hum Reprod 2002; 17: 2435–8
5. Burkitt HG, Young B, Heath JW. The female genital organs. In Young B, Burkitt HG, Heath JW, Wheater PR, eds. Wheater's Functional Histology. Edinburgh: Churchill Livingstone, 1993: 335–65
6. Valle RF, Sciarra JJ. Hysteroscopy: a useful diagnostic adjunct in gynecology. Am J Obstet Gynecol 1975; 122: 230–5
7. Baggish MS. Contact hysteroscopy: a new technique to explore the uterine cavity. Obstet Gynecol 1979; 54: 350–4
8. Valle RF, Sciarra JJ. Current status of hysteroscopy in gynecologic practice. Fertil Steril 1979; 32: 619–32
9. Barbot J, Parent B, Dubuisson JB. Contact hysteroscopy: another method of endoscopic examination of the uterine cavity. Am J Obstet Gynecol 1980; 136: 721–6
10. Taylor PJ, Hamou JE. Hysteroscopy. J Reprod Med 1983; 28: 359–89
11. Valle RF. Hysteroscopy for gynecologic diagnosis. Clin Obstet Gynecol 1983; 26: 253–76
12. Vercellini P, Colombo A, Mauro F, et al. Paracervical anesthesia for outpatient hysteroscopy. Fertil Steril 1994; 62: 1083–5
13. Lau WC, Lo WK, Tam WH, Yuen PM. Paracervical anaesthesia in outpatient hysteroscopy: a randomised double-blind placebo-controlled trial. Br J Obstet Gynaecol 1999; 106: 356–9
14. Zullo F, Pellicano M, Stigliano CM, et al. Topical anesthesia for office hysteroscopy. A prospective, randomized study comparing two modalities. J Reprod Med 1999; 44: 865–9
15. Bettocchi S, Selvaggi L. A vaginoscopic approach to reduce the pain of office hysteroscopy. J Am Assoc Gynecol Laparosc 1997; 4: 255–8
16. Soderstrom RM. Distending the uterus: what medium is best? Clin Obstet Gynecol 1992; 35: 225–8
17. Baker VL, Adamson GD. Intrauterine pressure and uterine distention. J Am Assoc Gynecol Laparosc 1996; 3: S53
18. Campo R, Van Belle Y, Rombauts L, et al. Office mini-hysteroscopy. Hum Reprod Update 1999; 5: 73–81
19. Loverro G, Bettocchi S, Cormio G, et al. Diagnostic accuracy of hysteroscopy in endometrial hyperplasia. Maturitas 1996; 25: 187–91
20. Clark TJ, Voit D, Gupta JK, et al. Accuracy of hysteroscopy in the diagnosis of endometrial cancer and hyperplasia. A systematic quantitative review. JAMA 2002; 288: 1610–21
21. Brill AI. What is the role of hysteroscopy in the management of abnormal uterine bleeding? Clin Obstet Gynecol 1995; 38: 319–45
22. Smith JJ, Schulman H. Current dilatation and curettage practice: a need for revision. Obstet Gynecol 1985; 65: 516–18
23. Grimes DA. Diagnostic dilation and curettage: a reappraisal. Am J Obstet Gynecol 1982; 142: 1–6

24. Dijkhuizen FP, Mol BW, Brolmann HA, Heintz AP. The accuracy of endometrial sampling in the diagnosis of patients with endometrial carcinoma and hyperplasia. Cancer 2000; 89: 1765–72

25. Valle RF. Office hysteroscopy. Clin Obstet Gynecol 1999; 42: 276–89

26. Stock RJ, Kanbour A. Prehysterectomy curettage. Obstet Gynecol 1975; 45: 537–41

27. Agostini A, Cravello L, Rojat-Habib MC, et al. Evaluation of two methods for endometrial sampling during diagnostic hysteroscopy. J Gynecol Obstet Biol Reprod 1999; 28: 433–8

28. Colafranceschi M, van Herendael B, Perino A, et al. Reliability of endometrial biopsy under direct hysteroscopic control. Gynaecol Endosc 1995; 4: 119–22

29. Bakour SH, Khan KS, Gupta JK. Controlled analysis of factors associated with insufficient sample on outpatient endometrial biopsy. Br J Obstet Gynaecol 2000; 107: 1312–14

30. Bettocchi S, Di Venere R, Pansini N, et al. Endometrial biopsies using small-diameter hysteroscopes and 5F instruments: how can we obtain enough material for a correct histologic diagnosis? J Am Assoc Gynecol Laparosc 2002; 9: 290–2

31. Gimpelson RJ. Hysteroscopic treatment of the patient with intracavitary pathology (myomectomy/polypectomy. Obstet Gynecol Clin North Am 2000; 27: 327–37

Müllerian duct anomalies

P Jadoul, C Pirard, J Donnez

INTRODUCTION

Uterine malformations are very common. Indeed, if we include minor malformations (hypoplastic and arcuate uterus), they are encountered in 7–10% of all women. If we take into account just the more widely known uterine malformations, they are observed in 2–3% of fertile women, 3% of infertile women and 5–10% of those suffering repeated miscarriage[1].

Three main principles govern the practical approach to malformations of the genital tract:

(1) The Müllerian and Wolffian ducts are so closely linked embryologically that gross malformations of the uterus and vagina are commonly associated with congenital anomalies of the kidney and ureter.

(2) The development of the gonad is separate from that of the ducts. Normal and functional ovaries are therefore usually present when the vagina, uterus and Fallopian tubes are absent or malformed.

(3) Müllerian duct anomalies are usually not associated with anomalies in the sex chromosome make-up of the individual.

EMBRYOLOGY

Gonadal development is not examined in this chapter, which is limited to Müllerian and Wolffian duct development.

Late in the fifth or sixth week of embryonic life, at the level of the third thoracic somite, a precise area of the celomic epithelium invaginates at several points on the lateral surface of the urogenital ridge, and coalesces to form a tube, termed the Müllerian or paramesonephric duct (Figure 43.1a). The duct extends caudally to the urogenital ridge, immediately lateral to the Wolffian duct. The paired Müllerian ducts give rise to the Fallopian tubes, uterus, cervix and upper vagina. For proper Müllerian duct migration to occur, it is essential that the Wolffian duct is present[2].

Each Müllerian duct, guided by its respective Wolffian duct, migrates and develops independently of the other, and one usually descends ahead of the other. Defects in development of the Wolffian duct lead to Müllerian anomalies. Initially lateral to the Wolffian ducts, the Müllerian ducts cross over to lie medial to them as they enter the pelvis. By the end of the seventh week of embryonic life, the Müllerian ducts fuse to form a single structure between the two Wolffian ducts. The two Müllerian ducts penetrate the posterior wall of the urogenital sinus, between the orifices of the Wolffian ducts, on a mound called Müller's tubercle. It is important that the point where the tip of the Müllerian duct abuts on the posterior wall of the urogenital sinus is within the patch of mesoderm inserted into the wall of the sinus by the Wolffian ducts. This point defines the site of the future vaginal orifice, the hymenal membrane (Figure 43.1b). Two solid

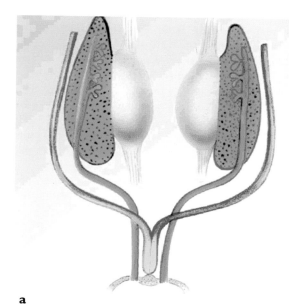

a

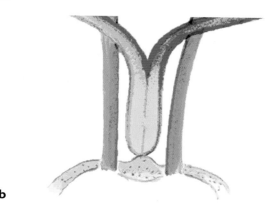

b

Figure 43.1 (a) The genital ducts in the female at the end of the second month of development. Note the Müllerian tubercle and the formation of the uterine canal: Müllerian ducts (orange), urogenital sinus (yellow). (b) Higher-power detail of the genital ducts in the female at the end of the second month of development

epithelial evaginations (sinovaginal bulbs) grow posteriorly from Müller's tubercle to meet the two solid tips of the fused Müllerian ducts. This epithelial proliferation of sinovaginal bulbs and the caudal ends of the Müllerian ducts form the solid vaginal plate (Figure 43.2a). The vaginal plate and the adjoining Müllerian ducts elongate, canalize and migrate from pelvic to perineal locations. At the same time, the urogenital sinus exstrophies into the vestibule, the urethra elongates and the plate canalizes (Figure 43.2b). The hymen remains as a membrane between the urogenital sinus and the canalized vaginal plate. The vaginal plate is first seen distinctly when the embryo is about 60–75 mm long, and its formation is complete at about 140 mm. Finally, when the cells of the plate desquamate, the vaginal lumen is formed[3] (Figure 43.2c).

As early as the end of the first trimester[4], there is a mesenchymal thickening around that portion of the fused Müllerian duct that is destined to become the endocervix. This mesenchymal thickening includes the Wolffian ducts, so that remnants of the latter, which persist into adulthood, are found within the body of the cervix. At all other levels of the genital canal, remnants of the Wolffian ducts are external to the wall of the adult Müllerian derivative. Smooth muscle appears in the walls of the genital canal between 18 and 20 weeks, and, by approximately 24 weeks, the muscular portion of the uterine wall is well developed[4]. Vaginal, uterine and tubal muscular walls develop around the Müllerian duct alone, so that the Wolffian duct remnants are external to the true wall of the canal. Cervical glands appear at about 15 weeks and rudimentary endometrial glands by 19 weeks, but the endometrium is not well developed even at term in most infants.

CLASSIFICATION OF MÜLLERIAN DUCT ANOMALIES

Müllerian duct anomalies can be classified into those of development and those of fusion (Table 43.1).

Development anomalies

Absence of both Müllerian ducts

Mayer–Rokitansky–Küster–Hauser syndrome is complete failure of the development of the Müllerian ducts resulting in an absence of the Fallopian tubes, uterus and most of the vagina. In such cases, the vulva is likely to be normal, and there may be a depression of variable depth representing the lower (urogenital sinus) part of the vagina. It is usual to find such a depression covered with a normal hymen[5,6] (Figure 43.3). In most cases, there is complete absence of the uterus and Fallopian tubes. In rare cases, the Fallopian tubes are present with or without associated rudimentary horns (Figures 43.4a and 43.4b). Myoma can develop on these rudimentary horns (Figure 43.4c).

This syndrome affects one in every 4000–5000 females. Although familial aggregates have been described, the defect usually appears sporadically.

Girls with Mayer–Rokitansky–Küster–Hauser syndrome present with primary amenorrhea associated with normal pubertal development. Although nothing can be done to restore fertility, vaginal construction or reconstruction has become well established as a method of permitting or restoring sexual function. A variety of procedures have been described.

The most natural techniques involve progressive dilatation of the vaginal cupula. Frank[7] reported graduated vaginal dilatation on a bicycle-seat tool, but this technique yielded favorable results in fewer than 50% of patients. Vecchietti[8] developed a technique whereby continuous traction (1 cm/day) is applied to an acrylic olive placed in the vaginal dimple. This olive is held by threads that are passed through the vaginal cupula and preperitoneal space, right through the skin, where they are fixed to a device on the abdomen (Figure 43.5).

This technique, first performed by laparotomy, has been modified by several authors and is now usually performed by laparoscopy[9–13].

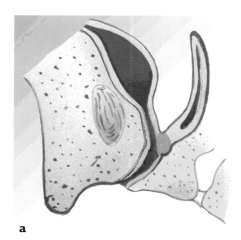
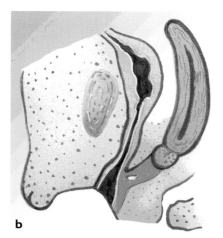
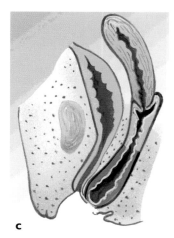

a b c

Figure 43.2 (a)–(c) Sagittal section showing the formation of the uterus and vagina during development

Table 43.1 Classification of Müllerian duct anomalies

Development anomalies

Absence of both Müllerian ducts

Absence of one Müllerian duct

Incomplete development of both Müllerian ducts

Incomplete development of one Müllerian duct

Fusion anomalies

Lateral fusion anomalies

    arcuate uterus

    uterus subseptus, uterus septus and uterus bicornis

    uterus didelphys

    septate and subseptate vagina

Vertical fusion anomalies

    cervical atresia

    vaginal atresia

    transverse vaginal septum

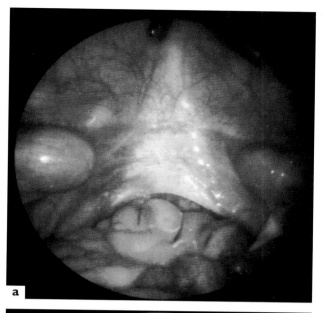

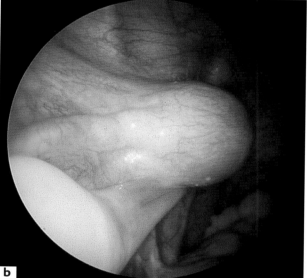

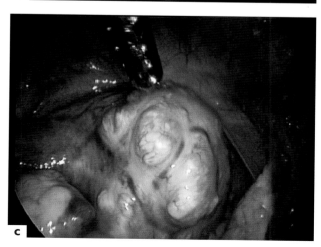

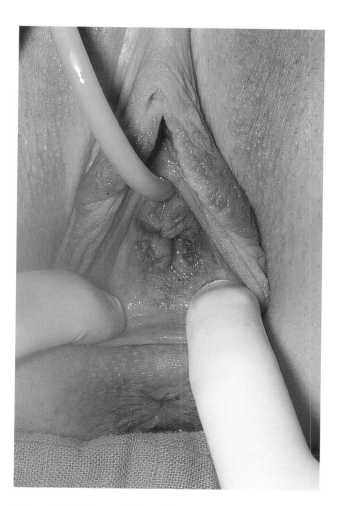

Figure 43.3 Mayer–Rokitansky–Küster–Hauser syndrome: external genital tract

Figure 43.4 (a) and (b) Mayer–Rokitansky–Küster–Hauser syndrome: presence of rudimentary horns; (c) a myoma can develop on these rudimentary horns

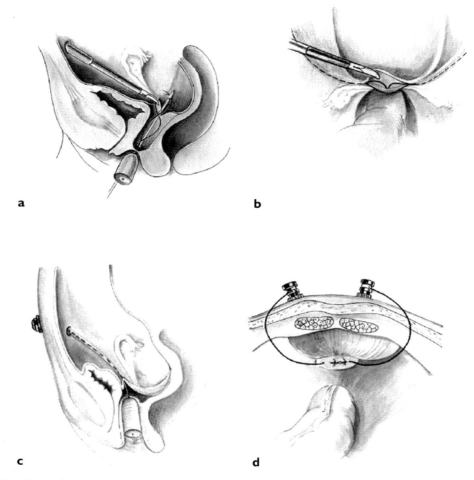

Figure 43.5 (a)–(d) Vecchietti procedure

Other techniques involve creating a tunnel in the vesicorectal space. Whether or not a graft is needed to cover this tunnel and which tissue should be used (skin, intestine, amnion, peritoneum) are still matters of debate.

The use of cecal or sigmoid bowel segments was reported by Baldwin[14], Turner-Warwick and Kirby[15] and O'Connor et al.[16]. Although some authors claimed good results, this method is a major surgical procedure with significant morbidity and mortality. Moreover, profuse secretions, persistent unpleasant odor and ulceration of the mucosal surface could be major side-effects.

McIndoe and Bannister[17] transplanted a split-thickness skin graft into a newly formed vaginal cavity, held in place by a vaginal mold. Great variations in success rate, a high incidence of postoperative infection, necrosis of the skin graft and scarring make this technique less acceptable. The patient also suffers considerable discomfort from the donor skin site, which may remain visible.

Myocutaneous flaps have been used by several surgeons. The gracilis myocutaneous flap has become very popular in recent years[18–21], but a serious disadvantage is the precarious vascularity of the flaps. In McCraw et al.'s series of 22 patients[22], six suffered catastrophic loss of the flap. The rectus abdominis flap is another popular flap, but creates a large abdominal donor site defect[23] and requires a long operative procedure. The neurovascular pudendal thigh flap procedure can be used reliably to reconstruct the vagina[24]. All flap techniques, however, are reported to be associated with an unacceptable failure rate due to partial flap loss and necrosis. Such dissections also cause major scars, and can only be indicated for vaginal reconstruction after pelvectomy for pelvic cancer, when subsequent irradiation must be carried out.

In order to overcome these difficulties, amnion alone, with the clean mesenchymal surface placed towards the host, has been used by several surgeons[25–30]. Faulk et al.[31] demonstrated microscopic evidence of new vessel formation, and suggested that an angiogenic factor is produced by amnion. There is no problem with immune rejection because amnion does not express histocompatibility anti-

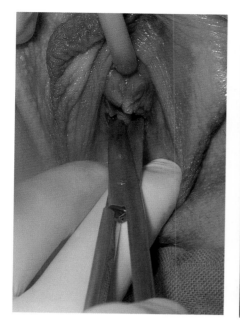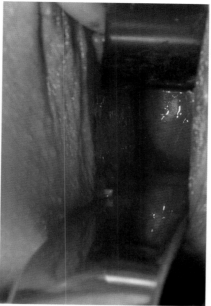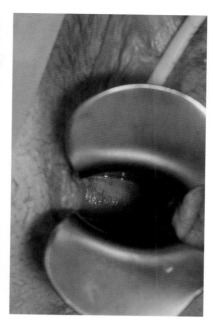

Figure 43.6 Dissection of the vesicorectal space

gens. Akle *et al.*[32] found no evidence of tissue rejection when amnion was implanted subcutaneously in volunteers.

Tancer *et al.*[33], Dhall[30] and Ashworth *et al.*[34] have all reported the successful use of amnion as a graft in vaginoplasties.

In our department, amniotic membranes were used between 1985 and 2002. They were taken immediately postpartum (< 6 h) and rinsed in sterile physiological solution.

Under general anesthesia, the patient is placed in the lithotomy position and vaginal dissection is performed (Figure 43.6). A vaginal pouch is created by blunt dissection using scissors. At the same time, a laparoscopy is performed to confirm the diagnosis and check the blunt dissection. When hemostasis has been achieved, a rigid vaginal mold (Figure 43.7) is selected, just large enough to ensure firm application of the amniotic membranes, with which it is covered (Figure 43.8). The labia majora are approximated with silk sutures to keep the mold in place (Figure 43.9). Laparoscopy is not necessary for the dissection but, when performed to ascertain the diagnosis, it permits visualization of the top of the mold between the bladder and the rectum (Figure 43.10).

The mold is removed under light sedation 7 days later, and the newly constructed vagina is inspected and cleaned. The amniotic membranes are found to be adherent to the vagina. A flexible mold (Figure 43.11) is then inserted and the patient discharged the following day, having been advised to refrain from sexual activity for an additional 2 weeks and to use the mold at night during this period.

All patients had greatly improved vaginal length and capacity as a result of this treatment. Excellent results were achieved in all cases. The vaginal tissue remained supple, with no evidence of fibrous tissue formation. Chronic granulation tissue was not observed and vaginal shrinkage did not occur.

Recently, we used a new product, Surgisis™ Enhanced Strength (Cook, Brussels, Belgium), in order to avoid the application of human tissue with the potential risk of viral transmission in young women (Figure 43.12). Small intestinal submucosa (SIS) is a new biomaterial for the replacement and repair of damaged tissue. It does not contain cells because it is extracted from the porcine small intestine in a manner that removes all cells, but leaves the complex matrix intact. The manufacturing process has been validated to ensure that any virus that might be present in source animals is completely inactivated. The cells of adjacent tissue invade the SIS material. Progressively, capillary growth and progressive degradation of the SIS material should be observed. This new tissue graft has already been used in animal surgery by several authors, and appears encouraging for use in human surgery[35,36].

Another way to create a new vagina is to pull down the peritoneum between the bladder and the rectum. The peritoneum is pushed down and sutured to the hymen after opening the vaginal cupula. A peritoneal purse-string is performed to close the neovagina (Figure 43.13). This technique, first performed by Davydov[37] in 1969 by laparotomy but nowadays done by laparoscopy[38–43], has the advantage of not causing sequelae to the donor site and

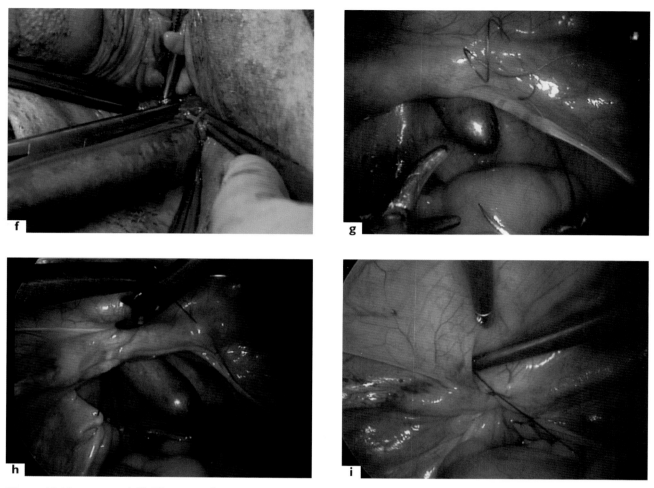

Figure 43.13 *continued* (f) The opened peritoneum is sutured to the hymen. (g)–(i) A purse-string is performed to close the peritoneum above the Hegar probe

and tubes. This may cause gross structural anomalies of the cervix, such as a cervical collar, pseudopolyp or hood, as well as uterine deformities such as a T-shaped endometrial cavity (Figure 43.15).

DES is a non-steroidal synthetic estrogen used between 1941 and 1977 to prevent miscarriage, gravidic hemorrhage and premature delivery[47]. In 1971, it was prohibited in the USA by the Food and Drug Administration (FDA) after Herbst and Scully[48] showed an increased risk of vaginal clear-cell adenocarcinoma in girls exposed *in utero* to DES. Cervicovaginal, tubal and uterine anomalies, infertility and obstetric complications have been related to DES exposure. Sixty-nine per cent of women exposed to DES present with uterine anomalies at hysterosalpingography[44]. The most frequently encountered anomaly is the T-shaped uterus (55%). Uterine hypoplasia occurs in 44–49% and supraisthmic stenosis in 26% of cases (Figure 43.16).

DES-exposed women have an increased risk of infertility[44,49] and an increased risk of obstetric complications

such as early and late miscarriage and premature delivery. In the case of a T-shaped uterus or supraisthmic stenosis, hysteroscopic uterine cavity enlargement can be proposed. A lateral 5–7-mm-deep incision is performed in the lateral sides of the myometrium (Figure 43.17). An intrauterine device (IUD) is left in place and high doses of estrogens and progesterone are prescribed for a duration of 2–3 months, allowing re-epithelialization of the incised myometrium. After removal of the IUD, hysterography allows evaluation of the anatomic results (Figure 43.18).

In the literature, we found four retrospective non-controlled studies of hysteroplasty in 82 patients exposed to DES[50–53]. Hysterosalpingography showed apparent improvement in all cases but no objective criteria were defined. Two postoperative synechiae and two cases of placenta acreta were described. These studies are too limited to allow conclusions to be drawn on the safety and efficacy of hysteroplasty for DES uterus. There are potential risks of intraoperative uterine perforation, cervical incompetence, uterine rupture during pregnancy,

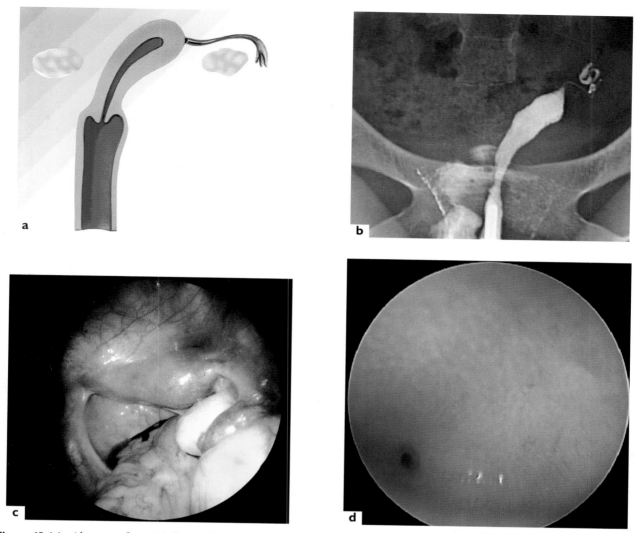

Figure 43.14 Absence of one Müllerian duct. (a) Unicornuate uterus; (b) view on hysterography; (c) laparoscopic view; (d) hysteroscopic view

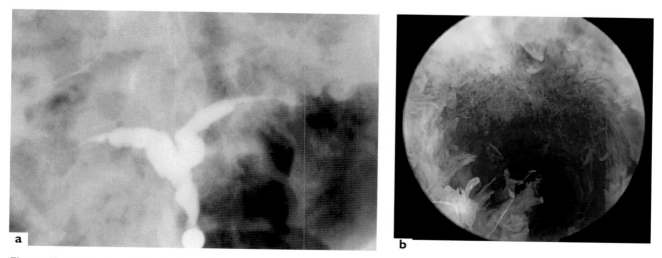

Figure 43.15 *In utero* diethylstilbestrol exposure: (a) T-shaped endometrial cavity at hysterography; (b) tunnelized cavity at hysteroscopy

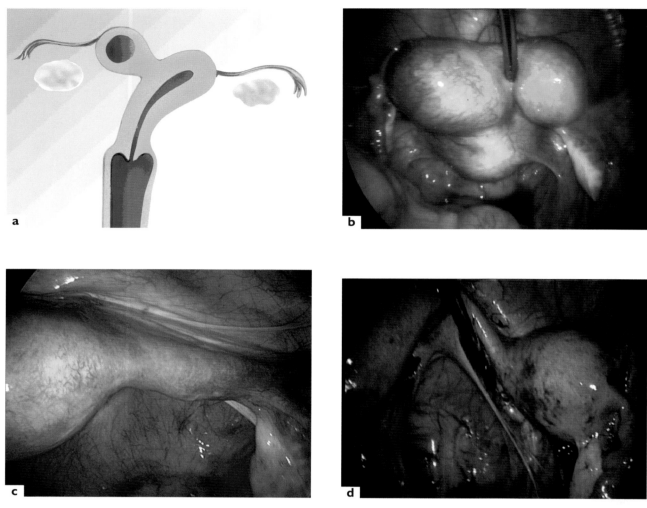

Figure 43.19 (a) Unicornuate uterus with rudimentary horn. (b) and (c) The size of the rudimentary horn can vary. (d) Associated endometriosis is frequently seen

a vaginal septum, the diagnosis is simple, because two distinct external cervical orifices are clearly visible. Opacification through these two orifices allows the diagnosis of a septate uterus with cervical duplication.

It is not clear why uterine anomalies are associated with reproductive failure. According to histological observations, the septum is described as 'fibroelastic tissue'[57]. Using scanning electron microscopy to compare endometrial biopsy specimens obtained from different areas of the uterine cavity, Fedele et al.[58] found that septal endometrium showed defective development, indicative of a reduction in sensitivity to steroid hormones. They subsequently postulated that endometrial septal defects could play a role in the pathogenesis of primary infertility in cases of uterine septa.

Another hypothesis that could explain reproductive failure is that spontaneous miscarriage may be the result of a poor blood supply to the septum, leading to poor implantation dynamics[59].

In a review published in 2000, Homer et al. reported the reproductive outcome of women with an untreated septate uterus[60]. Out of 1376 pregnancies, 1085 (79%) ended in miscarriage and 125 (9%) in preterm delivery. However, if we calculate the percentage of preterm deliveries among ongoing pregnancies, a hefty 42% of patients, who escaped the very high risk of miscarriage, delivered prematurely. It is clearly necessary to try to improve the situation.

In their review, Homer et al.[60] reported data from several series that compared the outcomes of pregnancies before and after hysteroscopic metroplasty in patients with a septate uterus. The miscarriage rate, preterm delivery rate and term delivery rate were 88%, 9% and 3%, respectively, before surgery, and 14%, 6% and 80% after hysteroscopic metroplasty.

More recently, other authors have published their findings on reproductive outcome after hysteroscopic metroplasty for a septate uterus. Hickok[61] reported his

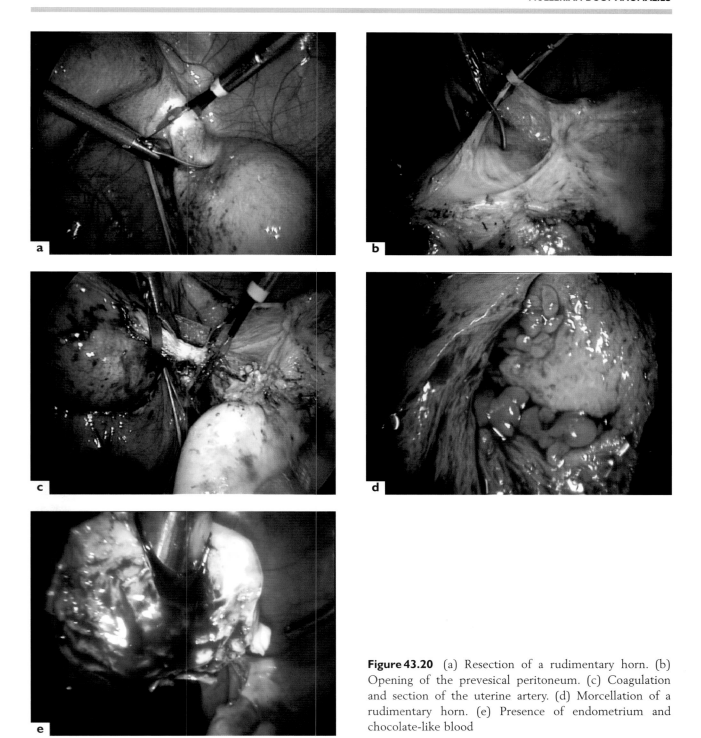

Figure 43.20 (a) Resection of a rudimentary horn. (b) Opening of the prevesical peritoneum. (c) Coagulation and section of the uterine artery. (d) Morcellation of a rudimentary horn. (e) Presence of endometrium and chocolate-like blood

experience with hysteroscopic treatment of uterine septa. The preoperative pregnancy loss rate was 77.4%, while the postoperative miscarriage rate was 18.2%. Patton et al.[62] reported a very similar result. In the specific case of complete uterine septum, duplicated cervix and vaginal septum, 12 out of 16 women conceived after surgery. The pregnancy loss rate was 81% before surgery and 18% after.

Litta et al.[63] reported their experience with hysteroscopic metroplasty under laparoscopic guidance for patients with a septate uterus. Of 35 patients treated, 26 (75%) achieved pregnancy. Only three patients delivered prematurely.

Table 43.2 summarizes the reproductive outcome after hysteroscopic metroplasty for septate uterus. After surgery, the miscarriage rate is 14.3% (88/617). Out of 529

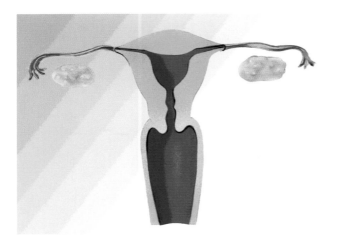

Figure 43.21 Arcuate uterus

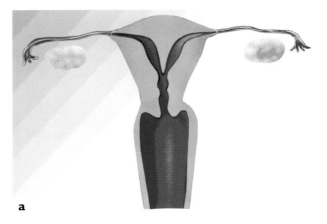

a

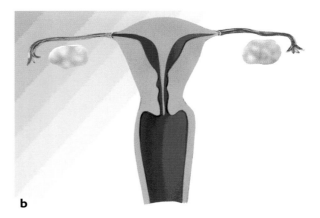

b

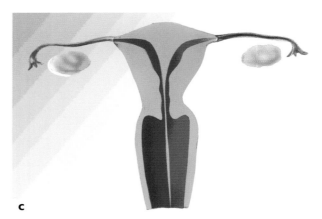

c

Figure 43.22 (a) Incomplete uterine septum, (b) complete uterine septum and (c) complete uterovaginal septum

ongoing pregnancies, the preterm delivery rate is 7.2% (38/529) and the term delivery rate 92.8% (491/529)

The endoscopic technique for the management of uterine septa was first proposed in 1970 by Edström and Fernström[77].

The basic concept involves transcervical observation of the uterine septum by means of hysteroscopy, followed by its resection[78–81]. The use of an operative hysteroscope allows the passage of surgical instruments.

Various instruments can be used for resection of the septum: miniature scissors or semirigid miniature scissors, which supply the required pressure but are small enough to pass through the hysteroscopic operating sheath and along the cervical canal with no difficulty or risk. The blades can be opened wide enough to allow resection of even thick septa. Other surgeons prefer to use the resectoscope[82–84]. High-frequency electrical sources are advised for safety reasons. The resectoscope has several advantages: it is inexpensive and readily available in most operating rooms, as well as being simple to operate and highly efficient at removing the septum. Finally, others have suggested the use of lasers for this type of hysteroscopic surgery[85–87]. Argon, krypton, KTP/532 (potassium–titanyl–phosphate) and Nd:YAG (neodymium:yttrium–aluminum–garnet) lasers have all been successfully employed in the resection of uterine septa.

Partial uterine septum: With the help of the 'bare fiber' or the L-shaped electrode of the resectoscope, the surgeon begins resection of the septum (Figure 43.25), continuing until it has been resected almost flush with the surrounding endometrium. Regardless of the type of medium employed, the surgeon must be able to see the right and left cornual regions completely, and keep the septum in view at all times. Concurrent laparoscopy at the time of hysteroscopic resection is recommended to confirm the

diagnosis, but is not mandatory if the diagnosis has previously been confirmed.

The most delicate part of the procedure is probably deciding exactly when the resection is sufficient, and when continuing would cause damage to the myometrium and immediate complications such as perforation, or more delayed complications such as uterine rupture during

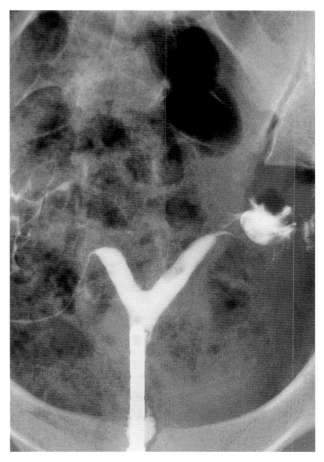

Figure 43.23 Partial uterine septum: hysterography

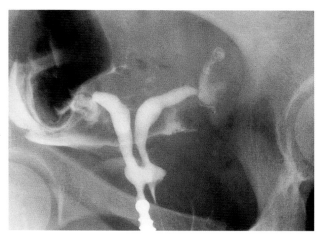

Figure 43.24 Complete uterine septum (uterocervical septum) with a fistula between the two uterine cavities

pregnancy. Almost all surgeons stop resection when the area between the tubal ostia is a line. In 1996, Fedele *et al.*[88] suggested that a remaining uterine septum of less than 1 cm after hysteroscopic metroplasty does not impair reproductive outcome and therefore does not require a second hysteroscopic surgical procedure.

Complete uterine septum: In some cases, not only may a double cervical canal be observed, but also a vaginal sagittal septum may be present in the upper vagina or throughout its length.

First, the vaginal septum (if present) is resected using scissors or unipolar coagulation (Figure 43.26). Both cervices are dilated (Figure 43.27), and the cervical septum is then incised with scissors (Figure 43.28) or with a CO_2 laser connected to a colposcope, until the lower portion of the uterine septum is seen. After section of the cervical septum, the external cervical os appears completely normal (Figure 43.29). The hysteroscope is advanced while visual contact is maintained with the right and left uterine ostia. Because the septum is poorly vascularized, bleeding is usually minimal.

Pre- and postoperative management: Although preoperative hormonal therapy causes atrophy of the endometrium

and reduces vascularization and intraoperative bleeding, it also reduces the depth of the myometrium and therefore increases the risk of perforation and/or myometrial damage. It is suggested that surgery be performed immediately after the end of menstrual bleeding. Postoperatively, a broad-spectrum antibiotic is administered for 3–4 days. In order to avoid the risk of synechiae, an intrauterine device (IUD; Multiload®) is inserted into the uterine cavity. Hormone replacement therapy with estrogens (100–200 µg of ethinylestradiol) and progestogens (5–15 mg lynestrenol) is given for 3 months. De Cherney *et al.*, however, use neither hormone replacement therapy nor IUDs[82]. Formerly, Perino *et al.*[68] administered estrogens and medroxyprogesterone and inserted IUDs, but they subsequently abandoned these measures and now administer no postoperative therapy at all. Hamou[84] performs a hysteroscopic procedure 1 month after surgery in order to separate synechiae, if necessary. Almost all authors agree that a follow-up examination should be performed 1–2 months after the operation, irrespective of the postoperative management. Inspection can be done by means of either hysterosalpingography or hysteroscopy.

In our department, the postoperative morphology of the uterine cavity is systematically evaluated 4 months after resection. One month after removal of the IUD, hysterosalpingography is carried out; the morphology of the uterine cavity almost always resembles an arcuate uterus (Figure 43.30). Indeed, it is preferable not to resect the septum too much, but to leave a sufficient depth of myometrium at the top of the uterus. Hysteroscopy was performed in a first series[89] to confirm that re-epithelialization of the resected endometrial area had occurred. Nowadays, this procedure is not performed systematically.

Results and complications: Operative hysteroscopy is a safe and effective method for the management of uterine septa associated with recurrent pregnancy loss, and makes future vaginal delivery possible. In one of our series of 17

Table 43.2 Reproductive outcome after hysteroscopic metroplasty for septate uterus

Author(s)	Patients (n)	Pregnancies (n)	Miscarriages (n (%))	Ongoing pregnancies (n)	Ongoing pregnancies with preterm deliveries (n)	Ongoing pregnancies with term deliveries (n)
Chervenak and Neuwirth[64]	2	2	0	2	0	2
De Cherney and Polan[65]	15	11	2 (18)	9	0	9
Fayez[66]	12	16	2 (13)	14	0	14
March and Israel[67]	57	56	8 (14)	48	4	44
Perino et al.[68]	24	15	1 (7)	14	0	14
Daly et al.[69]	55	75	15 (20)	60	5	55
Choe and Baggish[70]	14	12	1 (8.3)	11	1	10
Fedele et al.[58]	71	65	10 (16)	55	10	45
Cararach et al.[71]	62	41	12 (29)	29	0	29
Pabuccu et al.[72]	49	44	2 (4.5)	42	2	40
Valle[73]	115	103	12 (12)	91	7	84
Mencaglia and Tantini[74]	94	62	4 (6)	58	0	58
Patton et al.[62]	16	17	3 (18)	14	0	14
Hickok[61]	40	22	4 (18.2)	18	1	17
Jourdain et al.[75]	20	12	2 (16.6)	10	0	10
Colacurci et al.[76]	69	46	10 (21.8)	36	5	31
Litta et al.[63]	20	18	0	18	3	15
Total	735	617	88 (14.3%)	529 (85.7%)	38 (7.2%)	491 (92.8%)

complete uterine septa, ten out of 17 women became pregnant, and no signs of cervical incompetence were observed[56]. Prophylactic cerclage was never performed after resection of a complete cervical and uterine septum. Following hysteroscopic metroplasty, cesarean section should be performed only for obstetric reasons. In our series, intraoperative and postoperative complications were encountered in only three cases (1.8%).

Uterus didelphys If the two Müllerian ducts remain separate, the two halves of the uterus remain distinct and each has its own cervix (Figure 43.31). Some distinguish between uterus didelphys and uterus pseudodidelphys, according to the degree of separation between the two ducts.

Septate and subseptate vagina A sagittal septum with a crescentic lower edge may be present in the upper vagina or throughout its length. It can occur alone or in conjunction with a septate or bicornuate condition of the uterus,

and may have one or two cervices opening into it. This condition arises either because late fusion of the Müllerian ducts gives rise to two Müllerian tubercles, or because of failure of proper canalization of the two sinovaginal bulbs.

In some cases, the hemivagina is not patent, taking the form of a blind vaginal pouch (Figures 43.32 and 43.33). The obstructed hemivagina is associated with either a functioning double uterus or a degenerate remnant of the paramesonephric duct. This uterine remnant is lined with ciliated columnar cells with occasional papillary projections. It may also contain patches of endometrial and/or glandular epithelium that produce a mucoid and/or menstrual discharge. At the time of puberty, absence of the lower part of the hemivagina is responsible for the development of hematocolpos, while the opposite hemivagina is patent. The diagnosis is usually facilitated by magnetic resonance imaging or computed tomography scan (Figure 43.34), which reveals not only hematocolpos but also

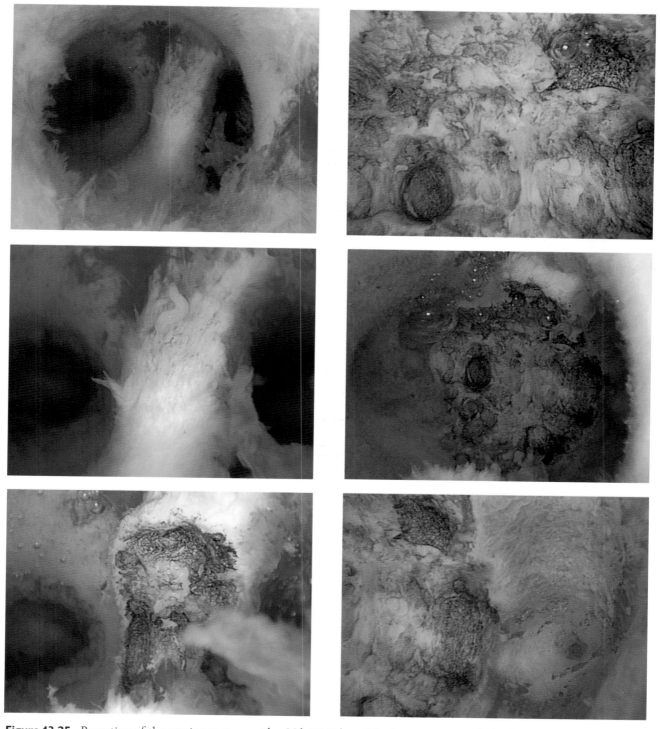

Figure 43.25 Resection of the uterine septum with a Nd : YAG laser. The hysteroscope with the laser fiber is advanced and the septum is melted away by simply advancing the fiber

hematometra and hematosalpinx. In childhood, an obstructed hemivagina is usually asymptomatic unless distended by mucus. In this case, a simple incision and resection of the vaginal septum will allow continued drainage. With menstruation, the resulting hematocolpos may be evacuated after complete resection of the septum. An obstructed hemivagina and double uterus are almost always associated with ipsilateral renal agenesis[90,91].

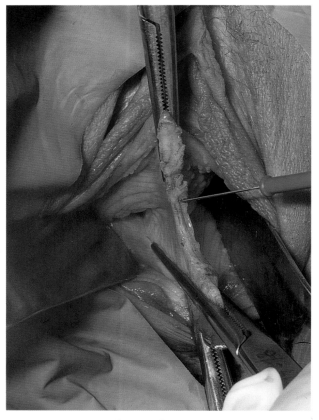

Figure 43.26 Vaginal sagittal septum. Resection of the septum using unipolar coagulation

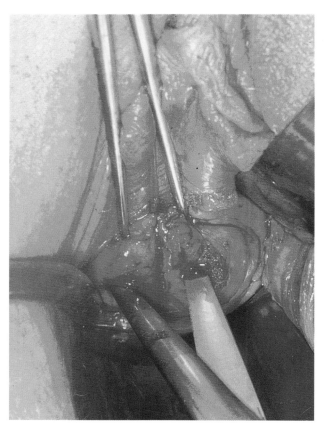

Figure 43.28 The cervical septum is incised with scissors

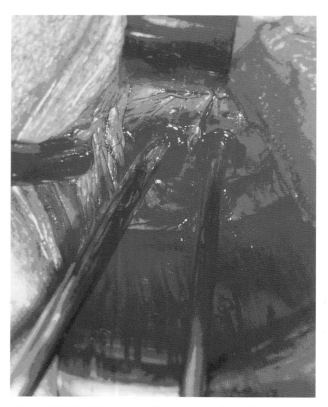

Figure 43.27 Dilatation of both cervical canals

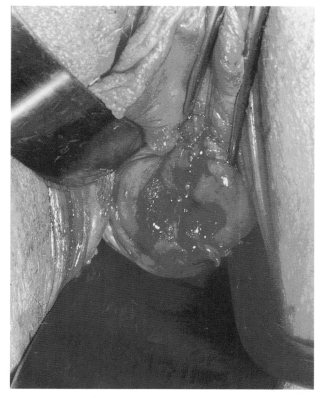

Figure 43.29 The external os is completely normal

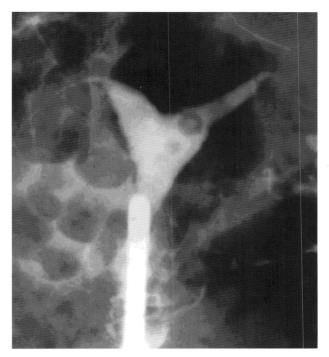

Figure 43.30 Postoperative hysterography: the morphology of the uterine cavity resembles an arcuate uterus

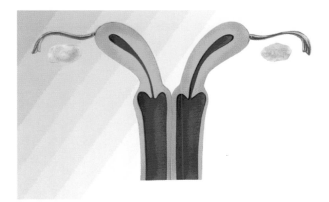

Figure 43.31 Uterus didelphys

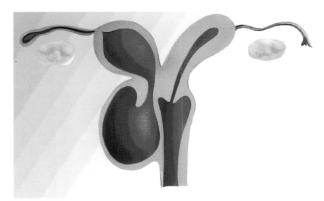

Figure 43.32 Septate vagina. The obstructed hemivagina is associated with a functioning double uterus

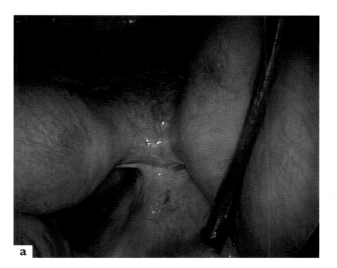

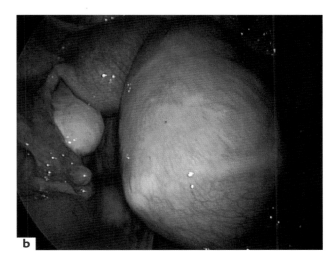

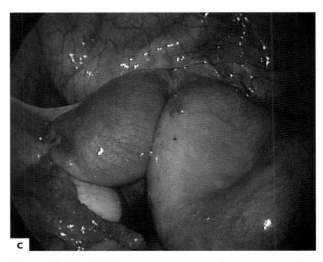

Figure 43.33 (a) Laparoscopic view of a septate vagina associated with uterus didelphys. (b) The right uterus is distended by hematometra. (c) After removal of the vaginal septum, the right uterus is emptied

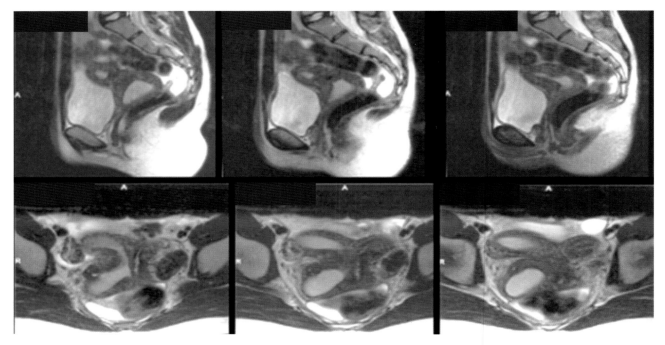

Figure 43.34 Magnetic resonance imaging of a septate vagina with hematocolpos and hematometra on the right side

Vertical fusion anomalies: incomplete canalization

The Müllerian buds have solid tips, behind which canalization takes place progressively. The Müllerian and sinovaginal bulb tissue, which forms the vagina, is also lumenless at first. Failure to canalize results in either solid organs or membranes of varying thickness obstructing the genital canal. Thus, a rudimentary uterus sometimes lacks a cavity and the vagina may be represented by an uncanalized column of tissue. Atresia may affect only one Müllerian duct, so that one horn of a bicornuate uterus may fail to communicate with the cervical canal, or one half of a septate vagina may be a closed cavity. Unilateral hematocolpos, mucocolpos and pyocolpos are not common.

Cervical atresia Congenital atresia of the cervix of an otherwise normal uterus or bicornuate uterus is rare (Figure 43.35). When it does occur, a reasonably normal vagina is invariably present. It is more common to encounter apparent cervical atresia in association with an absence of the lower vagina.

Vaginal atresia and transverse vaginal septum Disorders of vertical fusion result from defects in the union between the downward-progressing Müllerian tubercles and the upgrowing derivative of the urogenital sinus. Similar defects may also occur secondary to failure in canalization of the solid vaginal tube, either because of abnormal proliferation of paravaginal mesoderm or because of some form of intrauterine infection. Partial vaginal atresia is usually diagnosed in young patients at the time of puberty. Indeed, an

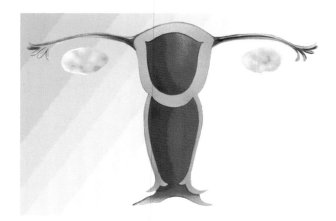

Figure 43.35 Cervical atresia

absence of the lower part of the vagina is responsible for the development of hematocolpos.

Progressive distension of the upper part of the vagina causes hypogastric pain, and, in the case of abundant hematocolpos (> 500 ml), dysuria or urinary retention may be associated. Vulvar and rectal examinations allow us to make the diagnosis of vaginal atresia. A computed tomography scan or magnetic resonance imaging reveal the hematocolpos, associated or not with a uterine malformation (uterine septum) (Figure 43.36).

Transverse vaginal septa are relatively rare, affecting approximately one in every 80 000 females. The septum consists of a central fibromuscular plate or ring of varying

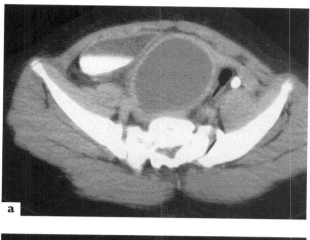

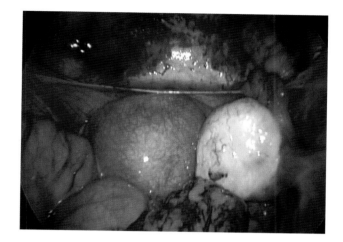

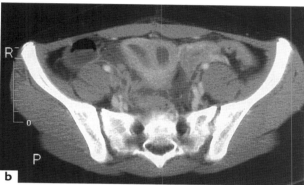

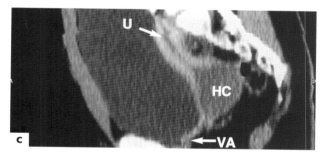

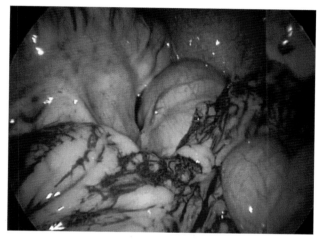

Figure 43.36 (a) Computed tomography reveals hemato-colpos. (b) It has been found to be associated with uterine septum. (c) Magnetic resonance imaging reveals partial vaginal atresia (VA), hematocolpos (HC) and the uterus (U)

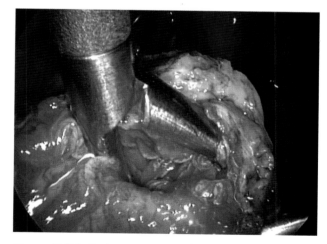

Figure 43.37 Endometriosis related to obstructive malformation

thickness. When the obstruction is complete, the outer surface is covered with stratified squamous epithelium, while the inner aspect is composed of glandular columnar epithelium. The interruption can occur at any level of the vagina, and may be multiple. The middle and lower zones of the vagina may be imperforate over a length of 0.5–6.0 cm. More frequently, the vagina is obstructed by a thinner membrane situated in the vagina, just above the hymen. Transverse vaginal septa usually go unnoticed in children unless mucocolpos develops or vaginal patency is tested. A rim of hymenal tissue will help to distinguish low transverse septa from an imperforate hymen. Distension of

the septum, as seen vaginally, will depend on its thickness and location. As in the case of imperforate hymen, the vulva may be very engorged and swollen. The obstruction of menstrual flow and subsequent endometriosis may result in infertility (Figure 43.37). In a study of 15 teenage patients with pelvic pain and endometriosis, six (40%)

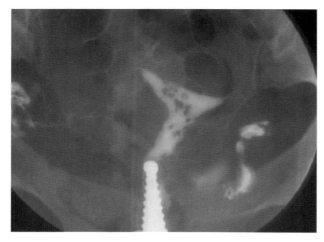

Figure 44.1 Intrauterine adhesions: degree Ia central adhesions (bridge-like adhesions)

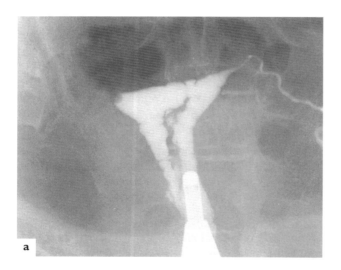

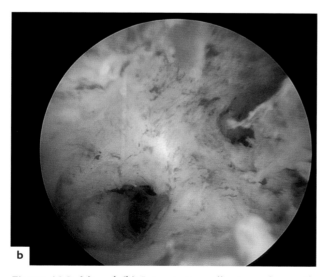

Figure 44.2 (a) and (b) Intrauterine adhesions: degree Ib myofibrous central adhesions

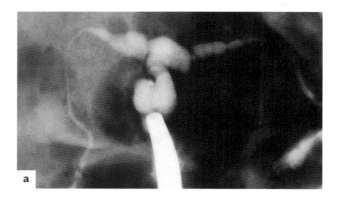

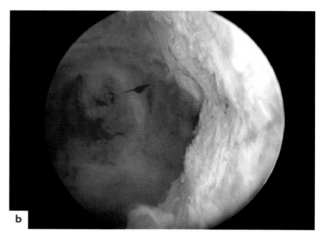

Figure 44.3 (a) and (b) Intrauterine adhesions: degree IIa marginal adhesions (always myofibrous or connective adhesions)

TREATMENT AND RESULTS

Hysterotomies for the division of adhesions and other blind transcervical manipulations are only of historical interest. Blind division of intrauterine adhesions by dilatation does not provide accurate and precise treatment. Thin or filmy endometrial adhesions are often easily removed by pushing with the tip of the hysteroscopic sheath. Myofibrous or connective adhesions require synechiotomy. The surgical treatment of intrauterine adhesions thus consists of dividing the adhesions mechanically, or using electrosurgery and/or fiberoptic lasers. The gynecological resectoscope with a modified knife electrode has been used to divide adhesions electrosurgically. Fiberoptic lasers, such as the argon, krypton (KTP)/532, and neodymium : yttrium–aluminum–garnet (Nd : YAG) laser with sculpted or extruded fibers, have also been used.

In our series, the Nd : YAG laser was used to remove endometrial adhesions, even when they were multiple and fibrous. Degree Ia and b adhesions were easily cut by the

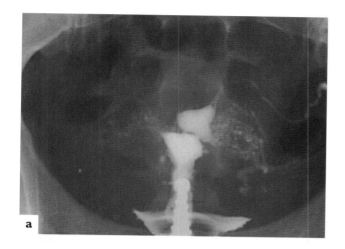

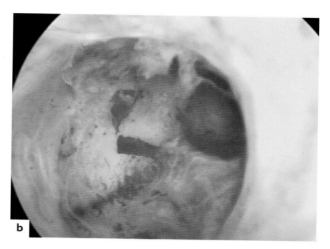

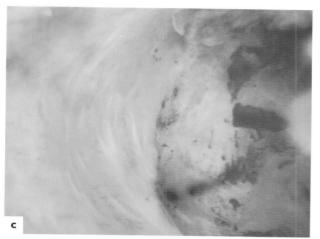

Figure 44.4 (a)–(c) Intrauterine adhesions: degree IIb right marginal adhesions, obliterating the horn

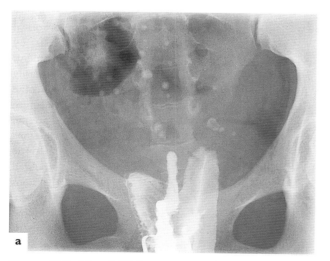

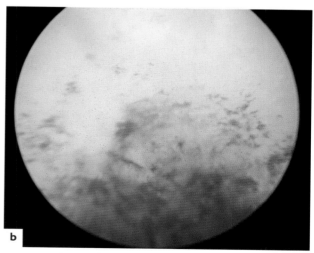

Figure 44.5 (a) and (b) Intrauterine adhesions: degree III. The cervical canal is visible. The uterine cavity is 'absent'. Only preoperative evaluation permits differentiation of pseudo-Asherman's syndrome

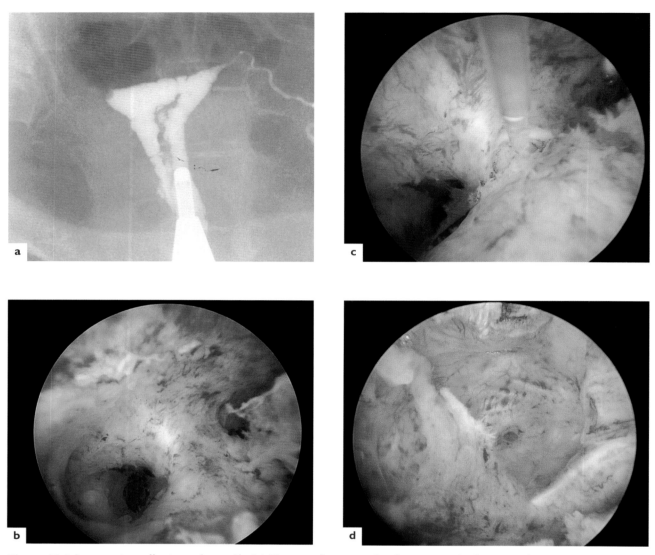

Figure 44.6 Intrauterine adhesions: degree Ib. (a) Hysterosalpingography determines the location. (b) Hysteroscopy determines the type (connective tissue). (c) The adhesion is divided with the laser (Nd : YAG) fiber. (d) Final view: the fundus of the uterine cavity (with tubal ostium)

laser fiber (Figure 44.6). Combined laparoscopy and hysteroscopy can be used, if indicated, to decrease the risk of uterine perforation. The lateral, back and front scattering of KTP and Nd : YAG laser beams may decrease the viability of the surrounding healthy endometrium. When the adhesions partially occlude the uterine cavity (degree Ib), their division is simple: they are divided in the middle, the remaining stumps retract and the uterine cavity distends, providing a panoramic view (Figure 44.6). Marginal or lateral adhesions (degree IIa and b) may be difficult to divide, particularly if they are extensive and fibromuscular or composed of connective tissue (Figures 44.7 and 44.8). The Nd : YAG laser may not be a good tool for the treatment of this type of adhesion. More severe adhesions may even develop, due to the scattering of the laser beam, decreasing the viability of the surrounding

healthy myometrium. For uterine adhesions of degree III (Figure 44.9), hysteroscopic observation of the uterine cavity should begin at the internal cervical os; if the adhesions extend to that area, their selective division begins there. As the adhesions are divided and the uterine cavity opens, the hysteroscope is advanced to the fundal area, and both uterotubal ostia are visualized. Sometimes, increased pressure in the uterine cavity, obtained by increasing the inflow pressure, can facilitate the dissection by distending the uterine cavity. However, although the plane of dissection is better exposed, this procedure can lead to excessive fluid intravasation if prolonged.

Low-viscosity fluids are frequently chosen for operative hysteroscopy because of their ability to remove debris and cleanse the uterine cavity, even in the presence of slight uterine bleeding. Normal saline and Ringer's

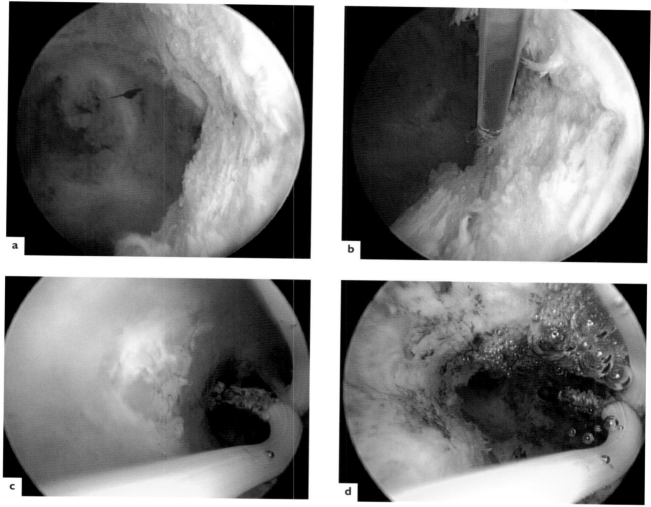

Figure 44.7 Intrauterine adhesions: degree IIa. (a) Left marginal adhesions. (b) Resection of adhesions with the Nd : YAG laser. (c) and (d) Resection of adhesions with an L-shaped electrode

lactate are excellent media for distending the uterine cavity when treating intrauterine adhesions with hysteroscopic scissors or with the Nd : YAG laser. Care must be taken to avoid solutions containing electrolytes when applying electrocoagulation, to control the volume of fluids not accounted for, and to prevent excessive fluid intravasation, particularly in the case of fluids without electrolytes. Intrauterine adhesions of the moderate and severe type require extensive dissection, increasing the risk of excessive intravasation. Prophylactic antibiotics are given 1 h prior to hysteroscopic treatment and for 2–3 days postoperatively, when an intrauterine device (IUD) is left in the uterine cavity. We have not found a second hysteroscopy to be of any particular value. A second therapeutic hysteroscopy is performed only if hysterosalpingography demonstrates residual adhesions. The subsequent insertion of an IUD and hormonal treatment have been associated with increasing success rates. In our department, estrogen and progestogen

replacement therapy is initiated after surgery for 3 months (ethinylestradiol 100 µg/day and lynestrenol 10 mg/day for 6 weeks). The doses are doubled for the following 6 weeks.

SUCCESS RATE

In collective series (Table 44.2), success rates of 74–94% have been obtained[7]. It is very difficult to compare different series because the results have not been evaluated according to the degree of severity. In a review[7], the pregnancy rate was found to be 60.5%, and 80% of those pregnancies reached term. In our series of 74 patients treated for intrauterine synechiae, eight patients were amenorrheic with an absent uterine cavity at hysterography. Four were classified as degree IIIa, and four as degree IIIb. Surgery was successfully performed in group IIIa, with a pregnancy rate of 100%. In group IIIb, however, adhesions recurred; second-look hysteroscopy showed only

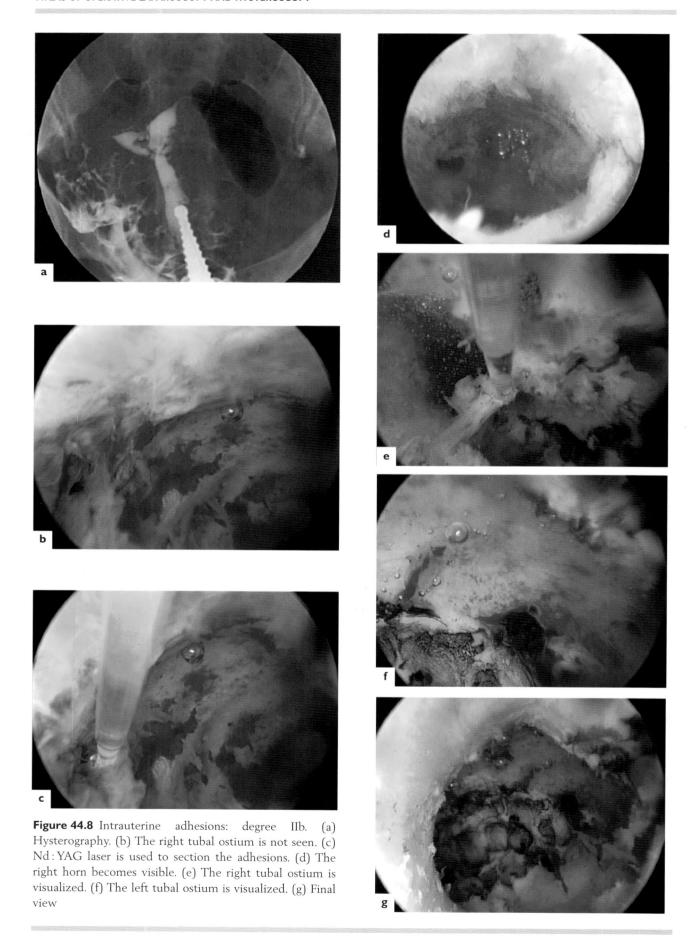

Figure 44.8 Intrauterine adhesions: degree IIb. (a) Hysterography. (b) The right tubal ostium is not seen. (c) Nd:YAG laser is used to section the adhesions. (d) The right horn becomes visible. (e) The right tubal ostium is visualized. (f) The left tubal ostium is visualized. (g) Final view

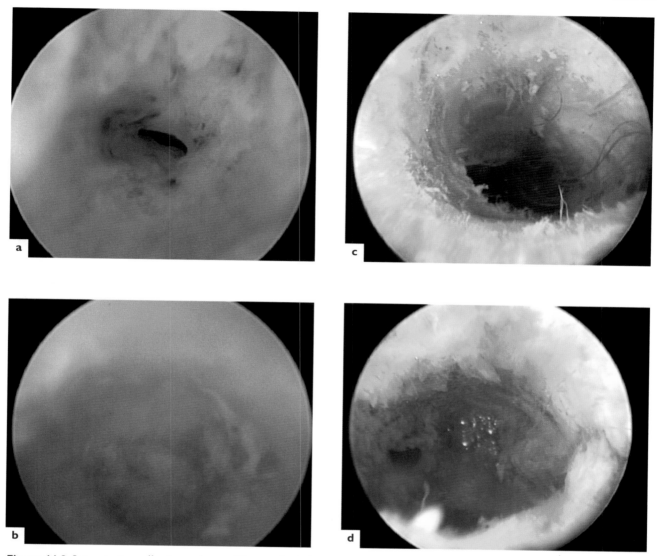

Figure 44.9 Intrauterine adhesions: degree III; pseudo-Asherman's syndrome. (a) Visualization of the internal cervical os. (b) The hysteroscope is advanced to the fundal area. (c) The adhesion is forced and the uterine cavity becomes visible. (d) Visualization of the right tubal ostium and normal endometrium

Table 44.2 Hysteroscopic lysis of intrauterine adhesions

Reference	Number of patients	Technique	Normal menses		Pregnancy		Term pregnancy	
			n	%	n	%	n	%
8	27	Scissors alongside hysteroscope	20	74	14	51.8	13	48.1
4	36	Scissors/biopsy forceps	34	94.4	17	62.9	12	44.4
5	187	Flexible/semirigid/rigid scissors	167	89.3	143	76.4	114	79.7

a tunnel-shaped uterine cavity with an absence of healthy endometrium. Hysterosalpingography, carried out 3 months after surgery, confirmed the presence of adhesions; some were more severe than the initial adhesions.

CONCLUSION

Hysteroscopic treatment of intrauterine adhesions restored normal menstruation in more than 80% of treated patients[7]. The results in terms of normal menses and pregnancy rates are excellent for those with adhesions of degrees Ia, Ib, IIa and IIIa. Degree IIb and IIIb adhesions tended to recur and to be more severe in six out of ten women, and no pregnancy occurred in this group. Patients treated for moderate or severe adhesions should be considered at risk during delivery. Following delivery, care must be taken to make an early diagnosis of any abnormalities, such as placenta accreta or percreta[5].

REFERENCES

1. Asherman JG. Amenorrhoea traumatica (atretica). J Obstet Gynaecol Br Emp 1948; 55: 23–30

2. Schenker JG, Margalioth EJ. Intrauterine adhesions; an updated appraisal. Fertil Steril 1982; 37: 593

3. Donnez J, Nisolle M. Operative laser hysteroscopy in Müllerian fusion defects and uterine adhesions. In Donnez J, ed. Operative Laser Laparoscopy and Hysteroscopy. Leuven, Belgium: Nauwelaerts Printing, 1989: 249–61

4. Wamsteker K. Hysteroscopy in the management of abnormal uterine bleeding in 199 patients. In Siegler AM, Lindemann HI, eds. Hysteroscopy, Principles and Practice. Philadelphia: JB Lippincott, 1984: 128–31

5. Valle RF, Sciarra JJ. Intrauterine adhesions: hysteroscopic diagnosis, classification, treatment, and reproductive outcome. Am J Obstet Gynecol 1988; 158: 1459–70

6. Valle R. Lysis of intrauterine adhesions (Asherman's syndrome). In Sutton C, Diamond M, eds. Endoscopic Surgery for Gynecologists. London: WB Saunders, 1993: 338

7. American Fertility Society. The American Fertility Society classifications of adnexal adhesions, distal tubal occlusion, tubal occlusion secondary to tubal ligation, tubal pregnancies, Müllerian anomalies and intrauterine adhesion. Fertil Steril 1988; 49: 944–55

8. Neuwirth RS, Hussein AR, Schiffman BM, et al. Hysteroscopic resection of intrauterine scars using a new technique. Obstet Gynecol 1982; 60: 111–13

Hysteroscopic myomectomy

J Donnez, P Jadoul, M Smets, J Squifflet

Laser energy has some advantages in precision of tissue destruction that are not shared by the electrical energy used in the resectoscope[1,2]. Since the most popular laser in gynecology has been the carbon dioxide (CO_2) laser, efforts have been made to adapt this for hysteroscopic use. However, several features of the CO_2 laser make it impractical for hysteroscopic use. The neodymium : yttrium–aluminum–garnet (Nd : YAG) laser, however, has three specific features, making it readily adaptable for hysteroscopic myomectomy:

- Its ability to transmit the beam of energy easily into the uterine cavity by means of a flexible quartz fiber

- Its ability to transmit laser energy to the tissue surface through a liquid distending medium

- Its ability to penetrate tissue to a controlled depth

The depth at which tissue destruction will occur can be controlled by varying the power used[3,4]; this physical quality can be applied for myomectomy and hysteroscopic myolysis[5,6]. This chapter describes the different techniques of hysteroscopic myomectomy.

HYSTEROSCOPIC EQUIPMENT

The fiber used to carry the laser light consists of quartz, surrounded by a thin plastic jacket, beyond which the tip of the fiber extends for several millimeters. The fiber is gas-sterilized or wiped with alcohol or Cidex® prior to use.

The deflecting arm is not of particular value, but allows the fiber to be stabilized. The hysteroscope is inserted into two different sheaths of varying diameter: one for inflow and the other for outflow. This resembles the classic resectoscope[7] and permits the constant cleaning of the uterine cavity. A Sharplan 2100 apparatus (Sharplan, Tel Aviv, Israel) is used for generating the laser. A power output of 80 W is used.

THE ROLE OF PREOPERATIVE GONADOTROPIN-RELEASING HORMONE AGONIST THERAPY

In one of our studies, we treated 376 women aged between 23 and 43 years (mean 33 years), with symptomatic submucous uterine fibroids, with a biodegradable gonadotropin-releasing hormone (GnRH) agonist (Zoladex® implant; ICI, Cambridge, UK). The implant was injected subcutaneously at the end of the luteal phase to curtail the initial gonadotropin stimulation phase always associated with a rise in estrogen. One implant was systematically injected at weeks 0, 4 and 8. Hysteroscopic myomectomy was carried out at 8 weeks. After the initial stimulation of estrogen secretion, GnRH agonist administration produced estrogen levels in the postmenopausal range (15 ± 6 pg/ml). Luteinizing hormone and follicle stimulating hormone levels were significantly suppressed within 2 weeks of treatment. The recovery of ovarian secretion occurred an average of 4–5 weeks after the last injection[6] (Figure 45.1).

Using the method previously described[5,6], the reduction in area of large submucous fibroids was calculated. When more than one fibroid was present, only the largest was evaluated. In all but four patients, the fibroid area decreased by an average of 38%[8] (range 4–95%). The fibroid area was found to decrease significantly ($p < 0.01$) from the baseline area (7.2 ± 4.7 cm^2), to 4.4 ± 3.5 cm^2 after 8 weeks of therapy. Figure 45.2 shows the mean fibroid area in patients with a pretreatment fibroid area of < 5 cm^2 versus those with an area of > 5 cm^2 to < 10 cm^2 and those with an area of > 10 cm^2. In all subgroups, a significant decrease ($p < 0.005$) was noted.

There was no significant difference between the different subgroups, but there was a significant difference between individual myomas (Figure 45.3). About 10% of myomas did not appear to respond very well to GnRH agonist treatment.

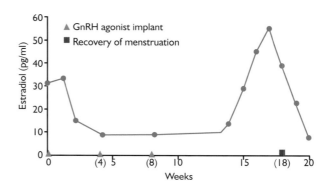

Figure 45.1 Hormonal levels (17β-estradiol) during gonadotropin-releasing hormone (GnRH) agonist therapy. An implant of Zoladex® was injected at weeks 0, 4 and 8

incomplete resection. A complete resection continues down to the cervical canal. The percentage of amenorrhea is higher with the latter technique.

Step six

The fundal and corneal areas are now treated (Figures 46.10–46.13). The fundal area can be treated with the loop by bringing the loop sideways over the fundal area.

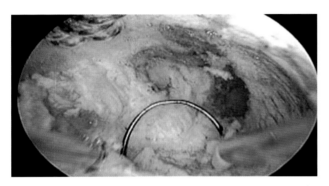

Figure 46.10 The tubal ostium, seen to the right in the middle of the picture with the dark red/crimson color scheme, is often difficult to treat with the classical resector loop

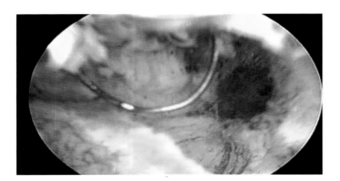

Figure 46.11 The combination of a deep-lying tubal ostium, a large resector loop and the bubbles makes it difficult to excise the osteal region precisely

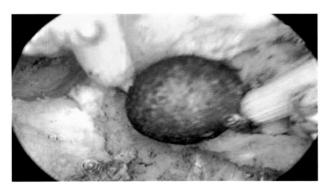

Figure 46.12 A small rollerball electrode can be useful in the treatment of these areas

The corneal areas can also be treated with the loop. If the loop is too large for the cornua, a small ball can be used to coagulate these areas.

Step seven

The fragments of tissue are grasped between the loop and the final lens of the resectoscope and brought out of the cavity (Figure 46.14).

Step eight

A last inspection of the uterine cavity is performed (Figure 46.15). If bleeding vessels are spotted, these are now coagulated. It can be useful to reduce the distension pressure in order to see the bleeding points (Figure 46.16).

Management of tissue fragments

If the uterus is large enough, the fragments of tissue should be 'parked' in the fundal area awaiting their removal at the end of the resection. If the uterus is small, resected fragments should be brought out whenever they interfere with good visibility.

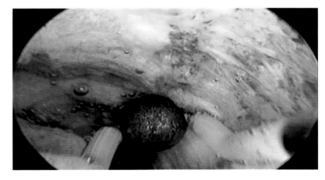

Figure 46.13 The rollerball electrode can also be used to treat the lower part of the resection in the cervix where deep resection is often dangerous as larger vessels can be opened inadvertently

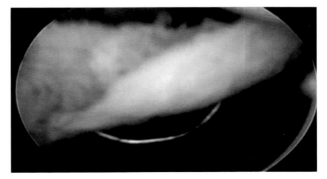

Figure 46.14 The fragments are grasped between the loop and the final lens and brought out of the uterine cavity

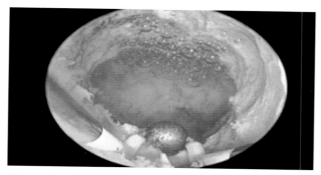

Figure 46.15 General view at the end of the resection

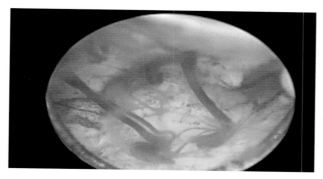

Figure 46.16 The pressure is reduced and the bleeding becomes visible so that the terminal part of the vessel can be coagulated

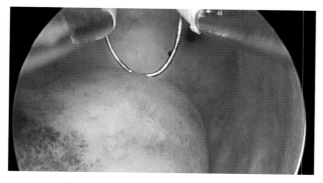

Figure 46.17 A polyp is removed at the same time as the endometrial resection

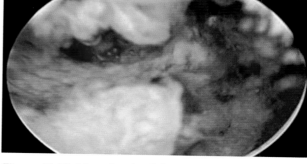

Figure 46.18 Note the glandular structure of the inside of the resected polyp

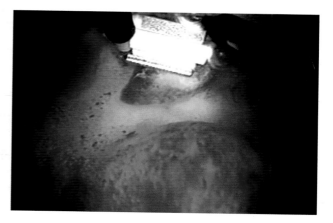

Figure 46.19 The electrode is brought in contact with the fundal area. Note that the visibility with normal saline is as good as with Glycine® when a through-flow resectoscope is used

caused by adenomyosis. This could be the reason why large uteri fare worse than their normal counterparts, as often there is the presence of adenomyosis alongside the myomas in these uteri.

If there are polyps in the uterine cavity, these should be treated during the same session (Figures 46.17 and 46.18). The outcome is the same as that for classical TCER.

If myomas are treated at the same time, the results seem slightly worse in the long-term follow-up. Our own long-term follow-up study (unpublished data) revealed that, after 5 years, 92% of the patients were still satisfied with the TCER and 96% would have the intervention again.

An alternative to unipolar high-frequency resection in Glycine distension medium is bipolar ablation in normal saline solution (Figures 46.19–46.21). It has to be said that fluid overload of the patient with normal saline has exactly the same consequences as overload with Glycine, except for the pharmacological effects of Glycine that do not

CONCLUSIONS

Provided that the uterine cavity is of a reasonable size, the author suggests a resection of 10 cm. TCER is a well-documented technique that should be used as a first approach in patients with menorrhagia provided that there are no other pathological conditions in the uterine wall or the endometrium. Most common problems or failures are

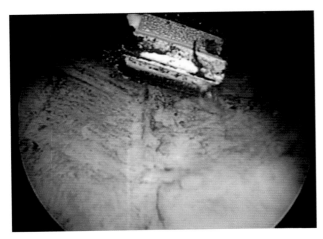

Figure 46.20 The action of the bipolar electrode is very powerful. The anatomical landmarks of the ablation are clearly visible. Note the different form of the electrode

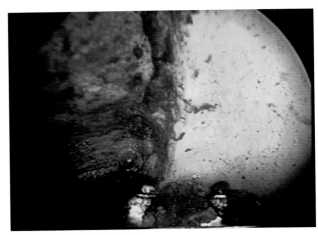

Figure 46.21 Both the posterior and the anterior wall must be treated. The bipolar electrodes are easier to manipulate than the classical resector loop

occur with normal saline. Ablation does not allow for pathological examination.

REFERENCES

1. Grainger DA, DeCherney AH. Hysteroscopic management of uterine bleeding. Baillieres Clin Obstet Gynaecol 1989; 3: 403–14

2. Wood C. Alternative treatment. Baillieres Clin Obstet Gynaecol 1995; 9: 373–97

3. Goldenberg M, Sivan E, Bider D, et al. Endometrial resection versus abdominal hysterectomy for menorrhagia. Correlated sample analysis. J Reprod Med 1996; 41: 333–6

4. Brumsted JR, Blackman JA, Badger GJ, et al. Hysteroscopy versus hysterectomy for the treatment of abnormal uterine bleeding: a comparison of cost. Feril Steril 1996; 65: 310–16

5. Donnez J, Polet R, Mathieu P-E, et al. Nd : YAG laser ITT multifiber device (the Donnez device): endometrial ablation by interstitial hyperthermia. In Donnez J, Nisolle M, eds. An Atlas of Laser Operative Laparoscopy and Hysteroscopy. Carnforth, UK: The Parthenon Publishing Group, 1994: 353–9

6. Mencaglia L. Hysteroscopy and adenocarcinoma. Obstet Gynecol Clin North Am 1995; 22: 573–9

7. Bhattacharya S, Cameron IM, Mollison J, et al. Admission-discharge policies for hysteroscopic surgery; a randomised comparison of day case with in-patient admission. Eur J Obstet Gynecol Reprod Biol 1998; 78: 81–4

8. van Herendael BJ. Hazard and dangers of operative hysteroscopy. In Sutton C, Diamond M, eds. Endoscopic Surgery for Gynaecologists. London: WB Saunders, 1998: 118–25

9. van Herendael BJ. Instrumentation in hysteroscopy. Obstet Gynecol Clin North Am 1995; 22: 391–408

47

Global endometrial ablation

G A Vilos

Abnormal uterine bleeding (AUB) from benign causes affects approximately 20–25% of premenopausal women. The prevalence increases with age, and peaks during women's fifth decade just prior to the menopause[1]. Traditionally, AUB has been treated medically, by dilatation and curettage (D&C) and/or hysterectomy. D&C has been widely used for the diagnosis and treatment of AUB; however, there are no randomized controlled clinical trials (RTCs) to demonstrate a sustained and prolonged therapeutic value. Hysterectomy has been the traditional and permanent treatment for AUB. However, the high hysterectomy rates and evaluation of risks and cost/benefit prompted the exploration of alternative therapies, one of which is endometrial ablation.

Hysteroscopic endometrial ablation or first-generation endometrial ablation technologies (FEATs) were introduced in the 1980s as an alternative to hysterectomy in women with AUB who failed medical management and/or D&C. Second-generation endometrial ablation technologies (SEATs), also called global endometrial ablation (GEA) technologies, were introduced in the 1990s as easier, possibly safer and equally effective alternatives to hysteroscopic endometrial ablation or FEATs[2].

Global endometrial ablation is defined as the automated destruction of the endometrium with an energy source without the use of operative hysteroscopy. The two exceptions to this rule include hydrothermablation (HTA), which can be performed under hysteroscopic observation, and microwave endometrial ablation (MEA), which is operator-dependent but performed without hysteroscopic visualization[3]. During the past decade several technologies have been introduced, some of which are extinct, but most remain available for clinical use, and others are still undergoing feasibility and/or comparative clinical trials. The technologies available for use are classified in Table 47.1.

All of these devices require minimal operator skills and no irrigant/distending solutions in the uterus, except for HTA which requires free circulating hot saline as the treating agent. All require thermal energy such as heat or cold to destroy the endometrium. Although all devices have produced good preliminary results, the long-term efficacy, complication rates and/or cost/benefit ratio, except for the hot liquid balloons, have not been established.

This chapter describes these devices as they appeared chronologically, and presents peer-reviewed publications and comparative randomized clinical trials with at least 12 months of follow-up. It is left up to the readers to assess the evidence and reach their own conclusions and preferences. Criteria in choosing any of the devices should take into account: (1) maximum safety, (2) user-friendliness, (3) patient convenience, (4) analgesia/anesthesia requirements, (5) menstrual reduction rates, (6) durability and avoidance of further treatment and (7) costs of treatment compared with the first-generation ablation treatments and/or hysterectomy.

ENDOMETRIAL ABLATION

Endometrial ablation is the destruction or elimination of the endometrium by coagulation, freezing or resection, offered as an alternative to hysterectomy to those patients with AUB and benign pathology who are unable or unwilling to tolerate traditional therapies. Dysfunctional uterine bleeding (DUB) is defined as menstrual blood loss greater than 80 ml per cycle occurring in the absence of genital tract anatomic lesions or systemic diseases. DUB can be the result of both ovulatory and anovulatory anomalies. The consequences of AUB are excessive menstrual blood loss (menorrhagia, hypermenorrhea, polymenorrhea, menometrorrhagia), which frequently leads to iron-deficiency anemia. These signs and symptoms are often serious, embarrassing and debilitating conditions for many women, adversely affecting their quality of life. AUB together with uterine fibroids account for up to 75% of all hysterectomies performed worldwide[1–5].

Patient assessment

By intent, the aim of endometrial ablation is to destroy/eliminate the endometrium. Therefore, it is imperative to exclude premalignant and malignant

Table 47.1 Classification of second-generation endometrial ablation technologies (SEATs)

Hot liquid balloons
    ThermaChoice® I, II and III
    Cavaterm™ and Cavaterm™ *plus*
    Thermablate™
Hydrothermablation (HTA)
Cryoablation (Her Option®)
Microwave endometrial ablation (MEA™)
Impedance-controlled ablation (NovaSure™)

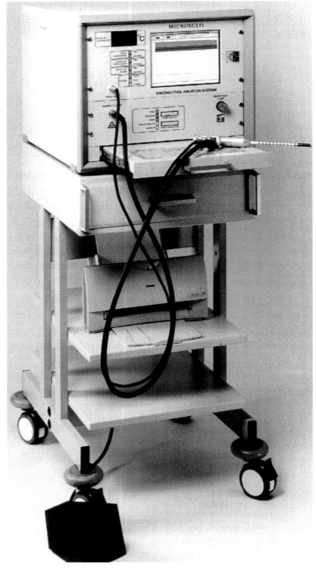

Figure 47.5 The microwave endometrial ablation (MEA™) system (Microsulis, Waterlooville, UK)

place the tip in the other cornual area to repeat the procedure. The probe is then gradually withdrawn while maintaining the probe temperature in the 80–95°C range to ensure even, complete endometrial destruction. The entire treatment is completed in 2–3 minutes. Prethinning of the endometrium is recommended.

Preliminary results after 6 months of treatment in 23 patients demonstrated: amenorrhea 57%, hypomenorrhea 26%, no improvement 12%. Three patients were retreated successfully. The overall results were 83% for single treatment and 96% after retreatment[76]. A randomized comparative clinical trial (MEA, $n = 129$) against transcervical resection (TCRE, $n = 134$) reported that at 12 months, 89 (77%) women in the MEA group and 93 (75%) in the

resection group were totally or generally satisfied with their treatment[78]. The menstrual pattern was similar in both groups, with a combined amenorrhea/hypomenorrhea rate of 89% in both groups and satisfaction rate of 90%. Repeat resection was performed in 1% and hysterectomy in 12–13% in both groups. The total operation time was 11 and 15 minutes in the MEA and TCRE groups, respectively[78]. After 2 years of treatment, the satisfaction rates were 79% vs. 67% in the MEA and TCRE groups, respectively[79].

A multicenter RCT compared MEA ($n = 215$) and rollerball endometrial ablation (REA, $n = 107$). By intent-to-treat analysis, the success rate of MEA at 12 months (87.0%) did not differ significantly from that of REA (83.2%). Among evaluable patients, the success rate was also similar in the MEA (96.4%) and REA (92.7%) groups. The amenorrhea rate in evaluable patients was 61.3% vs. 91.0% and the satisfaction rate was 98.5% vs. 99% in the MEA and REA groups, respectively[80]. At 3 years, the amenorrhea and satisfaction rates were 64% vs. 56% and 95% vs. 90% in the MEA and REA groups, respectively[81]. Success rates at 12 months in women with myomas and in those without myomas did not differ significantly between the MEA and REA groups. Among evaluable patients with myomas who underwent MEA, the success rate was 90.3%. These women attained an amenorrhea rate of 61.3%, compared with 38.5% of women with myomas treated by REA[80]. Although all three RCTs included intracavitary polyps and myomas up to 2 cm in diameter, only the last RCT reported a subgroup analysis of patients with myomas[80].

Advantages of MEA include a short treatment time (3–4 minutes), high success rate and applicability in a larger uterus (up to 14 cm cavity length) with or without intracavitary polyps and myomas. Disadvantages include reduced portability, requirement for pretreatment to thin the endometrium, cervical dilatation to 9 mm, ultrasonic measurement of myometrial thickness and lack of a perforation detection mechanism.

Although the technique is of short duration and easy to master, it is a blind procedure, and the relative safety has not been established. In 1433 cases performed in 13 centers in the United Kingdom and Canada, one burn of the small bowel was encountered with the MEA (frequency 0.7/1000)[82]. An additional bowel injury was reported at the Middlesbrough Consensus Meeting in the UK[2]. Furthermore, from November 2003 to March 2004, the FDA MAUDE database included three bowel burns and one case of peritonitis secondary to pyosalpinx, and no evidence of uterine perforation. One bowel burn occurred in the absence of obvious uterine perforation.

Cryoendometrial ablation

Cryosurgery of the endometrium using a probe to freeze the endometrium from –60°C to –100°C in six patients was first reported by Cahan and Brockunier in 1967[83].

Droegemueller *et al.* evaluated two types of cryoprobes using freon in 1970[84] (Frigitronics, Shelton, CT, USA). Ten of 16 patients with DUB developed amenorrhea during the 6–8-week interval between cryosurgery and a scheduled vaginal hysterectomy. In two patients, cryosurgery was accomplished under local anesthesia[85,86].

In two subsequent studies by Pittrof *et al.*, 18 patients underwent transcervical endometrial cryoablation using normal saline as a uterine distension medium[87,88]. The principle of this technique was to distend the uterine cavity with 3–15 ml of normal saline and then to freeze it with a nitrous oxide iceball, forming a mould of the uterine cavity, with a specially designed cryosurgical probe. The probe appeared similar to a number 8 Hegar dilator. After 5 minutes, the ice was allowed to melt, and the same procedure was repeated with the probe pointing toward the other uterine cornua. Of the 12 patients followed up to 3 or more months, eight were completely satisfied with their results. There were no operative complications, and 13 patients were discharged the day after their operation[87,88].

Rutherford *et al.*, in a pilot study involving 15 patients followed for 22 months, reported that amenorrhea was achieved in 50%. New equipment was able to freeze the endometrium to –170°C[89]. The cervix was dilated to 8 mm, and the bladder was filled with 300–400 ml of warm saline to act as a heat sink. The uterine cavity was filled with up to 10 ml of a water-soluble lubricant. An 8 mm × 27 cm conical-tip cryomedical freezing probe with a 4-cm freezing zone attached to a CMS 450 AccuProbe® system (Cryomedical Sciences, Rockville, MD, USA) was inserted to the uterine fundus. Once freezing of the uterine cavity was begun, iceball formation was monitored using a biplane 7.5-MHz transrectal transducer with an ultrasound scanner. Within 3–5 minutes after the probe reached –170°C, the front of the iceball was seen to be at least 50% through the myometrium. At this point, freezing was discontinued and thawing begun[89]. Fifteen patients underwent 16 procedures for DUB. Life-table calculations gave amenorrhea rates of 75.5% at 6 months and 50.3% at 22 months. One patient was retreated.

Her Option™ cryoablation   This cryosurgical system (CryoGen, San Diego, CA, USA) is compressor driven and uses a new mixed gas coolant to generate temperatures of –90° to –100°C. The cryoprobe is inserted into the uterine cavity and saline is injected to bath the cryoprobe (Figure 47.6). Freezing–thawing of the intrauterine iceball is monitored with transabdominal ultrasound. Endometrial cryoablation in ten women undergoing hysterectomy resulted in 9–12-mm depth of endomyometrial necrosis as determined by tetrazolium staining and electron microscopy[90–92].

A multicenter RCT compared Her Option ($n = 193$) with rollerball ($n = 86$) in women with menorrhagia. Women treated by cryoablation received significantly less general anesthesia (46%) than those treated by rollerball (92%). At 12 months of follow-up, the amenorrhea and overall success rates were 28% and 77% in the Her Option group compared with 56% and 84% in the rollerball group, respectively[93]. At 24 months, 77% of the cryoablation group reported that dysmenorrhea was non-existent or much improved, versus 81% of the rollerball group. Premenstrual symptoms were absent or mild in 64% of cryoablation and 79% of electrocoagulation patients. The satisfaction rates were 91% and 88% in the cryoablation and electrocoagulation groups, respectively. Of the cryoablation group, 7% proceeded to hysterectomy and 2.7% to repeat ablation, compared with 8.1% and 1.2% of the rollerball group, respectively[94].

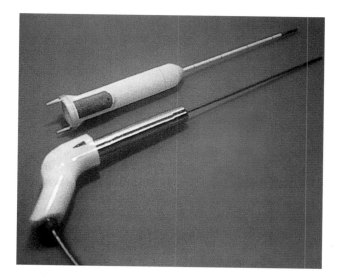 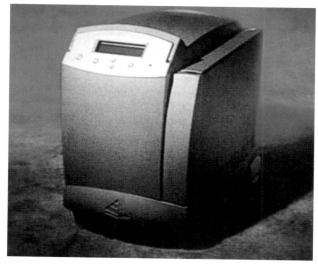

Figure 47.6 The Her Option™ cryoablation system (CryoGen, San Diego, CA, USA)

MAUDE database. Obstet Gynecol 2003; 102: 1278–82

52. Friberg B, Wallsten H, Henriksson P, Persson BRR. A new, simple, safe and efficient device for the treatment of menorrhagia. J Gynecol Tech 1996; 2: 103–8

53. Persson BRR, Friberg B, Olsrud J, et al. Numerical calculations of temperature distribution resulting from intracavitary heating of the uterus. Gynecol Endosc 1998; 7: 203–9

54. Hawe JA, Phillips AG, Chien PE, et al. Cavaterm thermal balloon ablation for the treatment of menorrhagia. Br J Obstet Gynaecol 1999; 106: 1143–4

55. Friberg B, Ahlgren M. Thermal balloon endometrial destruction: the outcome of treatment of 117 women followed up for a maximum period of 4 years. Gynecol Endosc 2000; 9: 389–95

56. Mettler L. Long-term results in the treatment of menorrhagia and hypermenorrhea with a thermal balloon endometrial ablation technique. J Soc Laparosc Surg 2002; 6: 305–9

57. Pellicano M, Guida M, Acunzo G, et al. Hysteroscopic transcervical endometrial resection versus thermal destruction for menorrhagia: a prospective randomized trial on satisfaction rate. Am J Obstet Gynecol 2002; 187: 545–50

58. Howe J, Abbott J, Hunter D, et al. A randomized controlled trial comparing the Cavaterm endometrial ablation system with the Nd : YAG laser for the treatment of dysfunctional uterine bleeding. Br J Obstet Gynaecol 2003; 110: 350–7

59. Abbott J, Howe J, Hunter D, et al. A double-blind randomized trial comparing the Cavaterm and the NovaSure endometrial ablation system for the treatment of dysfunctional uterine bleeding. Fertil Steril 2003; 80: 203–8

60. Cavaterm system. Wallsten Medical, Kvisgaard, Denmark. Available at www.wallstenmedical.com

61. Mangeshikar PS, Kopur A, Yackel D. Endometrial ablation with a new thermal balloon system. J Am Assoc Gynecol Laparosc 2003; 10: 27–32

62. Thomas JA, Leyland N, Durand N, Windrich RC. The use of oral misoprostol as a cervical ripening agent in operative hysteroscopy: a double-blind, placebo-controlled trial. Am J Obstet Gynecol 2002; 186: 876–9

63. Darwish AM, Ahmad AM, Mohammad AM. Cervical priming prior to operative hysteroscopy: a randomized comparison of laminaria versus misoprostol. Hum Reprod 2004; 19: 2391–4

64. Vilos GA. Endometrial ablation with a new balloon system (Thermablate EAS) to treat menorrhagia in high-risk surgical candidates. J Am Assoc Gynecol Laparosc 2003; 10: S36

65. Yackel D, Vilos GA. Thermablate EAS: a new endometrial ablation system. Gynecol Surg 2004; 1: 129–32

66. Vilos GA, Abu-Rafea B, Haque A. Endometrial thermablation: a two minute balloon treatment. Presented at the 7th World Congress on Controversies in Obstetrics and Gynecology and Infertility, Athens, Greece, April, 2005

67. Goldrath MH, Barrionuevo M, Husain M. Endometrial ablation with hysteroscopic instillation of hot saline solution. J Am Assoc Gynecol Laparosc 1997; 4: 235–40

68. Richart RM, Botacini das Dores G, Nicolau SM, et al. Histologic studies of the effects of circulating hot saline on the uterus before hysterectomy. J Am Assoc Gynecol Laparosc 1999; 6: 269–73

69. Bustos-Lopez HH, Baggish M, Valle RF, et al. Assessment of the safety of intrauterine instillation of heated saline for endometrial ablation. Fertil Steril 1998; 69: 155–60

70. Corson SL. A multicentre evaluation of endometrial ablation by HydroThermAblator and rollerball for treatment of menorrhagia. J Am Assoc Gynecol Laparosc 2001; 8: 359–67

71. Goldrath MH. Evaluation of HydroThermAblator and roller endometrial ablation for menorrhagia 3 years after treatment. J Am Assoc Gynecol Laparosc 2003; 10: 505–11

72. Glasser MH, Zimmerman JD. The HydroThermAblator system for management of menorrhagia in women with submucous myomas: 12-to-20-month follow-up. J Am Assoc Gynecol Laparosc 2003; 10: 521–7

73. Rosenbaum SP, Fried M, Munro MG. Endometrial hydrothermablation: a comparison of short-term clinical effectiveness in patients with normal endometrial cavities and those with intracavitary pathology. J Am Assoc Gynecol Laparosc 2005; 12: 144–9

74. Vilos GA, Harding PG, Sugimoto A, et al. Hysteroscopic endomyometrial resection of three uterine sarcomas. J Am Assoc Gynecol Laparosc 2001; 8: 545–51

75. Vilos GA, Ettler H. Atypical polypoid adenomyoma and hysteroscopic endometrial ablation. J Obstet Gynecol Can 2003; 25: 760–2

76. Sharp NC, Cronin N, Feldberg I, et al. Microwave for menorrhagia: a new fast technique for endometrial ablation. Lancet 1995; 346: 1003–4

77. Wallage S, Cooper KG, Graham WJ, Parkin DE. A randomized trial comparing local versus general anaesthesia for microwave endometrial ablation. Br J Obstet Gynaecol 2003; 110: 799–807

78. Cooper KG, Bain C, Parkin D. Comparison of microwave endometrial ablation and transcervical resection of the endometrium for treatment of heavy menstrual loss: a randomized trial. Lancet 1999; 354: 1859–63

79. Bain C, Cooper KG, Parkin DE. Microwave endometrial ablation versus endometrial resection: a randomized controlled trial. Obstet Gynecol 2002; 99: 983–7

80. Cooper TM, Anderson TL, Fortin CA, et al. Microwave endometrial ablation vs. rollerball electroablation for menorrhagia: a multicenter randomized trial. J Am Assoc Gynecol Laparosc 2004; 11: 354–403

81. Harris M, Anderson TL, Fortin C, et al. Microwave endometrial ablation: three year outcomes of a

multicenter trial [Abstract]. J Minim Invasive Gynecol 2005; 12 (Suppl 1): 8

82. Downes E, Cooper K, O'Donovan P, Sharp N. Microwave endometrial ablation is a safe technique [Abstract]. J Am Assoc Gynecol Laparosc 2000; 7: S13

83. Cahan WG, Brockunier A. Cryosurgery of the uterine cavity. Am J Obstet Gynecol 1967; 99: 138–53

84. Droegemueller W, Greer BE, Makowski EL. Preliminary observations of cryoablation of the endometrium. Am J Obstet Gynecol 1970; 107: 958–61

85. Droegemueller W, Greer B, Makowski E. Cryosurgery in patients with dysfunctional uterine bleeding. Obstet Gynecol 1971; 38: 256–8

86. Droegemueller W, Makowski E, MacSalka R. Destruction of the endometrium by cryosurgery. Am J Obstet Gynecol 1971; 110: 467–9

87. Pittrof R, Majid S, Murray A. Initial experience with transcervical cryoablation of the endometrium using saline as a uterine distension medium. Minim Invasive Ther 1993; 2: 69–73

88. Pittrof R, Majid S, Murray A. Transcervical endometrial cryoablation (ECA) for menorrhagia. Int J Gynecol Obstet 1994; 47: 135–9

89. Rutherford TJ, Zreik TG, Troiana RN, et al. Endometrial cryoablation, a minimally invasive procedure for abnormal uterine bleeding (pilot study). J Am Assoc Gynecol Laparosc 1998; 5: 23–8

90 Dobak JD, Willems J, Howard R, et al. Endometrial cryoablation with ultrasound visualized in women undergoing hysterectomy. J Am Assoc Gynecol Laparosc 2000; 7: 89–93

91. Dobak JD, Willems J. Extripated uterine endometrial cryoablation with ultrasound visualization. J Am Assoc Gynecol Laparosc 2000; 7: 95–101

92. Dobak JD, Ryba E, Kovalcheck S. A new closed-loop cryosurgical device for endometrial ablation. J Am Assoc Gynecol Laparosc 2000; 7: 245–9

93. Duleba AJ, Heppard MC, Soderstrom RM, Townsend DE. A randomized study comparing cryoablation and rollerball electroablation for treatment of dysfunctional uterine bleeding. J Am Assoc Gynecol Laparosc 2003; 10: 17–26

94. Townsend DE, Duleba AJ, Wilkes MM. Durability of treatment effects after endometrial cryoablation versus rollerball electroablation for abnormal uterine bleeding: two-year results of a multicenter randomized trial. Am J Obstet Gynecol 2003; 188: 699–701

95. Cooper J, Brill A, Fullop T. Is endometrial pre-treatment necessary in NovaSure 3-D endometrial ablation? Gynecol Endosc 2001; 10: 179–92

96. Gallinat A, Nugent W. NovaSure impedance-controlled system for endometrial ablation. J Am Assoc Gynecol Laparosc 2002; 9: 279–85

97. Rudowsky R, Gallinat A. NovaSure impedance controlled endometrial ablation system, long-term follow-up results in 107 patients [Abstract]. J Minim Invasive Gynecol 2005; 12 (Suppl 1): 76–7

98. Cooper J, Gimpelson R, Laberge P, et al. A randomized multicentre trial of safety and efficacy of the NovaSure system in the treatment of menorrhagia. J Am Assoc Gynecol Laparosc 2002; 9: 418–28

99. Bongers MY, Bourdrez P, Mol BW, et al. Randomized controlled trial of bipolar radiofrequency endometrial ablation and balloon endometrial ablation. Br J Obstet Gynaecol 2004; 111: 1095–102

100. Laberge PY, Sabbah R, Fortin C, Gallinat A. Assessment and comparison of intraoperative and postoperative pain associated with NovaSure and ThermaChoice endometrial ablation systems. J Am Assoc Gynecol Laparosc 2003; 10: 223–32

101. Bongers MY, Bourdrez P, Heintz PM, et al. Bipolar radiofrequency endometrial ablation compared with balloon endometrial ablation in dysfunctional uterine bleeding: impact on patients' health-related quality of life. Fertil Steril 2005; 83: 724–34

102. Pantaleoni D. On endoscopic examination of the cavity of the womb. Med Press Circ 1969; 8: 26

103. Kucuk M, Okman TK. Intrauterine instillation of trichloroacetic acid is effective for the treatment of dysfunctional uterine bleeding. Fertil Steril 2005; 83: 189–94

104. Garside R, Stein K, Wyatt K, et al. The effectiveness and cost-effectiveness of microwave and thermal balloon endometrial ablation for heavy menstrual bleeding: a systematic review and economic modeling. Health Technol Assess 2004; 8: 1–155

105. Della Badia C, Atogho A. Serious adverse events associated with the use of endometrial ablation devices [Abstract]. J Minim Invasive Gynecol 2005; 12 (Suppl 1): 15

106. Sharp H, Jardine G. Global endometrial ablation in 196 patients and associated risk factors [Abstract]. J Min Inv Gynecol 2005; 12 (Suppl 1): 8–9

107. Lethaby A, Hickey M, Garry R. Endometrial destruction techniques for heavy menstrual bleeding. Cochrane Database Syst Rev 2005; (4): CD001501

108. Bridgman SA, Dunn KM. Has endometrial ablation replaced hysterectomy for the treatment of dysfunctional uterine bleeding? National figures. Br J Obstet Gynaecol 2000; 107: 531–4

109. Lepine LA, Hillis SD, Marchbanks PA, et al. Hysterectomy Surveillance – United States, 1980–1993. MMWR Morb Mortal Wkly Rep 1997; 46: 1–15

110. Keshavarz H, Hillis S, Kieke B, et al. Hysterectomy Surveillance – United States, 1994–1999. MMWR Morb Mortal Wkly Rep 2002; 51: 1–8

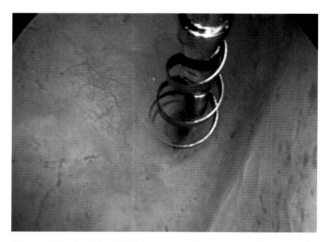

Figure 48.11 The STOP system: by turning the outside wheel counterclockwise, the device is now deployed so that it anchors itself in the intramural part of the tube

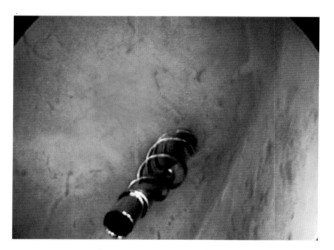

Figure 48.12 The STOP system: the device is now in place, the longer portion being left in the intramural part of the tube while the shorter part (approximately 1.5–2 cm) remains in the uterine cavity

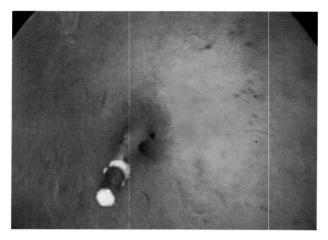

Figure 48.13 The STOP system: the right side of the same patient where a device had been installed exactly 1 month before. Because of an allergic reaction, the procedure had to be stopped at that time. Note the in-growths of the tissues at the tubal ostium and around the device blocking the intramural part of the tube

patent and of normal anatomic configuration. Bilateral placement at first attempt is around 85%. A second attempt brings the bilateral placement up to 92%. Over 800 women with a follow-up of more than 5 years have shown only one pregnancy, due to device malfunction. The fibers on the device causes a tissue reaction, which produces permanent occlusion of the intramural part of the tube.

In conclusion, we can state that a new era has begun as far as definitive contraception is concerned. Hysteroscopic placement, using thin-barrelled hysteroscopes, of small devices, causing occlusion of the intramural part of the tube, are the future of sterilization; the drawbacks are the difficulties of the hysteroscopic technique and the costs of the devices.

REFERENCES

1. Sokal DC, Zipper J, King T. Transcervical quinacrine sterilization: clinical experience. Int J Gynecol Obstet 1995; 51 (Suppl 1): S57–69
2. Sciarra JJ, Keith L. Hysteroscopic sterilization. Obstet Gynecol Clin North Am 1995; 22: 581–9
3. Donnez J, Malvaux V, Nisolle M, et al. Hysteroscopic sterilization. In Donnez J, Nisolle M, eds. An Atlas of Laser Operative Laparoscopy and Hysteroscopy. Carnforth, UK: Parthenon Publishing, 1994: 337–41
4. Brundin J. Hydrogel tubal blocking device: P-block. In Zatuchni GI, Shelton JD, Goldsmith A, eds. Female Transcervical Sterilization. Philadelphia: Harper & Row Publishers, 1983: 240
5. Ligt-Veneman NG, Tinga DJ, Kragt H, et al. The efficacy of intratubal silicone in the Ovabloc hysteroscopic method of sterilization. Acta Obstet Gynecol Scand 1999; 78: 824–5
6. Hamou J, Gasparri F, Scarselli GF, et al. Hysteroscopic reversible tubal sterilization. Acta Eur Fertil 1984; 15: 123

Complications of hysteroscopic surgery in gynecology

49

P Jadoul, J Donnez

INTRODUCTION

Hysteroscopic surgery has developed from a diagnostic tool into an effective surgical technique. It is now a standard investigational and therapeutic tool in gynecology, which, when implemented properly for the right indications in patients with no contraindications, has practically no complications. In retrospective studies, complication rates of 0.95–13.6% have been reported[1–4].

A members' survey of the American Association of Gynecologic Laparoscopists reported 17 298 operative hysteroscopies, with a complication rate of 3.8%[1]. Pasini and Belloni[3] reported 95 complications in a series of 697 operative hysteroscopies (13.6%), while Propst et al.[3] encountered 25 complications in 925 procedures (2.7%).

A more recent study by Agostini et al.[4] revealed a 3.5% complication rate (74/2116). In a prospective study conducted in The Netherlands in 1997, the complication rate among 2515 operative hysteroscopic procedures was just 0.95%[5]. Table 49.1 summarizes the published complication rates in prospective and retrospective studies. The wide variation is attributed to the varying experience of the gynecologists[2,5] and the range of pathologies treated.

In Pasini and Belloni's series[2], complication rates decreased progressively due to more extensive training and experience of the surgeons.

Complication risks increase when hysteroscopy is performed for the treatment of intrauterine synechiae[4,5], intrauterine myomas[2,3] and repeat endometrial resections[15]. Although complications are infrequent, their description helps us to understand their causes and thus take the necessary steps to avoid them. There are six groups of complications of operative hysteroscopy:

- Traumatic complications
- Hemorrhagic complications
- Distension medium complications
- Infection
- Thermal surgery damage
- Late complications

Less frequent complications, such as rupture of the tubes, rupture of the diaphragm leading to the patient's death, rupture of the uterine wall and trauma to pelvic vessels, have been reported.

Table 49.1 Reported complications of operative hysteroscopic procedures

Author(s)	Year	n	Perforation (%)	Bleeding (%)	Fluid (%)	Infection (%)	Urinary tract injury (%)	Bowel injury (%)
Magos et al.[6]	1991	234	2.0	0.4	3.0			
Hill et al.[7]	1992	850	0.8	0.8	0			
MISTLETOE study[8]	1994	10 686	1.48	2.38				0.06
Pinion et al.[9]	1994	105	1.0	6.0	11.0			
Scottish Hysteroscopy Audit Group[10]	1995	978	1.1	3.6	6.0			
O'Connor and Magos[11]	1996	525	2.0	0.6	4.0			
O'Connor et al.[12]	1997	116	3.0	0	3.0			
Nicoloso et al.[13]	1997	2757	1.5	0.11	0.11			
Jansen et al.[5]	2000	2515	1.3	0.16	0.2			
Propst et al.[3]	2000	925	0.4		0.7	0.2		
Pasini and Belloni[2]	2001	697	1.7	6.9	5.0			0.001
Ravi et al.[14]	2001	70	8.6		0.01		0.01	
Agostini et al.[4]	2003	2116	1.61	0.61	0.47	0.76		

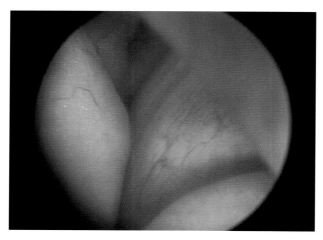

Figure 49.1 Visualization of the bowel through a uterine perforation

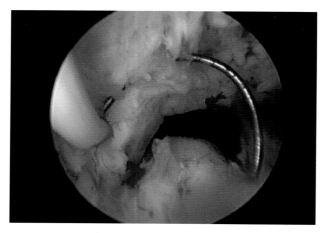

Figure 49.2 Perforation of the uterus with the resectoscope: hysteroscopic view

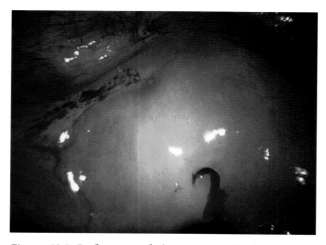

Figure 49.3 Perforation of the uterus with the resectoscope: laparoscopic view. Note the white aspect of the uterine serosa due to the thermal effect of the resectoscope

Our purpose is to describe the diagnosis, management and prevention of these complications.

TRAUMATIC COMPLICATIONS OF HYSTEROSCOPY

Traumatic complications of diagnostic hysteroscopy have been well documented. Hysteroscopic surgery, however, also involves some degree of blind manipulation. Dilating the cervix to accommodate wide-caliber operating instruments may cause cervical laceration and/or uterine perforation, with or without hemorrhage. The incidence of these complications has been estimated as 1–9%[16,17].

Diagnosis

Cervical laceration is diagnosed only if cervical bleeding occurs. Preoperative use of gonadotropin-releasing hormone (GnRH) analogs might render the cervix more resistant to dilatation.

Uterine perforation is suspected if the depth of passage of the sound or the dilator is greater than the apparent size of the uterus. Very rapid flow of liquid or very low distension pressure with CO_2 at the time of insertion of the hysteroscope should raise this suspicion.

Diagnosis is sometimes made by visualization of the bowel (Figure 49.1). Any hemorrhage before initiation of the surgical procedure is highly suggestive of traumatic damage.

Management

Cervical laceration is of little consequence, although sutures are occasionally required to prevent or stop cervical bleeding.

Uterine perforation does not usually need surgical repair. If perforation is diagnosed before the surgical procedure, surgery must be delayed and the patient observed for 24 hours. If perforation is diagnosed intra-operatively or after the surgical procedure, diagnostic laparoscopy is recommended to ensure that no thermal damage has been caused to adherent or adjacent structures, and that there is no unsuspected laceration of the large blood vessels (Figures 49.2 and 49.3).

Prevention

To prevent such complications, careful placement of the tenaculum and gentle dilatation of the cervix are recommended.

The hysteroscope must always be advanced under visual control, adapting the instrument axis to the direction of the cervical canal and the position of the uterus.

The use of *Laminaria* tents is favored by some hysteroscopists, but avoided by others, because of the possible risk of overdilatation, resulting in a loss of distension medium and intrauterine pressure, and causing poor visualization. Some hysteroscopists prefer pharmacological dilatation with vaginal prostaglandins[17]. Their action causes softening of the cervical stroma leading to dilatation of the canal. This is enhanced by contraction of the myometrium induced by the drug.

HEMORRHAGIC COMPLICATIONS OF HYSTEROSCOPY

Intraoperative bleeding, other than that due to cervical laceration or uterine perforation, is usually the result of inadvertent or intentional trauma to the uterine wall. The reported rate of bleeding requiring surgery or uterine tamponade ranges from 0 to 22.4%[18–21]. Hemorrhage can occur from false passages, with or without perforation, created either during dilatation or upon insertion of the hysteroscope. Bleeding can also occur after operative procedures, especially when the penetration of healthy myometrium is too deep. This can arise after using scissors or thermal energy (laser, resectoscope).

Diagnosis

Heavy and continuous vaginal bleeding during or after surgery must be investigated, to determine whether it is intrauterine or cervical bleeding. Management should be effected according to the origin of the hemorrhage.

Management

Intraoperatively, rapid bleeding can be controlled by coagulation, using either the tip of the laser fiber or the electrical loop. However, uncontrolled intraoperative or postoperative bleeding may sometimes require intrauterine tamponade. A Foley catheter is introduced into the uterine cavity and the balloon is inflated with 15 ml of liquid. After approximately 3 hours, half of the liquid is removed; if no bleeding recurs over the next hour, the catheter is removed and the patient is usually discharged. If active bleeding recurs, the balloon is reinflated and left in place overnight.

Prevention

Recommendations for avoiding trauma also apply to hemorrhagic complications. In addition, the entire surgical procedure must be carried out under strict visualization of the dissection plane. If large submucosal myomas or dense intrauterine synechiae are present, performing the procedure in two parts decreases the risk of such complications.

The use of intracervical vasopressin has been shown to reduce the risk of bleeding[19], but this drug must be used with consideration of its systemic effects. Preoperative medical therapy (GnRH agonists, danazol, progestins) has also been reported to decrease postoperative bleeding. Such therapy reduces the thickness and vascularity of the endometrium and shrinks myomas, and thus may be helpful in preventing this type of complication[18,22,23]. A randomized double-blind study (the AZTEC (Adjunctive Zoladex for Thinning the Endometrium Comparison) study) proved that the use of GnRH agonists was helpful during endometrial ablation owing to the significant reduction in endometrial thickness[24].

DISTENSION MEDIUM COMPLICATIONS

Complications specifically related to distension media occur in 0.14–4% of procedures, and vary according to the medium used.

Carbon dioxide and air embolism

Venous gas embolism is the most feared complication when using CO_2 as a distension medium[25–27]. This risk is low with the use of adequate hysteroflators. Most reports of fatal CO_2 embolism during operative hysteroscopy have been the result of using inadequate or faulty insufflators[28,29]. Carbon dioxide is not advised for operative procedures due to the presence of bubbles that become apparent with bleeding, and also due to the risk of CO_2 embolism.

Air embolism has also been described. It can occur while using a fluid distension medium, and is provoked by repeated introduction and removal of the hysteroscope, the use of pressure pumps without air detectors[30,31] and cervical trauma with subsequent dilacerated veins.

Diagnosis

Venous air embolism is marked by a sudden decrease in CO_2 pressure in the expired air. Clinical signs, such as decreased blood pressure, tachycardia, arrhythmia and increasing central venous pressure, come too late to be useful as warning signals. As soon as the end-tidal CO_2 drops in the expired air, insufflation must be stopped.

Management

The patient must be immediately ventilated with 100% oxygen[32]. If the patient is in the Trendelenburg position, this position must be maintained in order to prevent the passage of the air bubble into the pulmonary artery. If the patient is in normal decubitus, an anti-Trendelenburg position will keep the air bubble in the right atrium. A large catheter must be inserted into the right atrium through the internal jugular vein to aspirate the gas. Transesophageal ultrasound allows visualization of the gas embolism.

Prevention

The first rule of hysteroscopy with CO_2 is the use of adequate insufflators. The insufflation pressure must not exceed 100 mmHg. Faulty routes, especially submucosal passages, increase the risk of embolism. Cervical trauma with subsequent dilaceration of veins should be avoided to prevent air embolism. Repeated introduction of the hysteroscope must also be avoided, as must the use of CO_2 for cooling laser tips.

Fluid distension media

The ideal distending medium should be isotonic, non-hemolytic, non-conductive, non-toxic and rapidly eliminated from the body and must provide good visualization.

High-molecular-weight dextran The most feared complication of the use of dextran 70 (Hyskon®) is anaphylactic shock, although the incidence is rare at 1 in 10 000[33,34]. So-called dextran-induced anaphylactic reaction (DIAR) is not predictable, and does not depend on the amount used[35]. It can be prevented by performing an intravenous injection test with a small amount of 15% dextran, 2 minutes before using dextran 70. This distension medium also induces ascites and intravascular overload if a substantial volume is retained by the patient. Intravascular reabsorption of dextran has also been linked to non-cardiogenic pulmonary edema and to coagulation disorders[35–41].

Low-viscosity liquid complications These fluids (mainly sorbitol, glycine and dextrose in water) are primarily used during electrosurgical intrauterine procedures. When retained by the patient, they may cause hyponatremia and fluid overload.

Glycine solution has excellent optical and non-hemolytic properties during hysteroscopic surgery. Glycine is a non-essential amino acid which exists naturally in the body. Its normal plasma level is 120–155 μmol/l and it readily crosses the blood–brain barrier. Glycine functions as an inhibitory transmitter in the spinal cord and in the brainstem and retina. Its toxic effects on the central nervous system are also due to oxidative deamination in the liver and kidneys, and the formation of glycoxylic acid and ammonia[42].

Glycine overload results in fluid overload (hypervolemia and hyponatremia) and in neurological symptoms. Glycine and its metabolites may be a cause of visual disturbances and encephalopathy, independent of changes in serum sodium levels and osmolarity.

In order to study the metabolism of glycine after endoscopic uterine surgery, serum concentrations of the amino acid and its metabolites were measured in seven patients with artificially induced menopause scheduled for neodymium : yttrium–aluminum–garnet (Nd : YAG) laser endoscopic procedures in our department[43]. Fluid balance

was determined by a volumetric method (comparison of in- and outflow). The mean irrigant absorption was 1128 ± 673 ml. A significant increase in glycine concentration during and after the procedure (up to 100 times the normal value) correlated with a rise in serum ammonia levels (Figure 49.4). Recovery was uneventful in all cases. Serum sodium levels and osmolarity remained normal during and after surgery, and there was no increased oxaluria.

Diagnosis

Manifestations of fluid overload and glycine intoxication are treacherous, and can occur at any time postoperatively. Patients present with bradycardia and hypertension followed by hypotension, nausea, vomiting, headache, visual disturbances, agitation, confusion and lethargy. Other important factors are a decrease in serum osmolarity and a rapid drop in the serum sodium level. If untreated, the result may be seizures, coma, cardiovascular collapse and death.

Management

Monitoring of intake and output of liquids during and after the procedure is mandatory to assess fluid balance. A discrepancy of 1000 ml requires the assessment of serum electrolytes to permit diagnosis. If a discrepancy of 1500 ml is noted during surgery, the procedure must be immediately stopped. If the serum sodium level is normal and the patient has no particular complaints, no further treatment is necessary. In the case of decreased sodium levels and hemodilution, the patient should observe fluid restrictions and intravenous diuretics (furosemide) should be administered. In the case of severe hyponatremia causing neurological symptoms, perfusion of hypertonic

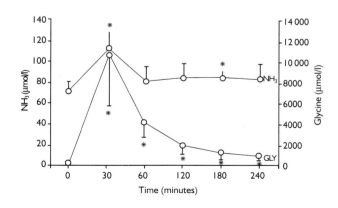

Figure 49.4 Concentrations of glycine and ammonia measured in the serum of seven patients with artificially induced menopause undergoing Nd : YAG laser endoscopic procedures

saline solution is required. If correction is too rapid, however, it may cause injury to the brain known as central pontine myelinolysis.

Prevention

During hysteroscopy with a liquid medium, monitoring of the inflow and outflow volumes is essential to prevent the retention of too much distension medium by the patient. An infusion pressure of more than 150 mmHg increases the risk of fluid absorption, but intravasation of the fluid often occurs through open uterine venous channels, or, in the presence of unrecognized perforation, with normal infusion pressure[44]. If uterine perforation and/or a fluid balance discrepancy of over 1500 ml is detected, the procedure must be stopped.

INFECTIOUS COMPLICATIONS

Infection is rare, with an incidence of 0.25–1%[19,45–50].

Usually, infection follows prolonged operative procedures, especially when repeated insertion and removal of the hysteroscope through the cervical canal have been necessary. It occurs about 72 hours postoperatively and manifests itself with fever, vaginal discharge and pelvic pain. It can be treated successfully with broad-spectrum oral antibiotics. Hospitalization is rarely required. To prevent this complication, the use of prophylactic antibiotics is recommended.

Postoperative infection can be the cause of late complications, such as synechiae and infertility.

THERMAL ENERGY COMPLICATIONS

There is little information in the gynecological literature on the occurrence and management of injury to the viscera during hysteroscopy. Ravi *et al.*[14] report one lesion to the bladder and ureter in 70 operative hysteroscopies, and Pasini and Belloni[2] one bowel injury after uterine perforation in a series of 697 operative hysteroscopies. The English MISTLETOE (Minimally Invasive Surgical Techniques – Laser, Endo-Thermal Or Endoresection) study of 10 686 endometrial resections from April 1993 to October 1994 reported a perforation rate of 0.64–2.47%, with 0.07% bowel injury[8]. Six visceral burns occurred, three with the loop associated with the rollerball and three with the loop alone. No visceral lesions were caused by the laser. Such injuries may be directly provoked by the electrical current or the thermal diffusion of energy. They often occur in the presence of uterine perforation. They can be induced by prolonged application of strong electrical or laser energy to the uterine wall, especially in the area of the tubal ostia.

Diagnosis

The diagnosis is missed intraoperatively in the majority of cases. Postoperative symptoms include fever, abdominal pain, leukocytosis and signs of peritonitis. Laparoscopy is helpful in suspect cases, but this may be insufficient to evaluate the bowel fully, and laparotomy is then required[51].

Management

Guidelines described in Chapter 39 relating to vessel injuries and bowel burns during laparoscopy apply to such injuries.

Prevention

The success of prevention depends on respecting the technical conditions of surgical hysteroscopy. If uterine perforation occurs, the procedure must be delayed for the patient's safety. In addition, the energy source must always be activated with completely clear visualization of the tip of the laser fiber or the resectoscope loop.

LATE COMPLICATIONS

Besides the commonly encountered acute complications, a number of late complications, such as uterine perforation during a subsequent pregnancy, incomplete resection and undesired pregnancy and post-resection pain (hematometra and postablation tubal sterilization syndrome) warrant attention.

Uterine perforation during subsequent pregnancy

Operative hysteroscopy has an important role in the correction of Müllerian anomalies such as uterine septa, and in the improvement of fertility in the case of uterine synechiae or uterine hypoplasia in women exposed to diethylstilbestrol. In women undergoing hysteroscopic metroplasty, the uterus is weakened, and several cases of uterine rupture during subsequent pregnancy have been described[52–59]. Some uterine ruptures even occurred after perforation during diagnostic hysteroscopy.

Undesired pregnancy

Endometrial ablation is not a method of contraception. Pregnancy rates of 0.2–1.6% have been described, but may be underreported[60–62]. Placenta accreta, increta and percreta, placental abruption and postpartum hemorrhage have all been reported[63].

50. McCausland VM, Fields GA, McCausland AM, et al. Tuboovarian abscesses after operative hysteroscopy. J Reprod Med 1993; 38: 198–200

51. Sullivan B, Kenne P, Seibel M. Hysteroscopic resection of fibroid with thermal injury to sigmoïd. Obstet Gynecol 1992; 80: 546–7

52. Creinin M, Chen M. Uterine defect in a twin pregnancy with a history of hysteroscopic fundal perforation. Obstet Gynecol 1992; 79: 879–80

53. Howe RS. Third-trimester uterine rupture following hysteroscopic uterine perforation. Obstet Gynecol 1993; 81: 827–9

54. Lobaugh ML, Bammel BM, Duke D, et al. Uterine rupture during pregnancy in a patient with a history of hysteroscopic metroplasty. Obstet Gynecol 1994; 83: 838–40

55. Yaron Y, Shenhav M, Jaffa AJ, et al. Uterine rupture at 33 weeks' gestation subsequent to hysteroscopic uterine perforation. Am J Obstet Gynecol 1994; 170: 786–7

56. Gabriele A, Zanetta G, Pasta F, et al. Uterine rupture after hysteroscopic metroplasty and labor induction. A case report. J Reprod Med 1999; 44: 642–4

57. Tannous W, Hamou J, Henry-Suchet J, et al. Uterine rupture during labor following surgical hysteroscopy. Presse Med 1996; 25: 159–61

58. Conturso R, Redaelli L, Pasini A, et al. Spontaneous uterine rupture with amniotic sac protrusion at 28 weeks subsequent to previous hysteroscopic metroplasty. Eur J Obstet Gynecol Reprod Biol 2003; 107: 98–100

59. Angell NF, Tan Domingo J, Siddiqi N. Uterine rupture at term after uncomplicated hysteroscopic metroplasty. Obstet Gynecol 2002; 100: 1098–9

60. Mints M, Radestad A, Rylander E. Follow up of hysteroscopic surgery for menorrhagia. Acta Obstet Gynecol Scand 1998; 77: 435–8

61. Baumann R, Owerdiek W, Reck C. Schwangerschaft nach Sterilisation und Endometriumablation. Gebürtshilfe Frauenheilkd 1994; 54: 246

62. Hill DJ, Mahrer P. Pregnancy following endometrial ablation. Gynaecol Endosc 1992; 1: 47

63. Rogerson L, Gannon B, O'Donovan P. Outcome of pregnancy following endometrial ablation. J Gynecol Surg 1997; 13: 155–60

64. Römer T, Campo R, Hucke J. Hämatometra nach hysteroskopischer Endometriumablation. Zentralbl Gynäkol 1995; 5: 278–80

65. Townsend DE, McCausland V, McCausland A, et al. Post-ablation tubal sterilization syndrome. Obstet Gynecol 1993; 82: 422–4

66. Bae IH, Pagedas AC, Perkins HE, et al. Postablation tubal sterilization syndrome. J Am Assoc Gynecol Laparosc 1996; 3: 435–8

Index

abdominal cerclage 403
  concerns in non-pregnant women 404
  see also laparoscopic abdominal cerclage
abdominal wall 2
abnormal uterine bleeding (AUB) *see* bleeding, uterine
abortion 465
accessory tube 120
adenomyosis *see* endometriosis
adhesiolysis 127–8, 151–3
adhesions 123, 151–2
  intratubal 146
  intrauterine 464, 507–14
    classification 507
    diagnosis 507
    etiopathogenesis 5–7
    treatment 508–14
  periadnexal 146–7
  postoperative 208, 234–5
  subovarian 32, 33
adnexal torsion 211–15
  etiology 212
    treatment 212
  follow-up 213–14
  ischemic lesion management 211–13
  postoperative fertility 214
adnexectomy 264, 315
  bilateral 315
  unilateral 315
Aesop™ laparoscope holder 413, 417
air embolism 442, 555–6
Allen–Masters syndrome 55
ampulla 122, 142
  dilatation 14
ampullary folds 142
  preservation of 144–6
ampullary–ampullary anastomosis 188
anastomosis *see* laparoscopic microsurgical tubal anastomosis
anesthesia
  fertiloscopy 117–18
  prolapse treatment 278
antibiotic therapy, prolapse treatment 281, 286
appendix 120
arcuate uterus 493
arterial relationships 5–6
Asherman's syndrome 464
atraumatic forceps 18, 20

biopsy
  forceps 20
  ovarian tissue 344–5
  targeted hysteroscopic biopsies 477–9
bipolar coagulation 268–70
bipolar resectoscope 456
bladder
  Burch bladder neck suspension 286
  catheter 278
  endometriosis 85–91
    diagnosis 85–6
    histology 89
    prevalence 85
    surgical technique 86–9
    symptoms 85, 86
  injury 111, 430–1, 436–7
    by secondary trocars 432
    diagnosis 432, 436–7
    management 432, 437
    prevention 432, 437
  mobilization 98
bleeding, uterine 533
  hysteroscopic evaluation 465–8
  postmenopausal 462–3
  see also hemorrhage
borderline ovarian tumors (BOT)
  diagnosis 311–14
    CA125 313–14
    CT 312
    laparoscopic staging 314
    MRI 314
    ultrasound 311–12
  epidemiology 307
  fertility preservation 317, 319
  histology 308–10, 317–18
    Brenner tumors 310
    clear cell tumors 310
    endometrioid tumors 310
    mucinous BOT 309–10
    peritoneal implants 310
    serous BOT 308–9
  molecular biology 310–11
  prognosis 307–8
  risk factors 308
  risk of 206
  surgical treatment 314–16
    adjuvant treatment 316
    HRT after 316

561

borderline ovarian tumors (BOT) (*cont.*)
   results 318–19
  symptoms 311
bowel injury 111–12, 429–30
  diagnosis 430, 434
  during surgical procedures 432–6
  management 430, 434–5
  prevention 430, 435–6
  subocclusion due to umbilical incision suture 445
bowel preparation 278
bowel surgery 107–9
breast cancer patient monitoring 463
Brenner tumors 310
broad ligament 3
Burch bladder neck suspension 286

CA125 369
  borderline ovarian tumor diagnosis 313–14
  ovarian cyst evaluation 195–7
cardiac surgery, fetal 399
Cavaterm™ system 537–8
  Cavaterm *Plus* 538
cerclage *see* abdominal cerclage
cervical atresia 502
cervical canal 471
  internal cervical os (ICO) 471, 472–3
cervical cancer 360–2, 375–87
  advanced-stage case management 385–6
  early-stage case management 384–5
  hysteroscopy 466–8
  laparoscopy-assisted hysterectomy 380–4
    Schauta operation 380
    Schauta–Amreich operation 380
    Schauta–Stoeckel operation 380–4
  lymphadenectomy 360–2, 375–80
    aortic 378–80
    pelvic 375–8
  sentinel node assessment 386–7
cervical laceration 554
cervical pregnancy 166–7
cervical sacrofixation 289–96
  see also prolapse
cesarean section 219
  ectopic pregnancy in scar 167–9
  scar dehiscence 219–20
    repair 220–5
chemotherapy
  effects on ovarian function 350
  IVF and 343–4
chorioangioma, placental 399
ciliation index 146
clear cell tumors 310
clips 201
CO_2 gas insufflator 21–2
  smoke evacuation 28
  see also insufflation

CO_2 laser 23, 24, 25–6
coagulation
  bipolar 268–70
  electrocoagulation of the endometrium 535, 542–3
  endometriosis 40
  instruments 19
  photocoagulation of the endometrium 535
  placental anastomoses 395–6
colpotomy 289–93
complications 425–6
  diaphragmatic injury 444
  distension medium complications 442, 555–7
  due to synthetic materials 445
  gastrointestinal injury 111–12, 428–30, 432–6, 445
  hysteroscopic surgery 553–8
  incisional hernias 442–3
  infection 557
  injury during surgical procedures 432–45, 554–5, 556
  pneumothorax 444
  port-site metastases 443–4
  secondary trocar injury 431–2
    bladder 432
    epigastric vessels 431–2
  spleen injury 444–5
  subcutaneous emphysema 426
  urinary tract injury 430–1, 432, 436–41
  vascular injury 426–8, 441–2, 555
  see also specific procedures
computed tomography (CT)
  borderline ovarian tumor diagnosis 312
  ovarian cyst evaluation 197
cord occlusion in abnormal twin pregnancy 397
cornual pregnancy 159–64
  intramyometrial implantation 162–3
  methotrexate treatment 162
  surgical management 160–2
  triplet pregnancy 162
  see also ectopic pregnancy
corpus, uterine 471
corpus luteum 120
cryoendometrial ablation 540–2
cryopreservation
  embryo 315–16, 333, 343
  oocyte 334–5
    in vitro maturation 334–5
    mature oocyte 334
  see also ovarian tissue cryopreservation
culdoplasty
  McCall 102–4
  prolapse and 283
culdoscopy 133
culdotomy, circumferential 101
cumulus–oocyte complex (COC) 335
cystectomy, ovarian 45–7, 199–202, 315
  clips 201
  complications 207–8

postoperative 208
  spillage 207–8
fibrin sealant 201–2
indications for 198–9
suturing 200–1
versus laser vaporization 47–53
see also ovarian cysts
cystoscopy 104, 286

da Vinci™ robotic system 417, 418–20
dextran 70 complications 556
diaphragmatic hernia, congenital 399
diaphragmatic injury 444
diethylstilbestrol (DES) exposure 489–93
digestive system 8–9
distension medium 453, 473–4
  complications 555–7
Doppler ultrasound, ovarian cyst evaluation 195
Douglas introducer 115–16, 119
Douglasectomy 59–60
drainage 272
dye test 118, 121
dysmenorrhea 55
  see also pain
dyspareunia 55
  see also pain

ectopic pregnancy 157
  diagnosis 157–8
  embryo transfer technique and 157
  future fertility prognosis 176–7
    ruptured ectopic pregnancy and 177
  laparoscopic management 181–6
    adjunctive therapy 184
    conservative treatment 181–3
    contraindications 183–4
    indications for 184–5
    postoperative work-up 184
    results 185
    salpingectomy 183
  risk after bilateral salpingectomy 158
  risk factors 157
  specific sites 159–69
    cervical pregnancy 166–7
    cesarean section scar 167–9
    cornual pregnancy 159–64
    ovarian pregnancy 164–5
  see also heterotopic pregnancy; methotrexate (MTX)
electrocoagulation of the endometrium 535
embryo cryopreservation 315–16, 333, 343
embryo transfer
  ectopic pregnancy and 157
  hydrosalpinx and 150–1
  salpingectomy before 151
embryoscopy 391
emphysema, subcutaneous 426
EndoAssist™ laparoscope holder 413

endometrial ablation 533–44
  complications 535
  contraindications 534
  first-generation technologies 535
  indications for 534
  patient assessment 533–4
  patient counseling 534
  preparation 534–5
  second-generation technologies (SEATs) 535–43
    classification 533
    cryoendometrial ablation 540–2
    hot liquid balloons 536–8
    HydroThermAblator 538–9
    impedance-controlled endometrial electrocoagulation 542–3
    microwave endometrial ablation 539–40
  third-generation technologies 543
  trichloroacetic acid 543
endometrial cancer 359, 369
  hysteroscopy 466
  laparoscopic hysterectomy 363
  lymphadenectomy 359, 369
    indications for 371–2
    medical advice 369–70
    rationale for 370
    which nodes to remove 370
  radiotherapy effectiveness 370–1
endometrial resection 527–32
  instruments 527–8
  technique 528–30
endometrioid tumors 310
endometriomas 43–4
  surgical treatment 44–53
    indications for 44
    risk of 47–53
    transvaginal laparoscopy 136
  see also endometriosis
endometriosis
  bladder 85–91
    diagnosis 85–6
    histology 89
    prevalence 85
    surgical technique 86–9
    symptoms 85, 86
  laparoscopic hysterectomy 95, 104–9
    bowel surgery 107–9
    surgical technique 105–7
  ovarian 43–53, 137
    indications for surgery 44
    laser vaporization 44–5, 47–53
    ovarian cystectomy 45–53
  pain in 55
  peritoneal 31–40
    black/bluish lesions 31
    coagulation 40
    diagnosis 31–7
    excision 38–40

endometriosis (*cont.*)
    laser vaporization 38
    non-visible endometriosis 34–7
    red lesions 31–2
    treatment modes 37–8
    white lesions 32
  rectovaginal 63–73
    diagnosis 65–6
    hormonal dependence 65
    recurrence 72–3
    surgical shaving 67–73
  retrocervical disease 63–4
    arguments for 64
  retroperitoneal disease 63–4
    arguments for 64
    classification of deep lesions 66–7
  transvaginal laparoscopy 136
  tubal surgery and 147
  ureteral 77–82
    left versus right 81–2
    prevalence 77, 81
    surgical treatment 78–80, 82
    symptoms and diagnosis 77–8
  uterine suspension 56–8
endometritis 465, 507
epigastric vessel perforation 431–2
  diagnosis 431
  management 431
  prevention 432
epithelial ovarian tumors of low malignant potential *see*
    borderline ovarian tumors (BOT)
ergonomics 409

Fallopian tubes
  intratubal adhesions 146
  mucosal evaluation 146
  tubal disease 465
  wall fibrosis and thickness 146
  see also tubal occlusion; tubal surgery
falloscopy 145
fertility preservation 333, 355–7
  borderline ovarian tumors 317, 319
  ovarian transposition 352, 355
  see also cryopreservation
fertility prognosis following treatment
  adnexal torsion 214
  hysteroscopic myomectomy 519
  laparoscopic myolysis 246–7
  laparoscopic myomectomy 235, 246–7
  methotrexate 177
  ovarian transposition 352
  salpingotomy 176–7
  see also fertility preservation
fertiloscope 116
  introduction 118, 119
fertiloscopy 115–30
  contraindications 128

instrumentation 115–16
operative procedure 119–28
  dye test 121
  hysteroscopy 125
  microsalpingoscopy 123–5
  operative fertiloscopy 125–8, 130
  pelvic exploration 119–21
  salpingoscopy 121–3
results 128–9
safety 130
technique 116–19
  anesthesia 117–18
  hydroperitoneum 118–19
  introduction of fertiloscope 118, 119
  patient preparation 116–17
  use of operative channel 119
fetal endoscopy 391–400
  complications 399
  contraindications 399
  diagnostic endoscopy 392–3
  techniques 391–2
  therapeutic endoscopy 393–9
    coagulation of placental anastomoses 395–6
    congenital diaphragmatic hernia 399
    cord occlusion in abnormal twin pregnancy 397
    fetal cardiac surgery 399
    myelomeningocele 399
    obstructive uropathies 397–8
    placental chorioangioma 399
    sacrococcygeal teratoma 399
    septostomy 396–7
    twin-to-twin transfusion syndrome (TTTS) 393–7
fetoscopy 391–2
  see also fetal endoscopy
fibrin sealant 201–2
fibroids *see* myomas
fibrosis, tubal wall 146
fimbria 119, 120
fimbrioplasty 147
FIPS laparoscope holder 413–14
Foley catheter 286
forceps
  atraumatic 18, 20
  biopsy 20
  bipolar 19
  grasping 18, 19
foreign bodies, intrauterine 468
funicular meso 3

gamete intrafallopian transfer (GIFT) 465
gastric perforation 428–9
gastrointestinal injury 111–12, 428–30, 432–6, 445
  see also bowel injury; stomach injury
genital ligament 5
genitofemoral nerve 9
global endometrial ablation (GEA) 533
  see also endometrial ablation

glycine solution 556
GnRH agonist therapy 273
   before endometrial ablation 534–5
   endometriosis 38, 45
   myomas 227–8, 246, 273, 515, 520–3
grasping forceps 18, 19

Hamou plug 549–51
hematometra 558
hemivagina 498–9
hemoglobin catabolism 36–7
hemorrhage 426–8, 441–2
   following hysteroscopy 555
   following laparoscopic hysterectomy 110
   following laparoscopic myomectomy 234, 246
   following lymphadenectomy 364–5
   see also bleeding, uterine
Her Option™ cryoablation 541–2
hernias, incisional 442–3
heterotopic pregnancy 158–9
   diagnosis 158
   incidence 158
   localization 158–9
   predisposing factors 158
   symptoms 158
   treatment 159
   see also ectopic pregnancy
hormone replacement therapy (HRT)
   hysterosonography and 462
   postoperative 316–17
human chorionic gonadotropin (hCG)
   ectopic pregnancy diagnosis 157–8
   persistent trophoblast diagnosis 173
hydatiform mole 467
hydrosalpinx
   diagnosis 141
   IVF–embryo transfer and 150–1
   physiopathology 141, 142
   see also tubal occlusion
hydrothermablation (HTA) 533, 538–9
   see also endometrial ablation
HydroThermAblator 538–9
hypermenorrhea 95–6
hypogastric plexi 10
hysterectomy 93, 263
   distension medium 453
   prolapse and 281, 282–3
   see also laparoscopic hysterectomy
hysterosalpingography 144
hysterosalpingosonography 144–5
hysteroscopic myomectomy 515–24
   equipment 515
   fertility and 519
   preoperative GnRH agonist therapy 515
   results 517–19
   techniques 516–17
      fibromatous uterus 517

submucosal fibroids 516
hysteroscopy 125, 126, 463–8, 471–2
   abnormal uterine bleeding evaluation 465–8
   complications 553–8
      distension media 555–7
      hemorrhagic 555
      late 557–8
      thermal energy 557
      traumatic 554–5
   infertility evaluation 463–5
      abortion 465
      endometritis 465
      GIFT 465
      intrauterine synechiae 464
      Müllerian anomalies 464
      sperm migration test 465
      submucous myomas 465
      tubal disease 465
      ZIFT 465
   instrumentation 453–6
      high-frequency generator 456
      resectoscopes 454, 456
      working elements 455
   internal cervical os as obstacle 472–3
   intrauterine foreign bodies 468
   myomectomy 515–24
   operative techniques 479–80
      bipolar surgery 479–80
      mechanical surgery 479
   targeted hysteroscopic biopsies 477–9
   uterine adhesion management 507–14
   uterine cavity distension 473–4
   uterine septum management 493–8
   vaginoscopic approach 472
hysterosonography 457–63
   breast cancer patient monitoring 463
   contraindications 458
   HRT and 462
   indications for 458
   infertility and 461–2
   postmenopausal bleeding evaluation 462–3
   results 458–61
   technique 457–8

iliac arteries 4, 5–6
iliac veins 7
ImagTrack laparoscope holder 414
impedance-controlled endometrial electrocoagulation 542–3
in vitro fertilization (IVF) 343–4
   chemotherapy and 343–4
   endometriomas and 44
   hydrosalpinx and 150–1
   hysterosonography 462
   stimulation protocols 344
infection
   following hysteroscopy 557

infection (*cont.*)
  following laparoscopic hysterectomy 110
infertility
  as risk factor for borderline ovarian tumors 308
  hysteroscopic evaluation 463–5
    endometritis 465
    GIFT 465
    intrauterine synechiae 464
    Müllerian anomalies 464
    sperm migration test 465
    submucous myomas 465
    tubal disease 465
    ZIFT 465
  hysterosonography 461–2
  myomectomy for 239–40
    outcome 240
  uterine displacement and 55
  see also fertility prognosis following treatment;
      fertiloscopy
innervation 9–11
installation
  laparoscopic myomectomy 229
  prolapse treatment 278
  see also preoperative preparation
insufflation 1–2
  CO_2 insufflators 21–2
  complications 442, 555–6
  smoke evacuation 28
  see also distension medium
internal cervical os (ICO) 471
  as obstacle in hysteroscopy 472–3
intestinal fixation 280
intestinal injury *see* bowel injury
intestinal probe 20, 21
introducers 115–16
irrigation–suction unit 22
isthmic–ampullary anastomosis 188
isthmic–isthmic anastomosis 188

KCl, ectopic pregnancy management 159, 162

laparoscope-holding systems 409–14
  active holders 413–14
  LapMan® project 409–12
    advantages 411
    indications in gynecological surgery 412
    solo surgery concept 412
  passive holders 412–13
laparoscopic abdominal cerclage 404
  technique 404–5
laparoscopic hysterectomy 93–112
  cervical cancer 380–4
    Schauta operation 380
    Schauta–Amreich operation 380
    Schauta–Stoeckel operation 380–4
  complications 109–12, 273, 274

bladder injury 111
bowel injury 111–12
hemorrhage 110
infection 110
urinary tract complications 110–11
definitions 94, 263
endometrial cancer and 363
endometriosis and 104–9
  bowel surgery 107–9
  surgical technique to remove endometriosis 105–7
in benign diseases 263–75
indications and contraindications 94–6, 263–4
postoperative considerations 109
preoperative GnRH agonist treatment 273
prolapse and 281, 282–3
techniques 264–6
  bipolar coagulation 268–70
  drainage 272
  ureter dissection 271
  uterine mobilizer 270–1
  vaginal closure 272
see also laparoscopic subtotal hysterectomy (LASH);
    total laparoscopic hysterectomy (TLH)
laparoscopic microsurgery 187
  digital enhancement 187
  instrumentation 187
  magnification 187
  needles 188
  prerequisites for surgery 188
  resolution 187
  sutures 188
  see also laparoscopic microsurgical tubal anastomosis;
      microsalpingoscopy
laparoscopic microsurgical tubal anastomosis
  indications for 187
  surgical technique 189–92
  types of 188–9
  see also laparoscopic microsurgery
laparoscopic myolysis 240–8
  fertility prognosis 246–7
  operative technique 242–5
laparoscopic myomectomy 227–36, 240–8
  conversion rate 234
  efficiency 246–8
  fertility prognosis 235, 246–7
  indications for 228
  installation 229
  instrumentation 229
  obstetric scars 235
  operation time 234
  operative technique 229–32, 242
    enucleation 230
    hysterotomy suture 230–1
    incision of myometrium 230
    myoma extraction 231
    uterine artery occlusion 231–2

postoperative adhesions 234–5
postoperative course 234
preoperative evaluation 227
preoperative treatment 227–8
safety 245–6
hemorrhage risk 234
second-look laparoscopy 232–4
technical principles 228–9
see also myomectomy
laparoscopic presacral neurectomy (LPSN) 61
laparoscopic sacrocolpexy 289–302
cervical/uterine sacrofixation 289–96
complications 297–300
vaginal vault sacrofixation 296–7
laparoscopic subtotal hysterectomy (LASH) 251–61
complications 258–60
results 257
surgical procedure 251–6
see also laparoscopic hysterectomy
laparoscopic supracervical hysterectomy (LSH) 94
see also laparoscopic hysterectomy
laparoscopic surgery
fully integrated operating room 415
human assistance 409
instrument manipulation 414–15
laparoscope holding systems 409–14
active holders 413–14
LapMan® project 409–12
passive holders 412–13
robotically assisted surgery 417–20
initial experience 417–18
preoperative planning 418
surgical training 418
technique 418–20
see also specific procedures
laparoscopy-assisted hysterectomy see laparoscopic
hysterectomy
laparoscopy-assisted vaginal hysterectomy (LAVH) 93–4
definition 94
see also laparoscopic hysterectomy
LapMan® project 409–12
advantages 411
indications in gynecological surgery 412
solo surgery concept 412
laser photocoagulation of the endometrium 535
laser treatment 22–7
CO_2 laser 25–6
endometriosis 38, 44–5, 47–53, 58–9
versus ovarian cystectomy 47–53
energy, power and power density 24–5
LUNA (laser uterine nerve ablation) 11, 58–9
Nd:YAG laser 27
physical effects on tissue 23–4
thermal effects 24
lateral ligaments 5
leiomyomas see myomas

LUNA (laser uterine nerve ablation) 11, 58–9
lymph nodes 12–13
lymphadenectomy 12–14, 363–7
cervical cancer 360–2, 375–80
aortic lymphadenectomy 378–80
pelvic lymphadenectomy 375–8
complications 364–5
endometrial cancer 359, 369–72
indications for 371–2
rationale 370
which nodes to remove 370
technique 363–4
vaginal cancer 359–60

McCall culdoplasty 102–4
magnetic resonance imaging (MRI)
borderline ovarian tumor diagnosis 314
endometrial cancer evaluation 369
ovarian cyst evaluation 197
matrix metalloproteinases (MMPs) 37
Mayer–Rokitansky–Küster–Hauser syndrome 484–9
menorrhagia 527
mesosalpinx 3
metastases, port-site 443–4
methotrexate (MTX) 162, 165, 166–7
adjunctive therapy 184
as first-line therapy 171–3
failure of treatment 172–3
follow-up 172
injection at laparoscopy 172
injection under ultrasonic guidance 171
systemic treatment 172
as second-line therapy 173–6
future fertility prognosis 177
mifepristone addition 176
versus conservative surgical treatment 185
microsalpingoscopy 123–5
results 129
microsurgery see laparoscopic microsurgery
microwave endometrial ablation (MEA) 533, 539–40
see also endometrial ablation
mifepristone 176
mobilization
bladder 98
uterine manipulator 270–1, 273, 279–80
morcellation 101–2, 286
morcellators 20–1
mucous cysts of the cervix 477, 478
Müllerian duct anomalies 464, 483–504
classification 485
development anomalies 484–93
absence 484–9
incomplete development 489–93
embryology 483–4
fusion anomalies 493–504
lateral 493–501
vertical 502–4

myelomeningocele 399
myolysis *see* laparoscopic myolysis
myoma holder 20
myomas 465, 475, 476
   assisted reproduction and 239–40
   classification 516
   preoperative evaluation 227
   preoperative treatment 227–8, 273, 515
   recurrence after laparoscopic myomectomy 235, 248
   see also myomectomy
myomectomy 479–80
   efficiency 246–8
   for infertility 239–40
      outcome 240
   indications for 239
   safety 245–6
   see also hysteroscopic myomectomy; laparoscopic myomectomy

Nd:YAG laser 23–4, 27
needle holders 20
needle placement 1–2
NovaSure™ electrocoagulation system 542–3

obstructive uropathies, fetal 397–8
obturator artery 6
obturator nerve 10
'one-stop fertility clinic' 135–6
oocyte cryopreservation 334–5
   in vitro maturation 334–5
   mature oocyte 334
oophorectomy 202–6
operating laparoscope 27
ovarian artery 6
ovarian cancer 362–3
   see also borderline ovarian tumors (BOT)
ovarian cysts 195
   borderline tumor risk 206
   laparoscopic oophorectomy 202–6
   patient selection 208
   preoperative evaluation 195–8
      CA125 195–7
      CT 197–8
      MRI 197–8
      ultrasound 195
   see also cystectomy, ovarian
ovarian drilling 126–7, 136–8
   results 129
ovarian plexus 10
ovarian pregnancy 164–5
ovarian suspension *see* ovarian transposition
ovarian tissue cryopreservation 316, 344–7, 355–7
   fragments of cortical ovarian tissue 335–7
   freezing procedures 345, 346
   oncological indications 336–7
   ovarian biopsy sample 344–5

primordial follicles 337
   isolation procedure 346–7
   reimplantation of ovarian tissue 323–30, 357
   thawing procedures 345, 346
   whole ovary 337–8, 345–6
ovarian transposition 350–2
   indications for 351–2
   ovarian function and fertility prognosis 352
   surgical technique 350, 355
ovarian tumors *see* borderline ovarian tumors (BOT); ovarian cancer
ovaries 119
   endometriosis 43–53, 137
      indications for surgery 44
      laser vaporization 44–5, 47–53
      ovarian cystectomy 45–53
      transvaginal laparoscopy 136
   radiotherapy effects on function 349–50
      chemotherapy and 350
   see also ovarian cancer; ovarian cysts; ovarian tissue cryopreservation
ovulation 119–20

pain
   anatomic basis 10–11
   dysmenorrhea 55
   dyspareunia 55
   endometriosis and 55
   therapeutic applications 11–12
      uterine suspension 56
papilloma 135
paratubal cyst 120
paravaginal repair 285–6
parietal disinfection 278
patient preparation *see* preoperative preparation
pelvic congestion syndrome 56
pelvic pain *see* pain
pelvis
   cellular tissue 4–5
   lymph nodes 12–13
periadnexal adhesions 146–7
perineal pain *see* pain
peritoneal implants 310
peritoneal lavage 286
peritoneum 3–4
   rectal 8
persistent trophoblast
   diagnosis 173
   prevalence 174
   treatment 174–5
phimosis 121
phlebitis prevention 286
photocoagulation of the endometrium 535
placental anastomoses 395–6
placental chorioangioma 399
pneumoperitoneal needle placement 1–2
pneumothorax 444

polycystic ovarian syndrome (PCOS) 127, 129
polymalformative syndromes 393, 394
polyps 125, 474–8
  removal 479
port-site metastases 443–4
postablation tubal sterilization syndrome 558
postmenopausal bleeding evaluation 462–3
pregnancy
  undesired 557
  uterine perforation 557
  see also ectopic pregnancy; fertility prognosis following
    treatment; fetal endoscopy
preoperative preparation
  endometrial ablation 534–5
  fertiloscopy 116–17
  prolapse treatment 277–8
  robotically assisted surgery 418
  total laparoscopic hysterectomy 96
  see also installation
prevesical neurectomy 61
primordial follicle cryopreservation 337
  isolation technique 346–7
probe
  intestinal 20, 21
  second-puncture 28
  third-puncture 28
prolapse 277–87, 289–302
  operating field organization 279–80
    intestinal fixation 280
    manipulator positioning 279–80
    uterosacral ligament identification 280
  operating strategy 280–1
  operating technique 281–6
    anterior prosthesis fixation 284
    Burch bladder neck suspension 286
    cervical/uterine sacrofixation 289–96
    culdoplasty 283
    hysterectomy 282–3
    opening the space of Retzius 285
    paravaginal repair 285–6
    peritonealization 284, 285, 286
    posterior prosthesis fixation 283
    promontofixation 284–5
    promontory dissection 281–2
    rectovaginal space dissection 282
    vaginal vault 296–7
  patient preparation 277–8
    installation 278
  postoperative care 286–7
  preoperative assessment 277, 278–9
  trocar positioning 279
  urinary function evaluation 277
promontofixation 284–5
promontory dissection 281–2
pseudomyxoma peritonei 316
pudendal nerve 11

surgical liberation 11–12
pudendal plexus 9, 10

radiotherapy
  effects on ovarian function 349–50
  endometrial cancer management 370–1
  ovarian transposition before 350–2
    indications for 351–2
    results 352
    surgical technique 350, 355
rectal arteries 6
rectal injury 433–4
  see also bowel injury
rectal ligament 5
rectovaginal adenomyosis 11, 63–73
  classification 66–7
  diagnosis 65–6
  hormonal dependence 65
  retrocervical and retroperitoneal disease 63–4
  shaving surgery 67–71
    complications 72
    recurrence 72–3
  see also endometriosis
rectovaginal space dissection 282
rectum 8–9
resectoscope 454
  bipolar 456
robotically assisted gynecological surgery 417–20
  initial experience 417–18
  preoperative planning 418
  surgical training 418
  technique 418–20

sacral arteries 6
sacral plexus 9
sacrococcygeal teratoma 399
sacrofixation
  cervical/uterine 289–96
  vaginal vault 296–7
  see also prolapse
sagittal ligaments 5
saline infusion sonohysterography (SIS) 457–8
  contraindications 458
  indications for 458
  see also hysterosonography
salpingectomy 149
  before IVF–embryo transfer 151
  contraindications 183
  ectopic pregnancy risk and 158
  ectopic pregnancy treatment 159, 183
  results 185
  versus conservative surgical treatment 184–5
salpingolysis 152, 153
salpingoscopy 118, 121–3
  microsalpingoscopy 123–5
  results 129

salpingostomy 147–8
    contraindications 184
salpingotomy 181–3
    future fertility prognosis 176–7
    indications for 184–5
        versus medical treatment 185
        versus salpingectomy 184–5
    results 185
scar dehiscence 219–20
    laparoscopic repair 220–5
Schauta operation 380
Schauta–Amreich operation 380
Schauta–Stoeckel operation 380–4
    laparoscopic step 381
    transvaginal step 381–4
scissors 19
second-puncture probe 28
sentinel node assessment 386–7
septate uterus see uterine septum
septate vagina see vaginal septum
septostomy 396–7
shaving surgery, endometriosis 67–71
    complications 72
    recurrence 72–3
smoke evacuation 28
sonohysterography see hysterosonography
space of Retzius opening 285
sperm migration test 465
spleen injury 444–5
sterilization, tubal 549–52
    postablation tubal sterilization syndrome 558
stomach injury 428–9
STOP® system 551–2
stress incontinence 14–15
subcutaneous emphysema 426
subovarian adhesions 32, 33
suturing 200–1, 230–1
synechiae, intrauterine 464
    see also adhesions
synthetic material complications 445

telescopes 17
tension-free vaginal tape (TVT) 14, 15
Thermablate endometrial ablation system 538
ThermaChoice® thermal balloons 536–7
thermal injuries 557
third-puncture probes 28
torus excision 59
torus uterinus ablation 11
total laparoscopic hysterectomy (TLH) 93–4
    definition 94
    technique 96–104
        bladder mobilization 98
        cervicovaginal attachment division 101
        cystoscopy 104
        exploration 97

incisions 96
morcellation 101–2
preoperative preparation 96
retroperitoneal dissection 97
skin closure 104
underwater examination 104
upper uterine blood supply 98–9
ureteral dissection 97–8
uterine vessel ligation 99–101
vaginal preparation 96
vaginal vault closure and suspension 102–4
    see also laparoscopic hysterectomy
transabdominal cervicoisthmic cerclage (TCC) 403
    see also abdominal cerclage
transcervical endometrial resection (TCER) 527–32,
    535
    instruments 527–8
    technique 528–30
transobturator tape (TOT) 14, 15
transvaginal laparoscopy 133–8
    evaluation 134–5
    instruments 133, 136
    'one-stop fertility clinic' 135–6
    operative procedure 136–8
        endometriosis 136
        ovarian capsule drilling 136–8
    technique 133
trichloroacetic acid, endometrial ablation 543
trocars 17–18
    insertion 1–2
        ancillary placement 2–3
    laparoscopic microsurgery 188
    secondary trocar injury 431–2
tubal anastomosis, types of 188
    see also laparoscopic microsurgical tubal
        anastomosis
tubal occlusion 143, 147–9
    classification 143, 144
    scoring systems 144, 145
tubal sterilization 549–52
tubal surgery
    prognostic factors 143–7
        ampullary dilatation 144
        ampullary fold preservation 144–6
        ciliation index 146
        endometriosis 147
        fibrosis 146
        intratubal adhesions 146
        periadnexal adhesions 146–7
        tubal mucosa 146
    techniques 147–9
tuberculosis
    genital 145
    uterine 478
tubo–cornual anastomosis 188
twin-to-twin transfusion syndrome (TTTS) 393–7

ultrasonography
    borderline ovarian tumor diagnosis 311–12
    methotrexate injection guidance 171
    ovarian cyst evaluation 195
    see also hysterosonography
umbilical artery 5
unicornuate uterus 489
    with rudimentary horn 493
ureter 7–8, 9
    blood vessel relationships 6
    dissection 271
    endometriosis 77–82
        diagnosis 78
        left versus right 81–2
        prevalence 77, 81
        surgical treatment 78–80, 82
        symptoms 77–8
    injury 437–41
        diagnosis 438
        following subtotal laparoscopic hysterectomy
            258–60
        location 8
        management 438–9
        prevention 439–41
    pelvic organ relationships 7
ureterolysis 78–9, 82
urinary tract injury 111, 430–1, 432, 436–41
uterine artery see uterine vessels
uterine cavity
    adhesions 464, 507–14
        classification 507
        diagnosis 507
        etiopathogenesis 507
        treatment 508–14
    distension 453, 473–4
    foreign bodies 468
    hysteroscopic examination 474–7
uterine introducer 115, 118
uterine manipulator 270–1, 273, 279–80
    laparoscopic microsurgery 188
    positioning 279–80
uterine perforation 554
    during subsequent pregnancy 557
uterine polyps 125
uterine sacrofixation 289–96
    see also prolapse

uterine septum 476, 478, 493–8
    complete 497
    partial 496–7
uterine suspension 56–8
    complications 57
    indications for 56
    operative technique 56–7
    results 57–8
uterine vessels 5–6
    ligation 99–101
    occlusion with laparoscopic myomectomy 231–2
uterosacral ligaments 5
    identification 280
uterus didelphys 498
uterus septus see uterine septum

vagina
    atresia 502
    closure 272
    disinfection 278
    estrogen treatment 278
    paravaginal repair 285–6
    reconstruction 484–9
vaginal cancer 359–60
vaginal septum 498–9
    transverse 502–4
    with uterine septum 493
vaginal vault prolapse 289
    sacrofixation 296–7
vascular injury 426–8, 441–2
    diagnosis 427, 428, 441
    epigastric vessel perforation 431–2
    management 427, 428, 441–2
    prevention 427–8
    see also hemorrhage
venous air embolism 442, 555–6
venous relationships 7
Veress needle 116, 117
vesical ligament 5
vesicouterine ligaments 5
visceral fascia 4, 5
visceral ligaments 4–5

Wolffian ducts 483–4

zygote intrafallopian transfer (ZIFT) 465